SANFORD GUIDE®

Thirty – third Edition

THE SANFORD

GUIDE TO

ANTIMICROBIAL

THERAPY

DI019634

David N. Gilbert, MD
Robert C. Moellering, Jr, MD
Merle A. Sande, MD

THE SANFORD GUIDE TO ANTIMICROBIAL THERAPY 2003
(33RD EDITION)

Jay P. Sanford, M.D.
1928-1996

EDITORS

David N. Gilbert, M.D.
Director of Medical Education and
Earl A. Chiles Research Institute
Providence Portland Medical Center
Professor of Medicine
Oregon Health Sciences University
Portland, Oregon

Robert C. Moellering, Jr., M.D.
Physician-in-Chief
Beth Israel Deaconess Medical Center
Herman L. Blumgart Professor of Medicine
Harvard Medical School
Boston, Massachusetts

Merle A. Sande, M.D.
Clarence M. and Ruth N. Birrer Professor of Medicine
University of Utah School of Medicine
Salt Lake City, Utah

The Sanford Guide to Antimicrobial Therapy is published annually by:

ANTIMICROBIAL THERAPY, INC.
P.O. Box 70, 229 Main Street
Hyde Park, VT 05655 USA
Tel 802-888-2855   Fax 802-888-2874
Email: info@sanfordguide.com

www.sanfordguide.com

PUBLISHER'S NOTE

You, the reader, should know that the SANFORD GUIDE is not sponsored by or prepared for any pharmaceutical company or distributor. Though copies are distributed by a variety of means, including pharmaceutical companies, the SANFORD GUIDE has been independently prepared and published since its inception in 1969. Decisions regarding the content of the SANFORD GUIDE are solely those of the editors and the publisher. Please feel free to contact us. Your comments and questions are encouraged and appreciated.

Our thanks to the Editors, Carolyn Wickwire for preparation of the manuscript, Gateway Graphics for printing and Delaware Valley Bindery and McCormick's Bindery for finishing of this edition of the SANFORD GUIDE.

Jeb C. Sanford, Publisher

—TABLE OF CONTENTS —

TABLE 1
CLINICAL APPROACH TO INITIAL CHOICE OF ANTIMICROBIAL THERAPY
Treatment based on presumed site or type of infection. In selected instances, treatment and prophylaxis based on identification of pathogens

ANATOMIC SITE/DIAGNOSIS/ MODIFYING CIRCUMSTANCES	ETIOLOGIES (usual)	SUGGESTED REGIMENS*		ADJUNCT DIAGNOSTIC OR THERAPEUTIC MEASURES AND COMMENTS
		PRIMARY	ALTERNATIVE†	
ABDOMEN: See Peritoneum, page 31; Gallbladder, page 10; and Pelvic Inflammatory Disease, page 16				
BONE: Osteomyelitis General Comment: **Regardless of the type of osteomyelitis, a specific microbiologic diagnosis is essential.** It is not possible to predict the microbial etiology based on epidemiology. In chronic osteomyelitis, organism(s) isolated from sinus tract drainage may not accurately reflect organisms present in bone. Ideally, empiric therapy is initiated after collection of blood and infected bone for culture. For review: NEJM 336:999, 1997.				
Hematogenous—Regimens refer to **EMPIRIC THERAPY** of acute disease				
Newborn (to 4 mos.)	S. aureus, Gm-neg. bacilli, Group B strep	[Nafcillin or oxacillin] + P Ceph 3 (Dosage in Table 16)	Vanco + P Ceph 3 (Dosage in Table 16)	Often afebrile. Localizing signs best predictor of osteo. Over 2/3 have positive blood cultures. Risk factors: Preterm and mechanical vent. PIDJ 14:1047, 1995. Treat for minimum of 21 days.
Children (>4 mos.) Often at or adjacent to epiphysis of long bones	S. aureus, Group A strep, coliforms rare	Nafcillin or oxacillin Add P Ceph 3 if Gm-neg. bacteria on Gram stain. Pediatric doses Table 16, adult below	Vanco or clinda See Comments	With immunization, H. influenzae almost disappeared. Vanco for nafcillin/oxacillin if pen-allergic or high prevalence of MRSA. IV rx initially. If bacterial etiology known, then po or IV rx at home for total of 2–3 wks.
Adult (>21 yrs) More often vertebral (Review: AJM 101:550, 1996) Vertebral osteo: CID 20:320, 1995 & AJM 100:85, 1996	S. aureus most common + variety other aerobic/ anaerobic cocci & bacilli; culture before empiric rx unless blood cultures pos	Nafcillin or oxacillin 2.0 gm q4h IV or cefazolin 2.0 gm IV q8h See Comments	Vanco 1.0 gm q12h IV	Rx regimens assume empiric rx and either no organism or Gm+ cocci on Gram stain. If high prevalence of MRSA, use vanco. Dx: MRI if spine. **Consider epidural abscess!** If proven MSSA, ceftriaxone another option (CID 30:205, 2000). Linezolid reported effective vs S. aureus osteo (AnIM 2002, in press).
Adult or child (special circumstances)				
Sickle cell anemia	Salmonella sp.	P Ceph 3		Stermoclavicular joint and ribs in addition to vertebral and long bones
IV drug abuse, hemodialysis pts	S. aureus, P. aeruginosa	[Nafcillin or oxacillin] + CIP	Vanco + CIP	
Contiguous Osteomyelitis Without Vascular Insufficiency				
Post-reduction & internal fixation of fracture	Coliforms, S. aureus, P. aeruginosa	Nafcillin 2.0 gm q6h IV + CIP 750 mg bid po	Vanco 1.0 gm q12h IV + P Ceph 3 AP	Usually necessary to remove "hardware" to achieve bone union. Revascularization if needed, e.g. pedicle muscle flaps, myocutaneous flaps.
Post-op sternotomy	S. aureus, S. epidermidis	Vanco 1.0 gm q12h IV	Vanco 1.0 gm q12h IV + RIF 600–900 mg qd po	Sternal debridement establishes microbial etiology & removes necrotic bone. Use of internal mammary artery (esp. in diabetics) for CABG increases risk of sternal osteo.
Post-nail puncture of foot through tennis shoe	P. aeruginosa	Ceftazidime 2.0 gm q8h IV or CFP 2.0 gm q12h IV	CIP 750 mg bid po (not in children)	Osteo evolves in 1–2% plantar puncture wounds in children. P. aeruginosa causes 93%. Debridement necessary to remove foreign body (CID 21:194, 1995). See Lung, cystic fibrosis, page 29, for CIP use in children
Contiguous Osteomyelitis With Vascular Insufficiency				
Pts with neuromuscular deficit & decubitus ulcers; atherosclerotic peripheral vascular disease; diabetic with neuropathy (see Diabetic foot, page 10)	Usually polymicrobic (Gm+ cocci [aerobic & anaerobic] and Gm-neg. bacilli (aerobic & anaerobic)	**Mild disease—outpatient therapy:** AM/CL 500 mg po tid. **Severe—hospitalized:** IMP or MER or TC/CL or PIP/TZ or AM/SB or trova or (CFP + metro) or (aztreonam + vanco + metro) (Dosage in footnote *)		Metal probe to bone correlates with presence of osteomyelitis (JAMA 273:721, 1995). **In extremity, determine extent of atherosclerotic vascular disease and revascularize if possible.** MRI helpful in documenting extent of infection. Surgical debridement for culture and removal of necrotic tissue. If neuropathy, avoid weight bearing. **Aggressive treatment** (debridement + antibiotics ± revascularization) in diabetic decreases need for amputation (CID 23:286, 1995).

* Drug dosage: **IMP** 0.5 gm q6h IV, **MER** 1.0 gm q8h IV (not licensed indication but should be effective), **TC/CL** 3.1 gm q6h IV, **PIP/TZ** 3.375 gm q6h or 4.5 gm q8h IV, **AM/SB** 3.0 gm q6h IV, **CFP** 2.0 gm q12h IV, **metro** 1.0 gm loading dose and then 0.5 gm q6h IV or po or 1.0 gm q12h IV, **vanco** 1.0 gm q12h IV, **trova** 200 mg/d po.

† Footnotes and abbreviations on page 45

NOTE: All dosage recommendations are for adults (unless otherwise indicated) and assume normal renal function

TABLE 1 (2)

ANATOMIC SITE/DIAGNOSIS/ MODIFYING CIRCUMSTANCES	ETIOLOGIES (usual)	SUGGESTED REGIMENS* PRIMARY	ALTERNATIVE†	ADJUNCT DIAGNOSTIC OR THERAPEUTIC MEASURES AND COMMENTS
BONE (continued) **Chronic Osteomyelitis** Ref.: JAMA 1(450), 1996) By definition, implies presence of dead bone	S. aureus, Enterobacteriaceae, P. aeruginosa	Empiric rx not indicated. Base systemic rx on results of culture, sensitivity testing.		Important adjuncts to be considered: removal of orthopedic hardware, surgical debridement, vascularized muscle flaps, distraction osteogenesis (Ilizarov) technique. Antibiotic-impregnated cement & hyperbaric oxygen adjunctive. NOTE: RIF + (vanco or β-lactam) very effective in animal models + one clinical trial of S. aureus chronic osteo (SM/ 79:947, 1986). Quinolone rx chronic osteo (CID 25:1327, 1997.
BREAST **Mastitis** Postpartum	S. aureus	**Dicloxacillin** 500 mg po or **cefazolin** 1.0 gm q8h I.V.	**Clinda** 300 mg q8h po	If no abscess, increased frequency of nursing may hasten response.
		Nafcillin or oxacillin 2.0 gm q4h I.V or **cefazolin** 1.0 gm q8h I.V.	**Vanco** 1.0 gm q12h I.V.	
Abscess				With abscess, d/c nursing. I&D standard; needle aspiration reported successful (Am J Surg 182:117, 2001).
Non-puerperal abscess	S. aureus, Bacteroides sp., peptostreptococcus	**Clinda** 300 mg q6h po or IV + (**nafcillin/oxacillin** IV as above or **cefazolin** IV as above) + **metro** 7.5 mg/kg q12h IV	**AMCL** 875/125 mg q12h po or **AM/SB** 1.5 gm q6h IV or (**vanco** + **metro**)	If subareolar, most likely anaerobes. If not subareolar, staph. Need pretreatment aerobic/anaerobic cultures. Surgical drainage for abscess.
CENTRAL NERVOUS SYSTEM **Brain abscess**				
Primary or contiguous source Ref.: CID 25:763, 1997	Streptococci (60–70%), bacteroides (20–40%), Enterobacteriaceae (25–33%), S. aureus (10–15%). Rare: Nocardia (Table 10A, page 77)	**P Ceph 3** (**cefotaxime** 2.0 gm IV q4h or **ceftriaxone** 2.0 gm IV q12h) + **metro** 7.5 mg/kg q6h or 15 mg/kg q12h IV	**Pen G** 20–24 mU IV qid + **metro** 7.5 mg/kg q6h IV or 15 mg/kg q12h IV Duration rx unclear: rx until response by neuroimaging (CT/MRI)	If CT scan suggests cerebritis (JNS 59:972, 1983), abscesses <2.5 cm and pt neurologically stable and conscious, start antibiotics and observe. Otherwise, surgical drainage necessary. Neurologic deterioration usually mandates surgery. Experience with Pen G (HD) + metro without P Ceph 3 or nafcillin/oxacillin has been good. We use P Ceph 3 because of frequency of isolation of Enterobacteriaceae. S. aureus rare without positive blood culture and/or signs of endocarditis; Strep. milleri group esp. prone to produce abscess.
Post-surgical, post-traumatic	S. aureus, Enterobacteriaceae	(**Nafcillin or oxacillin** 2.0 gm q4h IV + **P Ceph 3**)	**Vanco** 1.0 gm q12h IV + **P Ceph 3**	If hospital-acquired and MRSA a consideration, substitute vanco for nafcillin or oxacillin. P Ceph 3 dose as for brain abscess, primary
HIV-1 infected (AIDS)	Toxoplasma gondii	See Table 12, page 94		
Subdural empyema. In adult 60–90% are extension of sinusitis or otitis media. Rx same as primary brain abscess. Surgical emergency: must drain (CID 20:372, 1995).				
Encephalitis/encephalopathy (See Table 14, page 106, and for rabies, Table 20C, page 135)	Herpes simplex, arboviruses, rabies, listeria, cat-scratch disease	Start IV **acyclovir** while awaiting results of CSF PCR for H. simplex.		Newly recognized strain of tick rabies. May not require a break in the skin. Eastern equine encephalitis causes focal MRI changes in basal ganglia and thalamus (NEJM 336:1867, 1997). Cat-scratch ref.: PIDJ 14:866, 1995)
Meningitis, "Aseptic": Pleocytosis of 100s of cells, CSF glucose normal; not culture for bacteria (see Table 14, page 102)	Enteroviruses, HSV-2, LCM, HIV, other viruses, drugs (NSAIDs, metronidazole, carbamazepine, TMP/SMX, IVIG), rarely leptospirosis	For all but leptospirosis, IV fluids and analgesics. D/C drugs that may be etiologic. For lepto: (**doxy** 100 mg q12h IV po) or (**Pen G** 5 mU q6h IV) or (**AMP** 0.5–1.0 gm q6h IV). Repeat LP if suspect partially-treated bacterial meningitis.		If readily available, culture or PCR of CSF for enterovirus. HSV-2 unusual without concomitant genital herpes. Drug-induced aseptic meningitis: AIM 159:1185, 1999. For lepto, positive epidemiologic history and concomitant hepatitis, conjunctivitis, dermatitis, nephritis.

(Footnotes and abbreviations on page 45)   NOTE: All dosage recommendations are for adults (unless otherwise indicated) and assume normal renal function

TABLE 1 (3)

ANATOMIC SITE/DIAGNOSIS/ MODIFYING CIRCUMSTANCES	ETIOLOGIES (usual)	SUGGESTED REGIMENS* PRIMARY	ALTERNATIVE§	ADJUNCT DIAGNOSTIC OR THERAPEUTIC MEASURES AND COMMENTS
CENTRAL NERVOUS SYSTEM (continued)				
Meningitis, Bacterial, Acute: Goal is empiric therapy, then CSF exam within 30 min. If focal neurologic deficit, give empiric rx, then do head CT, then do LP - (NEJM 345:1727, 2001 & 346:1248, 2002). If CSF culture & Gram stain neg and CSF cultures to ↓um neg. in 2 hrs with immunocompetent & partial response with pneumococco in 4 hrs (Peds 108:1169, 2001)				
Empiric Therapy—CSF Gram stain is negative—immunocompetent (modified from NEJM 336:708, 1997)				
Age: Preterm to <1 month	Group B strep 49%, E. coli 18%, listeria 7%, misc. Gm- neg. 10%, misc. Gm-pos. 10%	**AMP + cefotaxime** Intraventricular use not recommended. Repeat CSF exam/culture 24–36 hrs after start of rx. *For dosage, see Table 16*	**AMP + gentamicin**	Primary & alternative regimens active vs Group B strep, most coliforms, & listeria. If premature infant with long nursery stay, S. aureus, enterococci, and resistant coliforms are potential pathogens. Optional empiric regimens: (nafcillin + cefotaxime or ceftazidime) or (nafcillin + gentamicin). If high risk of MRSA, use vanco + cefotaxime. Alter regimen after culture/sensitivity data available
Age: 1 mo.– 50 yrs 1999–2000 respiratory disease season, 34.1% of S. pneumo in U.S. were either intermediate in susceptibility or resistant to concentrations of Pen G achieved in CSF (CID 34 (Suppl.1):S4, 2002]. **See footnote³ for empiric treatment rationale.**	S. pneumo, meningococci, H. influenzae now very rare, listeria unlikely if young & immunocompetent. Statement from Am. Acad. of Peds.: Peds 99:289, 1997	Adult dosage: ((Cefotaxime 2.0 gm q4-6h IV OR ceftriaxone 2 gm IV q12h]) + (dexametha- sone) + **vanco** (see footnote³). Peds: see footnote³	((Cefotaxime (Peds: 40 mg/kg IV q8h]) + **vanco** (see footnote³) Peds: see footnote³	**For pts with severe pen. allergy: Chloro** 50 mg/kg IV q6h (max. 4 gm/d.) (for meningococcus) + **TMP/SMX.** 15–20 mg/kg/d div. q6-8h (for listeria (if immuno- compromised) + vanco. Rare meningococcus isolates chloro-resistant (NEJM 339:868, 1998). The standard alternative for pts with severe pen. allergy was chloro. However, high failure rate in pts with DRSP (Ln 342:240, 1993). **Value of dexamethasone** over than H. influenzae uncertain, but we recom- mend if evidence of ↑ intracranial pressure, e.g., obtundation (NEJM 345:1727, 2001; & 346:1248, 2002). Give 1st dose 15–20 min. Prior to or concomitant with 1st dose of antibiotic. **Dose: Either (0.4 mg/kg q12h IV x2 d.) OR (0.15 mg/kg IV q6h x4 d.).** Steroid risks: NEJM 336:708, 1997. **For meningococcal immunization, see Table 20, page 134.**
Age: 1 mo – 50 yrs		**Dexamethasone** 0.4 mg/kg q12h IV x2 d. (Ln 342:457, 1993) or 0.15 mg/kg IV q6h x4 d. (JAMA 278:925, 1997). Give with or w/o 1st dose of antibiotic (see Comment). *See footnote³ regarding drug-resistant S. pneumo. See footnote³ for best ref. dosage*		
Age: >50 yrs or alcoholism or other debilitating associated diseases or impaired cellular immunity	S. pneumo, listeria, Gm-neg bacilli. Note ↑ prevalence of meningo- coccus	(AMP 2.0 gm IV q4h) + (ceftriaxone 2.0 gm IV q12h or cefotaxime 2.0 gm IV q8h) + **vanco** (see Comment). For vanco dose, see footnote³	**MER** 1.0 gm q8h IV + vanco (see footnote³). **Dexamethasone** see Comment	**Severe penicillin allergy: Vanco** 500–750 mg q6h IV + **TMP/SMX** 15–20 mg/kg/d div. q6-8h (avoid listeria) + vanco. Chloro has failed vs DRSP (Ln 342:240, 1993). **MER** active vs listeria in vitro (JAC 36(Suppl. A):1, 1995); CSF levels appear ade- quate (JAC 34:175, 1994) but no clinical data (PIDJ 18:581, 1999).
Post-neurosurgery or post-head trauma	S. pneumoniae most common, esp. if CSF leak MRSA (until known neg.). Other: S. aureus, coliforms, P. aeruginosa	(**Vanco** until known neg. MRSA 1.0 gm q12h IV + cefotaxime 2.0 gm IV q4-8h or ceftazidime 2.0 gm IV q8h (see Comment)	**MER** 2.0 gm q8h IV + **vanco** 1.0 gm IV q12h, but not an FDA- approved indication	**Vanco** not optimal for S. pneumo. If/when suscept. S. pneumo identified, quickly switch to **ceftriaxone** or **cefotaxime.** If culture-proven coliform or pseudomonas meningitis, some add intrathecal gentamicin (4 mg q12h into lateral ventricles). **Vanco** does not have seizure potential of IMP.

---

¹ **Rationale:** Hard to get adequate CSF concentrations of anti-infectives, hence MIC criteria for in vitro susceptibility are lower for CSF isolates (AIM 161:2538, 2001). Cefotaxime/ceftriaxone selected for activity vs meningococci, Hemophilus spp., & pen-sens. S. pneumo. For pen-resistant S. pneumo, total of intermediate susceptibility + resistance to cefotaxime/ceftriaxone 88.1% (CID 34(Suppl.1):S4, 2002). Hence, added vanco empirically pending in vitro susceptibility of known or.

² Low CSF penetration of vanco into the CSF (PIDJ 16:895, 1997). Recommended dose in children is 15 mg/kg q6h IV. Limited clinical data in adults given 15 mg/kg q6h (double the standard dose). **In adults,** a maximum dose of 2-3 gm/day is suggested: 500–750 mg q6h IV.

³ **Dosage of drugs used to rx children ≥1 mo. of age:** Cefotaxime 200 mg/kg/d IV div. q6-8h; ceftriaxone 100 mg/kg/d IV div. q12h; vanco 15 mg/kg IV q6h. *(Footnotes and abbreviations on page 45   NOTE: All dosage recommendations are for adults (unless otherwise indicated) and assume normal renal function*

TABLE 1 (4)

ANATOMIC SITE/DIAGNOSIS/ MODIFYING CIRCUMSTANCES	ETIOLOGIES (usual)	SUGGESTED REGIMENS* PRIMARY	ALTERNATIVE§	ADJUNCT DIAGNOSTIC OR THERAPEUTIC MEASURES AND COMMENTS
CENTRAL NERVOUS SYSTEM (continued)				
Meningitis, Bacterial/Empiric Therapy/Negative CSF Gram Stain (continued)				
Ventriculitis/meningitis due to infected ventriculo-peritoneal (atrial) shunt	S. epidermidis, S. aureus, coliforms, diphtheroids (rare), P. acnes	**Vanco** 1.0 gm q8–12h IV or **ceftriaxone** 50 mg/kg q8h IV or **cefotaxime** 50 mg/kg q12h IV]		Early shunt removal usually necessary for cure. Refs.: Adv PID 11:29, 1996; IDCP 4:277, 1995. For adults, can use P Ceph 3 alone if positive Gram stain for Gm-neg. bacilli
Empiric Therapy—Positive CSF Gram Stain				
Gram-positive diplococci	S. pneumoniae	Either (**ceftriaxone** 2.0 gm IV q12h or **cefotaxime** 2.0 gm IV q6h) + **vanco** 15 mg/kg IV q6–12h* + **dexa-methasone** 0.4 mg/kg q12h IV x2 d		**For severe penicillin allergy: vanco + RIF 600 mg qd (po or IV).** Dexamethasone should (1) decrease penetration of vanco into CSF of **children**, so ceftriaxone + vanco OK; (2) in **adults**, probably OK based on animal model data (AAC 43:876, 1999)
Gram-negative diplococci	N. meningitidis[1]	**Pen G** 4 million units IV q4h x5–7 d; if pen. allergic, **chloro** 50 mg/kg IV (up to 1.0 gm) IV q6h		No clinical data to support use of dexamethasone (CID 20:685, 1995)
Gram-positive bacilli or coccobacilli	Listeria monocytogenes	**AMP** 2.0 gm IV q4h + **gentamicin** 2 mg/kg loading dose then 1.7 mg/kg q8h		Listeria ref.: CID 24:1, 1997. **If pen.-allergic, use TMP/SMX 15–20 mg/kg/d. div. q6–8h.**
Gram-negative bacilli	H. influenzae, coliforms, P. aeruginosa	**Ceftazidime** 2.0 gm IV q8h + **gentamicin** 2 mg/kg loading dose then 1.7 mg/kg q8h		Other possible drugs: aztreonam, CIP, MER, trova. CIP rx success: CID 25:936, 1997
Specific Therapy—Positive culture of CSF with in vitro susceptibility results available				
H. influenzae		**Ceftriaxone** (peds): 100 mg/kg/d IV div q12h		**Pen. allergic: Chloro** 50 mg/kg/d IV div q6h (max. 4 gm/d)
Listeria monocytogenes		**AMP** 2.0 gm IV q4h + **gentamicin** 2 mg/kg loading dose, then 1.7 mg/kg q8h		**Pen. allergic: TMP/SMX** 15–20 mg/kg/d div. q6–8h. One report of greater efficacy of AMP + TMP/SMX as compared to AMP + gentamicin (JID 33:79, 1996)
N. meningitidis		**Pen G** 4 million units IV q4h x7 d; if pen. allergic, **chloro** 50 mg/kg IV (up to 1.0 gm) IV q6h		Rare isolates chloro-resistant (NEJM 339:868 & 917, 1998)
S. pneumoniae	Pen G MIC < 0.1 μg/ml	**Aq. pen G** 4 mU IV q4h x10–14 d.		For severe pen. allergy: (Vanco + 600 mg RIF/d) or chloro 50 mg/kg/d (po or IV)/6h.
S. pneumoniae	Pen G MIC > 0.1 μg/ml and/ or ceftriaxone MIC > 0.5 μg/ml	**Children** [(Ceftriaxone 50 mg/kg IV q12h to max. of 4 gm/d or cefotaxime 50–75 mg/kg IV q6h) + vanco 15 mg/kg IV q6h] + dexamethasone 0.4 mg/kg q12h IV x2 d. **Adults** [(Ceftriaxone 2.0 gm IV q12h) + (vanco 15 mg/kg q6–12h*)] + dexamethasone		In experimental S. pneumo meningitis, vanco + ceftriaxone synergistic; even with high ceftriaxone MIC (AAC 37:1630, 1993). In children, dexamethasone does not ↓ vanco penetration of CSF (AAC 39:1988, 1995). MER may work but little clinical experience. **Rx if severe penicillin allergy: vanco IV + [RIF 600 mg qd (po or IV)].**
A.2° CSF exam after 24–48 hrs is suggested both because of difficulty treating resistant S. pneumo & because dexamethasone (if used) may impair clinical assessment		Treat for 10–14 days		
Prophylaxis for H. influenzae and N. meningitidis				
Hemophilus influenzae type b Household and/or day care contact: residing with index case or ≥4 hrs. Day care contact: same day care as index case for 5–7 days before onset		**RIF** 20 mg/kg po (not to exceed 600 mg) qd x4 doses		**Household:** If there is one unvaccinated contact ≤4 yrs in the household, RIF prophylaxis for all household contacts except pregnant women. **Child Care Facilities:** With 1 case, if attended by unvaccinated children ≤2 yrs, consider prophylaxis + vaccinate susceptibles. If all contacts attend, prophylaxis in 60 days & unvaccinated children immunized. **Child Care** (Am Acad Ped Red Book 1997, page 222).
Prophylaxis for meningococcal				

[1] For meningococcal prophylaxis, see Table 15, page 117
(Footnotes and abbreviations on page 45)   NOTE: All dosage recommendations are for adults (unless otherwise indicated) and assume normal renal function

TABLE 1 (5)

ANATOMIC SITE/DIAGNOSIS/ MODIFYING CIRCUMSTANCES	ETIOLOGIES (usual)	SUGGESTED REGIMENS* PRIMARY	SUGGESTED REGIMENS* ALTERNATIVE§	ADJUNCT DIAGNOSTIC OR THERAPEUTIC MEASURES AND COMMENTS
CENTRAL NERVOUS SYSTEM/Meningitis, Bacterial/Prophylaxis *(continued)*				
Neisseria meningitidis exposure (close contact) [MMWR 46(RR-5):1, 1997] CDC recommends informing college freshmen living in dormitories & residence halls of available vaccine [MMWR 46(RR-7):1, 2000 & 50:23-487, 2001]		[**RIF** 600 mg po q12h x 4 doses. (Children >1 mo. age 10 mg/kg po q12h x4 doses, <1 mo. age 5 mg/kg q12h x4 doses)] **or** [**CIP** (adults) 500 mg po single dose]. **or** [**Ceftriaxone** 250 mg IM x1 dose (child <15 yrs 125 mg IM x1)]. **Spiramycin** 500 mg po q6h x5 d. Children 10 mg/kg po q6h x5 d		N. meningitidis spread by respiratory droplets, not aerosols, hence close contact required. ↑ risk if close contact for at least 4 hrs during week before illness onset (e.g., housemates, day care contacts, cellmates) or exposure to pt's naso-pharyngeal secretions (e.g., via kissing, mouth-to-mouth resuscitation, intubation, nasotracheal suctioning). Azthro 500 mg x1 as effective as RIF 600 mg bid x2 d (PID 17:816, 1998). Ceftriaxone equivalent to RIF (JAC 45:909, 2000). Primary prophylactic regimen in many European countries.
Meningitis, chronic Defined as symptoms + CSF pleocytosis for ≥4 wks	M. tbc 40%, cryptococcosis 7%, neoplastic 8%, Lyme, syphilis, Whipple's disease	Treatment depends on etiology. No urgent need for empiric therapy.		Long list of possibilities: bacteria, parasites, fungi, viruses, neoplasms, vasculitis, and other miscellaneous etiologies—see chapter on chronic meningitis in latest edition of Harrison's Textbook of Internal Medicine
Meningitis, eosinophilic (See Table 12A, page 94)	Angiostrongyliasis, gnatho-stomiasis, rarely others	Corticosteroids	Not sure antihelminthic rx works	1/3 lack peripheral eosinophilia. Need serology to confirm dx. Steroid ref.: CID 31:660, 2001. Recent outbreak: NEJM 346:668, 2002.
Meningitis, HIV-1 infected (AIDS)	As in adults, >50 yrs: also consider cryptococci, M. tuberculosis, syphilis, HIV aseptic meningitis, Listeria monocytogenes	If etiology not identified: rx as adult >50 yrs + obtain CSF/serum crypto-coccal antigen (see Comments)	For crypto rx, see Table 10A, page 75	C. neoformans most common etiology in AIDS (for H. influenzae, pneumococci). Tbc, syphilis, viral, histoplasma & coccidiodes also need to be considered. Obtain blood cultures. L. monocytogenes risk >60x ↑, ¾ present as meningitis (CID 17:224, 1993).
EAR				
External otitis "Swimmer's ear"	Pseudomonas sp., Entero-bacteriaceae, Proteus sp. (Fungi rare.) Acute infection usually 2° S. aureus	Eardrops: {[**polymyxin B + neomycin + hydrocorti-sone**] (qid)} or {ofloxacin (3% susp) bid}. For acute disease: **dicloxacillin** 500 mg po 4x/d.		Rx should include gentle cleaning. Recurrences prevented (or decreased) by drying with alcohol drops (1/3 white vinegar, 2/3 rubbing alcohol) after swimming, then antibiotic drops of 2% acetic acid solution. Ointments should not be used in ear. Ofloxacin ref.: PIDJ 20:108, 2001
Chronic	Usually 2° to seborrhea	Eardrops: {[**polymyxin B + neomycin + hydrocorti-sone**] qid} + **selenium sulfide**}		Control seborrhea with dandruff shampoo containing selenium sulfide (Selsun) or (ketoconazole shampoo) + (medium potency steroid solution, triamcinolone 0.1%)
Diabetes mellitus, acute "malignant otitis externa"	Pseudomonas sp.	**IMP** 0.5 gm q6h IV or **MER** 1.0 gm q8h IV or **CIP** 400 mg q12h IV or 750 mg q12h po) or **ceftaz** 2.0 gm q8h IV or **CFP** 2 gm q12h or [**PIP** 4-6 gm q4-6h IV + **APAG**] (dose depends on drug) or {**TC** 3.0 gm q4h IV + **APAG**}		CIP po especially useful for outpatient rx with early disease. Surgical debridement usually required, but not radical excision. R/O osteomyelitis. CT or MRI scan more sensitive than x-ray. If bone involved, rx for 4–6 wks.

NOTE: All dosage recommendations are for adults (unless otherwise indicated) and assume normal renal function

TABLE 1 (6)

ANATOMIC SITE/DIAGNOSIS/ MODIFYING CIRCUMSTANCES	ETIOLOGIES (usual)	SUGGESTED REGIMENS†		ADJUNCT DIAGNOSTIC OR THERAPEUTIC MEASURES AND COMMENTS
		PRIMARY	ALTERNATIVE†	
EAR (continued)				
Otitis media—infants, children, adults				
Acute otitis media (AOM)	S. pneumo 40–50%, H. influ-enzae 20–25%, M. catar-rhalis 10–15%.	**If NO antibiotics in prior month:** Amox po UD¹ or HD¹	**Received antibiotics in prior month:** Amox-clav, AM/CL, HD¹ or (clinically vs DRSP) cefprozil or cefuroxime axetil¹	If allergic to β-lactam drugs ?: High failure rate with TMP/SMX if etiology is DRSP or H. influenzae (PIDJ 20:260, 2001); azithro x5 d. or clarithro x10 d. (both have ↑ activity vs DRSP). Increased risk macrolide resistance < age 5 (JAMA 286:1857, 2001).
Initial empiric therapy of acute otitis media (AOM) NOTE: Pending new data, recommend Amox po UD¹ or HD¹ as primary rx x 1–2 d. if child < 2 yrs old. 1/3 have **no bacterial pathogen** (NEJM 340:260 & 312 & 2001; NEJM 347:1169, 2002).	Note: In 48%, RSV & rhino-viruses. 1/3 have **no bacterial pathogen** (NEJM 340:260 & 312 & 2001; NEJM 347:1169, 2002).		For dosage, see footnotes¹ and ² **All doses as pediatric**	Spontaneous resolution: 90% pts infected with M. catarrhalis, 50% with H. influenzae, and 10% with S. pneumoniae.
				Selection of drug based on (1) risk of drug-resistant S. pneumo (DRSP). Risk of DRSP ↑ with age <2 yrs, antibiotics last 3 mos, and/or daycare attendance.
		Duration of rx: <2 yrs old x10 d, ≥2 yrs old x5–7 d. Appropriate duration unclear. 5 d. may be inadequate for severe disease NEJM 347:1169, 2002)		(2) effectiveness against H. influenzae & M. catarrhalis and (2) effectiveness against DRSP, including **Cefaclor, loracarbef, cefixime, & ceftibuten less active vs DRSP** than other agents listed. Taste/smell of cefdinir well-received in children (~8-3 y.o. (PIDJ 19 (Suppl 2):S174, 2000).
Treatment for clinical failure after 3 days rx	Drug-resistant S. pneu-moniae main concern	**NO antibiotics in month prior to last 3 days:** AM/CL HD¹ or cefdinir or cefpodoxime or cefprozil or cefuroxime axetil or IM ceftriaxone x3 d.	**Antibiotics in month prior to last 3 days:** ((if allergy) clindamycin) and/or tympanocentesis) **All doses as pediatric**	**Clindamycin** not active vs H. influenzae or M. catarrhalis. Definition of failure: no change in ear pain, fever, bulging TM or otorrhea after 3 days of rx. Tympanocentesis will allow culture. **Newer FQs active vs DRSP, but not approved for use in children. Vanco is active vs DRSP.** Ceftriaxone IM x3 d. superior to 1 d. treatment vs DRSP (PIDJ 19:1040, 2000). AM/CL HD reported successful for pen-resistant S. pneumo AOM (NEJM 344:1188, 2001).
After >48 hrs of nasotracheal intubation	Pseudomonas sp. klebsiella, enterobacter	Ceftazidime or CFP or IMP or MER or TC/CL or CIP (For dosages, see Ear, malignant otitis externa)		With nasotracheal intubation >48 hrs, about ½ pts will have otitis media with effusion.
Prophylaxis: acute otitis media	Pneumococci, H. influenzae M. catarrhalis, Staph aure-us, Group A strep (see **Comments**)	Sulfisoxazole 50 mg/kg po at bedtime or **amoxicillin** 20 mg/kg po qd	**Use of antibiotics to prevent otitis media is a major contributor to emergence of antibiotic-resistant S. pneumo!** Pneumococcal protein conjugate vaccine ↓ freq. AOM due to vaccine serotypes ↓ need for future hospitalization for AOM (NEJM 344:188, 2001). Adenoidectomy at time of tympanostomy tubes ↓ need for future hospitalization for AOM (NEJM 344:1188, 2001).	

¹ **Amoxicillin UD or HD** = amoxicillin usual dose or high dose; **AM/CL HD** = amoxicillin/clavulanate high dose **Dosages in footnote 2.**
² **Drugs and peds dosage (all po unless specified) for acute otitis media: Amoxicillin UD** = 40 mg/kg/d div q12h or q8h. **Amoxicillin HD** = 90 mg/kg/d div q12h or q8h. **AM/CL HD** = 90 mg/kg/d div of amox component. Extra-strength AM/CL oral suspension (Augmentin ES-600) available with 600 mg AM & 42.9 mg CL per 5 ml—dose: 90/6.4 mg/kg/d div bid. **Cefuroxime axetil** 30 mg/kg/d div q12h. **Ceftriaxone** 50 mg/kg IM x3 d. **Clindamycin** 30 mg/kg/d div q8h (may be effective vs DRSP but no activity vs H. influenzae). **Other drugs suitable for otitis media (e.g., penicillin-sensitive S. pneumo: TMP/SMX** 8 mg/kg/d div q12h. **Erythro-sulfisoxazole** 50 mg/kg/d of erythro div q6–8h. **Clarithro** 15 mg/kg/d div q12h; **azithro** 10 mg/kg x1 d. & then 5 mg/kg qd on days 2–5. Other drugs only for penicillin-intermediate or penicillin-sensitive S. pneumo: **Cefprozil** 30 mg/kg/d div q12h; **cefpodoxime proxetil** 10 mg/kg/d div q24h. **Cefdinir** 7 mg/kg q12h or 14 mg/kg q24h.
Cefaclor 40 mg/kg/d div q8h; **loracarbef** 30 mg/kg/d div q12h. NOTE: All dosage recommendations are for adults (unless otherwise indicated) and assume normal renal function
(Footnotes and abbreviations on page 45)

TABLE 1 (7)

ANATOMIC SITE/DIAGNOSIS/ MODIFYING CIRCUMSTANCES	ETIOLOGIES (usual)	SUGGESTED REGIMENS* PRIMARY	ALTERNATIVE†	ADJUNCT DIAGNOSTIC OR THERAPEUTIC MEASURES AND COMMENTS
EAR (continued) **Mastoiditis** **Acute** Outpatient	Strep. pneumoniae 22%, S. pyogenes 16%, Staph. aureus 7%, H. influenzae 4%, P. aeruginosa 4%, others <1%	Empirically, same as Acute otitis media, above; need **nafcillin/oxacillin** if culture + for S. aureus.		Has become a rare entity, presumably as result of the aggressive rx of acute otitis media. ↑ in incidence in Netherlands where use of antibiotics limited to children with complicated course or high risk (PIDJ 20:140, 2001).
Hospitalized		**Cefotaxime** 1-2 gm IV q4-6h (depending on severity) or (**ceftriaxone** 2 gm q24h IV < age 60, 1 gm q24h IV > age 60)		
Chronic	Often polymicrobic: anaerobes, S. aureus, Enterobacteriaceae, P. aeruginosa	Treatment for acute exacerbations or perioperatively, usually, no treatment until surgical cultures obtained. Examples of empiric regimens: **IMP** 0.5 gm q6h IV or **TC/CL** 3.1 gm q4-6h or **PIP/TZ** 3.375 gm q4-8h or 4.5 gm q8h IV		May or may not be associated with chronic otitis media with drainage via ruptured tympanic membrane. Antimicrobials given in association with surgery. Mastoidectomy for chronic drainage and evidence of osteomyelitis by MRI or CT, evidence of spread to CNS (epidural abscess, suppurative phlebitis, brain abscess).
EYE—General Reviews: CID 21:479, 1995; IDCP 7:447, 1998				
Eyelid Blepharitis	Etiol. unclear. Factors include Staph. aureus & Staph. epidermidis, seborrhea, rosacea, & dry eye	Lid margin care with baby shampoo & warm compresses bid. Artificial tears if assoc. dry eye (see Comment)		Usually topical ointments of no benefit. If associated rosacea, add doxy 100 mg po bid x2 wks and then qd.
Hordeolum (Stye) External (gland of Zeis)	Staph. aureus	Hot packs only. Will drain spontaneously.		Infection of superficial sebaceous gland
Internal (Meibomian gland)	Staph. aureus	Oral **nafcillin/oxacillin** + hot packs		Also called acute meibomianitis. Rarely drain spontaneously.
Conjunctiva: General Reviews: NEJM 343:345, 2000				
Conjunctivitis of the newborn (**ophthalmia neonatorum**) by day of onset post-delivery—all doses pediatric Onset 1st day	Chemical due to AgNO₃	None		Usual prophylaxis is erythro ointment; hence, AgNO₃ irritation rare.
Onset 2-4 days	N. gonorrhoeae	**Cefriaxone** 25-30 mg/kg IV x1 dose (see Comment)		Treat mother & her sexual partners. Hyperpurulent. Topical rx inadequate. **Treat neonate for concomitant Chlamydia trachomatis.**
Onset 3-10 days	Chlamydia trachomatis	**Erythro syrup** 50 mg/kg/d (po in 4 div doses x14 d.)	No topical rx needed.	Diagnosis by antigen detection. Azithro susp 20 mg/kg po qd x3 d. reported efficacious (PIDJ 17:1049, 1998). Treat mother & sexual partner.
Onset 2-16 days	Herpes simplex types 1, 2	See keratitis, below.		Consider IV acyclovir if concomitant systemic disease.
Ophthalmia neonatorum prophylaxis: **Silver nitrate** 1% x1 or **erythro** 0.5% ointment x1 or **tetra** 1% ointment x1 application				
Pink eye (viral conjunctivitis) Usually unilateral	Adenovirus types 3 & 7 in children; 8, 11 & 19 in adults)	No treatment. If symptomatic, cold artificial tears may help.		Highly contagious. Onset of ocular pain and photophobia in an adult suggests associated keratitis—rare.
Inclusion conjunctivitis (**adult**) Usually unilateral	Chlamydia trachomatis	**Doxy** 100 mg bid po x1-3 weeks		Oculoglandular. Diagnosis by culture or antigen detection or PCR—availability varies by region and institution. Treat sexual partner.
Trachoma	Chlamydia trachomatis	**Azithro** 20 mg/kg po single dose—78% effective	**Doxy** 100 mg bid po x14 d. or **tetracycline** 250 mg qid po x14 d	Starts in childhood and can persist for years with subsequent damage to cornea. Topical therapy of marginal benefit. Avoid doxy/tetracycline in young children. Ref.: CID 24:363, 1997.
Suppurative conjunctivitis Non-gonococcal; non-chlamydial	Staph. aureus, S. pneumoniae; H. influenzae	Ophthalmic **bacitracin-polymyxin B** or **TMP** or **erythro** or **FQ** (**CIP, levo, or oflox**)	Ophthalmic **gentamicin** or **tobra** (see Comment)	Often self-limited. Eye drops preferred for adults and ointments for infants or young children. Topical gel, tobra, or neomycin may cause punctate staining of cornea. Avoid chloro. In children 2 mos – 6 yrs old, topical rx less effective than cefixime (PIDJ 20:1039, 2001).
Gonococcal	N. gonorrhoeae	**Ceftriaxone** 125 mg IM or IV (single dose). See Genital, page 15		

(Footnotes and abbreviations on page 45)   NOTE: All dosage recommendations are for adults (unless otherwise indicated) and assume normal renal function

TABLE 1 (8)

ANATOMIC SITE/DIAGNOSIS/ MODIFYING CIRCUMSTANCES	ETIOLOGIES (usual)	SUGGESTED REGIMENS* PRIMARY	ALTERNATIVE§	ADJUNCT DIAGNOSTIC OR THERAPEUTIC MEASURES AND COMMENTS
EYE (continued)				
Cornea (keratitis): Usually serious and often sight-threatening. Prompt ophthalmologic consultation essential. Herpes simplex most common etiology in developed countries; bacterial and fungal infections more common in underdeveloped countries.				
Viral				
H. simplex, types 1 & 2	H. simplex, types 1 & 2	**Trifluridine** one drop qh, 9x/d, for up to 21 days	**Vidarabine** ointment—useful in children. Use 5x/d for up to 21 days	Fluorescein staining shows topical dendritic figures. 30–50% rate of recurrence within 2 years. 400 mg acyclovir po bid ↓ recurrences, p 0.005 (N.EJ.M 339:300, 1998). If child fails vidarabine, try trifluridine.
Varicella-zoster ophthalmicus	Varicella-zoster virus	**Famciclovir** 500 mg tid or **valacyclovir** 1.0 gm tid x10 days	**Acyclovir** 800 mg po 5x/day x10 days	Clinical diagnosis most common: dendritic figures with fluorescein staining in patient with varicella-zoster of ophthalmic branch of trigeminal nerve.
Bacterial		*All rx listed for bacterial, fungal, & protozoan is topical*		
Contact lens users	P. aeruginosa	**Tobra** or **gentamicin** (14 mg/ml) + **piperacillin** or **ticarcillin** eye drops (6-12 mg/ml) q15–60 min. around clock x24–72 hrs, then slow reduction	**CIP** or **oflox** 0.3% drops q15–60 min. around clock q×24–72 hrs	Pain, photophobia, impaired vision. Recommend alginate swab for culture and sensitivity testing.
Dry cornea, diabetes, immunosuppression	Staph. aureus, S. epidermidis, S. pneumoniae, S. pyogenes, Enterobacteriaceae, listeria	**Cefazolin** (50 mg/ml) + **gentamicin** or **tobra** (14 mg/ml) q15–60 min. around clock x24–72 hrs, then slow reduction. See Comment	**Vanco** (50 mg/ml) + **cef-tazidime** (50 mg/ml) q15–60 min. around clock x24–72 hrs, then slow reduction. See Comment	Specific therapy guided by results of alginate swab culture and sensitivity. CIP 0.3% found clinically equivalent to cefazolin + tobra, only concern was efficacy of CIP vs S. pneumoniae (Ophthalmology 163:1854, 1996).
Fungal	Aspergillus, fusarium, candida. No empiric therapy—see Comment	**Natamycin** (5%) drops q4–3 hrs with subsequent slow reduction	**Ampho B** (0.05–0.1%) drops q4–3 hrs with subsequent slow reduction	No empiric therapy. Wait for results of Gram stain or culture in Sabouraud's medium.
Protozoan Soft contact lens users (over-night use ↑ risk 10–15 fold)	Acanthamoeba, hartmannella	**Propamidine** 0.1% + **polymyxin/neomycin/gramicidin/ polymyxin** Eyedrops q waking hour x1 week and then slow taper	**Polyhexamethylene biguanide** 0.02% or **chlorhexidine** 0.02%	Uncommon. Trauma and soft contact lenses are risk factors. Corneal scrapings stained with calcofluor white show characteristic cysts with fluorescent microscopy. Ref: CID 35:434, 2002
Lacrimal apparatus				
Canaliculitis	Actinomyces most common. Rarely, Arachnia, fusobacterium, nocardia, candida	Remove granules & irrigate with **pen G** 100,000 u/ml **Child: AMCL or O Ceph**	If turbid, irrigate with **nystatin** approx. 5 μg/ml + 1 gtt tid	Digital pressure produces exudate at punctum; Gram stain confirms diagnosis. Hot packs to punctal area qid.
Dacryocystitis (lacrimal sac)	S. pneumo, S. aureus, H. influenzae, S. pyogenes, P. aeruginosa	Empiric rx based on Gram stain of aspirate—see Comment		Often consequence of obstruction of lacrimal duct. Need ophthalmologic consultation. Can be acute or chronic.
Early, acute onset	Staph. aureus, S. epidem, Pseudomonas sp.			
Low grade, chronic	Propionibacterium acnes, S. epidermidis, S. aureus	May require removal of lens material. Intraocular **vanco**.		

Endophthalmitis: For etiologic agents of post-endophthalmitis, see Am J Ophthal 122:1, 1996
Bacterial: Haziness of vitreous (of both vitreous and aqueous humor for culture prior to therapy. Intravitreal administration of antimicrobials essential.
Postoperative surgery (cataracts) Injection/needle aspirate of both vitreous and aqueous humor for culture prior to therapy. Intravitreal administration of antimicrobials essential. As S. aureus or P aerugi-nosa eye may be destroyed within 24 hrs. Rx must be aggressive: early vitrectomy and then intravitreal antibiotics (**vanco** 1 mg + **amikacin** 0.4 mg/each in 0.1 ml). Repeat intravitreal injection after several days. Parenteral therapy not necessary unless infection outside globe. Possible risk of amikacin-induced macular infarction (Br J Ophthal 86:359, 2002); could substitute ceftazidime 2 mg (0.1 ml of 20 mg/ml solution) for amikacin.

Footnotes and abbreviations on page 45)   NOTE: All dosage recommendations are for adults (unless otherwise indicated) and assume normal renal function

TABLE 1 (9)

ANATOMIC SITE/DIAGNOSIS/ MODIFYING CIRCUMSTANCES	ETIOLOGIES (usual)	SUGGESTED REGIMENS* PRIMARY	ALTERNATIVE†	ADJUNCT DIAGNOSTIC OR THERAPEUTIC MEASURES AND COMMENTS
EYE/Endophthalmitis/Bacterial (continued)				
Post filtering blebs for glaucoma	Strep. species (viridans & others), H. influenzae	Intravitreal and topical agent and consider systemic **AM/CL, AM/SB** or **P Ceph 2**		
Post-penetrating trauma	Bacillus sp., S. epidermi-	Intravitreal agent as above + systemic **clinda** or **vanco**. Use topical antibiotics post-surgery (fotrax & cefazolin drops)		Intravitreal antibiotics as with early post-operative.
Hematogenous	dis, Staph. aureus	**P Ceph 3** (**cefotaxime** 2.0 gm q4h IV or meningi-	**vanco** 2.0 gm q24h IV) + **vanco** 1.0 gm q12h IV pending cultures.	
IV heroin abuse	Bacillus cereus, Candida sp.	Intravitreal agent + systemic **clinda** (or **vanco**)		
Mycotic (fungal)	Candida sp., Aspergillus sp.	Intravitreal **ampho B** 0.005–0.010 mg in 0.1 ml. Also see Table 10, pages 71, 72 for concomitant systemic therapy. See Comment.		With moderate/marked vitritis, options include systemic rx + vitrectomy ± intravitreal ampho B (CID 27:1130 & 1134, 1998). Report of failure of ampho B lipid complex (CID 28:1177, 1999).
Retinitis				
Acute retinal necrosis	Varicella zoster, Herpes simplex	IV **acyclovir** 10–12 mg/kg IV q8h x5–7 d, then 800 mg po 5x/d x6 wks. See Table 14, page 105		Strong association of VZ virus with atypical necrotizing herpetic retinopathy (CID 24:603, 1997).
HIV-1 (AIDS) CD4 usually < 100/mm³	Cytomegalovirus			Occurs in 5–10% of AIDS patients
Orbital cellulitis (see page 36 for erysipelas, facial)	S. pneumoniae, H. influen- zae, M. catarrhalis, S. aureus, anaerobes, group A strep, occ. Gm-neg. bacilli post-trauma	**P Ceph 2/3** (**cefuroxime** 1.5 gm q8h IV, **cefoxitin** 2.0 gm q8h IV, **cefotetan** 2.0 gm q12h IV or **ceftriaxone** 2.0 gm q24h IV, **AM/SB** 1.5 gm q6h IV	**TC/CL** or **PIP/TZ** (see foot- note† for dosages) or **cefo- taxime** 2.0 gm q4h IV or **ceftriaxone** 2.0 gm q24h IV	See mucor/rhizopus, Table 10, page 77. H. influenzae becoming a rare etiology.
FOOT				
"Diabetic". Reviews: CID 25:1318, 1997; NEJM 341:1906, 1999.				
Extent, no osteomyelitis	Aerobic Gm+ cocci; S.	Non-limb-threatening:	NEJM 343:787, 2000.	Clinda 300 mg po or cephalexin 500 mg qid x14 d, 90% cure (AnM 150:790,
Previously untreated, limited in extent, no osteomyelitis	aureus, enterococcus	**Clinda** or **O Ceph 1**	**Clinda** (see footnote¹ and Comment on dosage¹)	1990) (AHCL 98:1964, 1998).
Chronic, recurrent, limb-threatening (see Bone, page 3, for associated osteomyelitis)	enterococci, aerobic Gm+/ cocci, anaerobic Gm+ cocci, aerobic Gm-neg. bacilli (e.g. E. coli) & strict	Non-limb-threatening: **TC/CL** or **AM/CL**	**TC/CL** or **PIP/TZ** (see footnote²) or **levo** or (**cefoxime**/**cefotaxime** or **CIP** or **levo** or (**aztreonam**)	Osteomyelitis unless ulcers unreliable. R/O necrotizing fasciitis and R/O osteo. X-ray to R/O gas and concomitant osteomyelitis. Ability to insert probe to bone suggests concomitant osteomyelitis (JAMA 273:721, 1995). MRI cannot distinguish marrow edema from osteo (Radiol 203:849, 1997).
NOTE: Prognosis depends on blood supply; assess for arterial insufficiency early	anaerobes (e.g. B. fragilis)	Limb-threatening: [(**IMP** or **MER** or **ertapenem** or **trova**) + **vanco²**]	Limb-threatening: [(**IMP** or **MER** or **ertapenem** or **trova**) + **vanco²**] Dosages in footnote²	Avoidance of weight-bearing is key (NEJM 331:854, 1994). NOTE: **Ertapenem** less active vs P. aeruginosa than IMP or MER.
Onychomycosis. See Table 10, page 76, fungal infections				
GALLBLADDER				
Cholecystitis, cholangitis, biliary sepsis, common duct obstruc- tion (partial: 2° to tumor, stones, stricture)	Enterobacteriaceae 68%, enterococci 14%, bacteroi- des 10%, Clostridium sp. 7%	**PIP/TZ** or **AM/SB** or **TC/CL** If life-threatening: **IMP** or **MER**	**P Ceph 3** + (**metro** or **clinda**) OR **Aztreonam** + **clinda** OR **AMP** + **gent** ± **metro** Dosages in footnote²	For severely ill pts, antibiotic rx is complementary to establishment of adequate biliary drainage (CID 19:279, 1994). 15–30% pts will require decompression: surgi- cal, percutaneous or ERCP-placed stent. Whether empirical rx should always cover pseudomonas & anaerobes is uncertain (CID 19:279, 1994). Ceftriaxone associated with biliary sludge (by ultrasound) 50%, symptomatic 3%, NEJM 322:1821, 1990); clinical relevance still unclear but has led to surgery (MMWR 42:39, 1993).

¹ **Cefotaxim** 2.0 gm q6h IV, **CIP** 750 mg bid po or 400 mg bid IV, **clinda** 300 mg po or 450–900 mg q8h IV, **IMP** 0.5 gm q6h IV, **MER** 1.0 gm q8h IV, **AM/CL** 875/125 mg q12h or 500/125 mg tid po, **TC/CL** 3.1 gm q4-6h IV, **PIP/TZ** 3.375 gm q6h IV or 4.5 gm q8h IV, **aztreonam** 2.0 gm q8h IV, **FQ IV** (**CIP** 400 mg q12h, **levo** 500 mg q24h, **gati** 400 mg q24h, **ofllox** 400 mg q12h, **trova** 200 mg), **APAG**: see Table 9C, page 71 for dosing of aminoglycosides.
² **Pen** **ticarcillin**-11.0 gm q6h IV, **PIP** 4.0 gm q6h IV, **metro** 1.0 gm IV loading dose then 0.5 gm q6h IV or 1.0 gm q12h IV, **gent and gent** and other **aminoglycosides**, see Table 9C, page 71, **IMP** 0.5 gm q6h IV, **MER** 1.0 gm q8h IV, **CIP** 400 mg q12h IV, **levo** 750 mg IV q24, **trova** 300 mg IV q24. **clinda** and **aztreonam** dosage, **P Ceph 3** dose in Table 9B, pages 65, 66. **CIP** 400 mg IV q12h, **levo** 750 mg IV q12h. NOTE: All dosage recommendations are for adults (unless otherwise indicated) and assume normal renal function.
(Footnotes and abbreviations on page 45)

TABLE 1 (10)

ANATOMIC SITE/DIAGNOSIS/ MODIFYING CIRCUMSTANCES	ETIOLOGIES (usual)	SUGGESTED REGIMENS* PRIMARY	SUGGESTED REGIMENS* ALTERNATIVE§	ADJUNCT DIAGNOSTIC OR THERAPEUTIC MEASURES AND COMMENTS
GASTROINTESTINAL				
Gastroenteritis—Empiric Therapy (laboratory studies not performed or culture, microscopy, toxin results NOT AVAILABLE) (Ref. *CID 32:331, 2001*)				
Premature infant with necrotizing enterocolitis	Associated with intestinal flora	Treatment and rationale is for diverticulitis/peritonitis, page 14. See Table 16, page 126 for pediatric dosages		Pneumatosis intestinalis on x-ray confirms dx. Bacteremia-peritonitis in 30–50%. If Staph. epidermidis isolated, add vanco (IV).
Mild diarrhea (≤3 unformed stools/day, minimal associated symptomatology)	Bacterial (see Severe, below), minimal associated symptomatology. Viral usually causes mild to moderate disease. (See A/M)	Fluids only + lactose-free diet, avoid caffeine		**Rehydration: For po fluid replacement, see Cholera, page 12.**
Moderate diarrhea (≥4 unformed stools/day and/or systemic symptoms)		Antimotility agents (see Comments) + fluids		**Antimotility:** Loperamide (Imodium) 4 mg po, then 2 mg after each loose stool to max. of 16 mg/day (daily dose ≤6 mg/day if mild disease), no antiperistaltic (po/IV) or bismuth subsalicylate (Pepto-Bismol) 2 tablets (262 mg) po qid. Do not use if suspect hemolytic uremic syndrome.
Severe diarrhea (≥6 unformed stools/day, and/or temperature ≥101°F, tenesmus, blood, or fecal leucocytes) **NOTE: Severe afebrile bloody diarrhea ↑ suspicion of E. coli 0157:H7 infection**—causes only 1–3% all cases diarrhea in U.S.—but causes up to 36% cases of bloody diarrhea (*CID 32:573, 2001*)	Shigella, salmonella, C. jejuni, E. coli 0157:H7, toxin-positive C. difficile, E. histolytica. For typhoid fever, see page 44	**FQ (CIP** 500 mg q12h po) x3–5 days *If recent antibiotic therapy (C. difficile possible) add:* **Metro** 500 mg tid po x10–14 days	**TMP/SMX-DS** bid po x3–5 days. Resistance to TMP/SMX common throughout tropics. **Vanco** 125 mg tid po x 14 days	**Hemolytic uremic syndrome (HUS):** Risk in **children** infected with E. coli 0157:H7 is 8–10%. Early treatment with TMP/SMX ↑ risk of HUS (*NEJM 342:1930 & 1990, 2000*). **Other potential etiologies:** Cryptosporidia—no treatment in immunocompetent host (see Table 12A & JID 170:272, 1994), Cyclospora—usually chronic diarrhea. Responds to TMP/SMX (see Table 12A & AIM 123:409, 1996). **Severe diarrhea** was treated with CIP 500 mg bid po or placebo, CIP ↓ duration of diarrhea and other symptoms without changing duration of fecal carriage. 10% campylobacter in Minn. resistant to FQs (*NEJM 340:1525, 1999*).
Gastroenteritis—Specific Therapy (results of culture, microscopy, toxin assay AVAILABLE), Ref. *CID 32:331, 2001*				
Aeromonas/plesiomonas		**CIP** 500 mg po bid x3 d.	**TMP/SMX-DS** po bid x3 d.	Although no absolute proof, increasing evidence as cause of diarrheal illness.
Campylobacter jejuni Fever in 53–83%,† bloody stools 37%	See Comment	**Azithro** 500 mg po qid x3 d. or **CIP** 500 mg po bid x5 d.	**Erytho stearate** 500 mg qid x5 d.	† worldwide resistance to FQs varies by region from 10% (USA) to 84% (Thailand) (*CID 32:1201, 2001; EID 7:24, 2001*). Risk of Guillain-Barré syndrome is less than 1/1000 infections (*JID 176:S125, 2007*).
C. difficile toxin positive antibiotic-associated colitis (Ref.: *MMWR 46:334, 2002*) **Remember: enteric isola-tion indicated** Fever in 28%		**Metro** 500 mg tid or 250 mg qid po x10–14 d. Rare reports of resistance to metro (*AAC 46:1647, 2002*)	**Vanco** 125 mg qid po) or **(bactracin** 25,000 u qid po) x10–14 d or **cholestyramine** 4 gm bid po x5–10 d **Teicoplanin**§,§ 400 mg bid po x10 d.	**DC antibiotic if possible; avoid antimotility agents; hydration; enteric isolation.** For refractory disease, vanco po + RIF reported effective (*IChE 16:459, 1995*). metro + RIF should work also but no published data. • If relapse (occurs in 10–20%, retreat with metro x10 d, then (cholestyramine 4 gm po) bid + (lactobacillus po) x10 d. If effective, not established. When po or metro po not possible, use IV metro + vanco 500 mg/L saline via small bowel tube and/or via nasogastric tube and/or IV (metro 500 mg q6h or vanco 125 mg q6h) po x10 d. Rare reports of relapses: metro x10 d. then (cholestyramine 4 gm po) bid + (lactobacillus po) x10 d. When po or metro not possible, use IV metro + vanco 500 mg/L saline via small bowel tube and/or via N-G or naso-small bowel tube (cecal tube) and/or retrograde cecal catheter and/or vanco enemas (see Comment)	Relapse occurs in 10–20%, retreat with metro x10 d, then (cholestyramine 4 gm po) bid + (lactobacillus po) x10 d. If effective, not established. When po or metro po not possible, use IV metro + vanco 500 mg/L saline via small bowel tube and/or via nasogastric tube at ≥2.0 ml/min via small bowel tube max. of 2.0 gm; see *NEJM 329:583, 1993 & DCI 35:690, 2002*. Perfuse at 1 ml/min to daily max. of 2.0 gm; see *NEJM 329:583, 1993 & DCI 35:690, 2002*. **NOTE: IV vanco not effective.** In hospital pts, exposure to P Ceph 3 have ↑ risk (*Aliment Pharm Ther 12:1217, 1998*). C. difficile toxin from community-acquired diarrhea; use of antibiotic exposure (*IDCP 6:385, 1997*).
Amebiasis (Entamoeba histolytica, cyclospora and cryptosporidia), see Table 12A				

NOTE: All dosage recommendations are for adults (unless otherwise indicated) and assume normal renal function

TABLE 1 (11)

ANATOMIC SITE/DIAGNOSIS/ MODIFYING CIRCUMSTANCES	ETIOLOGIES (usual)	SUGGESTED REGIMENS*		ADJUNCT DIAGNOSTIC OR THERAPEUTIC MEASURES AND COMMENTS
		PRIMARY	ALTERNATIVE⁵	
Gastrointestinal/Gastroenteritis—Specific Therapy (continued)				
E. coli 0157:H7 Fever in 16–45%, H/O¹ bloody stools 63%		**NO TREATMENT** with antimicrobials, as may enhance toxin release and ↑ risk of hemolytic uremic syndrome (HUS) (NEJM 342:1930 & 1990, 2000). Avoid anti-motility drugs.		Natural history: 95% resolve, 5% develop HUS. Toxin terminology: O: 351:1003, 1998. Anecdotal report of safety and efficacy of [testimony] (Dig Dis Nephr 52:367, 1999).
Listeria monocytogenes		AMP 200 mg/kg/d IV q6h	TMP/SMX 20 mg/kg/d IV div. q6-8h	Recently recognized cause of food poisoning, manifest as febrile gastroenteritis. Percentage with complicating bacteremia/meningitis unknown. Not detected in standard stool culture (NEJM 336:100 & 130, 1997).
Salmonella, non-typhi— For typhoid fever, see page	If pt asymptomatic or illness mild, antimicrobial therapy not indicated. (Also see Typhoid fever, page 43)			
Fever in 71–91%, H/O¹ bloody stools in 34%	If pt septic or immunocompromised, or pt ill enough to hospitalize, antimicrobial agents indicated. **CiP** 500 mg po bid x5-7 d. or **Kluvo** 10 gm po once d. Resistance ↑ (Ln 353:1590, 1999)	**TMP/SMX** and chloro. Cefriaxone, cefotaxime usually active (see footnote, page 16, for dosage), APAG and aztreonam **not** effective. Primary treatment of enteritis is fluid and electrolyte replacement. No adverse effects from FQs in children (Ln 348:547, 1996). If immunocompromised, rx 14 d.		**Peds doses:** TMP/SMX 5/25 mg/kg po x3 d. For severe disease: ceftriaxone 50–75 mg/kg/d x2–5 d. CiP suspension 10 mg/kg bid x5-7 (Ln 352:522, 1998). **Immunocompromised children & adults: Treat for 7–10 d.**
Shigella Fever in 58%, H/O¹ bloody stools 51%		**FQs po (CiP 500 mg)** or **(dfox 300 mg)]—bid x3 d.** See Comment	**TMP/SMX-DS** bid po x3 d.) or **(azithro** 500 mg po x1, then 250 mg x4 d.)	Sensitive in vitro to FQ, doxy. Often history of seafood ingestion.
Vibrio cholerae Treatment decreases duration of disease, vol. losses, and duration of excretion		**CiP** 1.0 gm po x1 + fluids **Primary rx is hydration** (see Comment)	**Doxy** 300 mg po x1 + fluids (see Comment) For children ≤ 8 yr, in pregnancy, give **TMP/SMX-DS**, one bid po x3 d	**Rehydration.** 1 level teaspoon table salt + a heaping teaspoon sugar + 1 liter H₂O—5.4 gm Na lactate, 8 gm glucose. **PO** use (per liter potable water): 1 level teaspoon table salt + a heaping teaspoon sugar (JTM 84:73, 1981). Volume given—fluid loss. Mild dehydration, give 5% body weight. For moderate, 7% body weight. (Refs. CID 20:1485, 1995; TRSM 89:103, 1995).
Vibrio parahaemolyticus		Antimicrobial rx does not shorten course.		Tetra & TMP/SMX resistance reported (Ln 349:924, 1997). Review. Ln 349:1825, 1997.
Yersinia enterocolitica Ref. PIDJ 14:771, 1995 Fever in 68%, bloody stools in 26%		**CiP** 1.0 gm po x1 for Shigella **CiP** eq for Shigella **TMP/SMX** or **doxy** if severe (CID 17:405, 1993)	**Ceftriaxone** 2.0 gm po and IV. **TMP/SMX-DS**, one bid po x3 d	Mesenteric adenitis can mimic acute appendicitis. Dx diagnosis difficult, requires "cold enrichment" and/or yersinia selective agar. Desferrioxamine rx ↑ severity, discontinue if pt on it. Iron overload states predispose to yersinia (CID 27:1362 & 367, 1998).
Gastroenteritis—Specific Risk Groups—Empiric Therapy				
Anoreceptive intercourse				
Proctitis (distal 15 cm only)	Herpes viruses, gonococci, chlamydia, syphilis. See Genital Tract, page 15		**FQ** (e.g., **CiP** 500 mg q12h po) x3 d.	See Table 12A
Colitis	Shigella, salmonella, campylobacter, E. histolytica (see Table 12A)			See Table 12A
HIV-1 infected (AIDS): >10 days diarrhea	[G. lamblia			See Table 12A
Acid-fast organisms:	Cryptosporidium parvum, Cyclospora cayetanensis			For influence of highly active antiretroviral therapy, see CID 27:695, 1999 and Table 14, page 113
Other:	Microsporidia, Isospora belli, microsporidia Enterocytozoon bieneusi, Septata intestinalis)			
Neutropenic enterocolitis or "typhlitis" (CID 27:695 & 700, 1998)	Mucosal invasion by Clostridium septicum. Occasionally caused by C. sordelli or P. aeruginosa		As for perirectal abscess. Ensure empiric regimen includes drug active vs Clostridia species; e.g., **pen G**, **AMP** or **clinda**. Empiric regimen should have predictive activity vs P. aeruginosa also.	Tender right lower quadrant. Surgical resection controversial but may be necessary.

¹ H/O = history of

NOTE: All dosage recommendations are for adults (unless otherwise indicated) and assume normal renal function

(Footnotes and abbreviations on page 45)

TABLE 1 (12)

ANATOMIC SITE/DIAGNOSIS/ MODIFYING CIRCUMSTANCES	ETIOLOGIES (usual)	SUGGESTED REGIMENS*		ADJUNCT DIAGNOSTIC OR THERAPEUTIC MEASURES AND COMMENTS
		PRIMARY	ALTERNATIVE†	
Gastrointestinal/Gastroenteritis—Specific Risk Groups—Empiric Therapy *(continued)*				
Traveler's diarrhea, self-medication. Patient usually afebrile *(NEJM 342:1716, 2000)*	**Acute:** Toxigenic E. coli, shigella, salmonella, campylobacter, C. difficile, amebiasis *(see Table 12)*. If **chronic:** cyclospora, cryptosporidia, giardia, isospora	**Mild—non-dysenteric: loperamide** (Imodium) + **one dose of CIP** 750 mg. Severe—**dysenteric diarrhea: loperamide + CIP** bid x3 d. If temp >102°F or blood in stool: **loperamide** 4 mg x1, then 2 mg after each loose stool to max. 16 mg/d. For FQ dosage, see footnote†	non-dysenteric: **loperamide** (Imodium) + **one azithro** 500 mg x1, then 250 mg x4 d. or 1000 mg x1 dose. Peds & pregnancy: avoid FQs. Peds dose of azithro 5–10 mg/kg/d x1 dose. No loperamide under age 2.	If can't use FQ: **azithro** 500 mg x1, then 250 mg x4 d. or 1000 mg x1 dose. Peds & pregnancy: avoid FQs. Peds dose of azithro 5–10 mg/kg/d x1 dose. No loperamide under age 2. Changing susceptibility of bacterial enteropathogens: AAC 45:212, 2001.
Prevention		Not routinely indicated. Current recommendation is to take **FQ + Imodium** with 1st loose stool *(NEJM 328:1821, 1993)*	Alternative during 1st 3 weeks only if activities are essential. Options: **Bismuth subsalicylate** (Pepto-Bismol) 2 tabs (262 mg) qid or **FQ**—**CIP** 500 mg po qd.	**Bismuth subsalicylate** can cause black tongue and dark stool
Gastrointestinal Infections by Anatomic Site				
Esophagitis	Candida albicans, HSV, CMV	[See SANFORD GUIDE TO HIV/AIDS THERAPY]		
Duodenal/Gastric ulcer, chronic (type B antral gastritis (not 2° NSAIDs). Prevalence of pretreatment resistance increasing *(NEJM 347:1175, 2002)*	**Helicobacter pylori** *See Comment*	**Rx 2x/day for 14 days: Omeprazole** 20 mg + **amox** 1 gm + **clarithro** 500 mg. Efficacy 80–95%	**Rx po for 14 days: Bismuth** (see footnote³) 4x/d. + **metro** 500 mg 4x/d. + **tetracycline** 500 mg 4x/d. + **metro** 500 mg 3x/d. + **omeprazole** 20 mg 2x/d. Efficacy 90–99%	**Dx gold standard:** positive urease on biopsy specimen, histology, or ¹⁴C or ¹³C labeled urea breath test (UBT). Can use antigen-based stool assay, esp. in children—compared to UBT: sens. of 94%, spec. of 90% *(PID J 19:364, 2000; Hepato-Gastro 49:576, 2002).* False-pos. stool antigen can occur—other Helicobacter species (BMJ 320:148, 2000). Confirm cure with UBT or stool antigen 8 wks after end of treatment. Rx failure usually 2° to resistance to metronidazole or clarithro; can overcome metro resistance with 14 d. (longer) rx.
Whipple's disease *(CID 32:457, 2001)*	Tropheryma whippleii	**Initial 10–14 days:** Pen G 24 mill. U/IV qd + **streptomycin** 1.0 gm IM/IV qd OR **ceftriaxone** 2.0 gm IV qd Then, for approx. 1 year **TMP/SMX-DS** 1 tab po bid	**TMP/SMX-DS** 1 tab po bid for approx. 1 year **Doxy** 100 mg po bid) or (**cefixime** 400 mg po qd).	Rx regimen based on impression and retrospective analyses. TMP/SMX: CNS relapses during TMP/SMX rx reported.
Infective endocarditis, culture-negative, page 20			**Cent VK** 500 mg po qid.	
Inflammatory bowel disease: Ulcerative colitis, Crohn's disease	Unknown	**Sulfasalazine** 1.0 gm q6h po or **mesalamine** (Asacol) 800 mg q8h po. See NEJM 334:841, 1996		Continued rx if response after initial response *(AJM 93:199, 1992).* Check stool for E. histolytica overgrowth with metro before steroid enemas; cause mucormycosis in 0.7–10% in 1st 3 months of rx with sulfasalazine, may respond to G-CSF.
Mild to moderate *Rx: NEJM 334:1091, 1996*		**Sulfasalazine** 1.0 gm q6h po or **mesalamine** (SASA) 1.0 gm q6h po.	Asacol) 800 mg q8h—all equally effective (AnIM 124:204, 1996). Corticosteroid enemas	
Severe Crohn's	Unknown	Etanercept	Unlabeled	Risk of disseminated TBc [see Table 11A] & other serious infections.

---

* **FQ** dosage for self-rx traveler's diarrhea—mild disease: **CIP** 750 mg x1; severe: 500 mg bid x3 d. **Oflox** 300 mg po bid x3 d. Once daily, **Levo** 500 mg, **gati** or **moxi** 400 mg x3 d. probably would work but not FDA-approved indication.

² Can substitute another proton pump inhibitor for omeprazole—all bid: esomeprazole 20 mg, lansoprazole 30 mg, pantoprazole 40 mg, rabeprazole 20 mg

³ **3 bismuth preparations:** (1) In U.S., bismuth subsalicylate (Pepto-Bismol) 262 mg tabs; adult dose for helicobacter is 2 tabs (524 mg) 4x/day. (2) Outside U.S., colloidal bismuth subcitrate (De-Nol) 120 mg chewable tablets, dose is 1 tablet 4x/day (3) Another treatment option: Ranitidine bismuth citrate 400 mg; give with metro 500 mg and clarithro 500 mg—all bid x7 d. Worked despite metro/clarithro resistance (Gastro 114:A923, 1998)

(Footnotes and abbreviations on page 45) NOTE: *All dosage recommendations are for adults (unless otherwise indicated) and assume normal renal function*

TABLE 1 (13)

ANATOMIC SITE/DIAGNOSIS/MODIFYING CIRCUMSTANCES	ETIOLOGIES (usual)	SUGGESTED REGIMENS*		ADJUNCT DIAGNOSTIC OR THERAPEUTIC MEASURES AND COMMENTS
		PRIMARY	ALTERNATIVE†	
GASTROINTESTINAL/Gastrointestinal infections by anatomic site (continued)				
Diverticulitis, peritoneal abscess, peritonitis Also see *Peritonitis, page 31*	P. aeruginosa, Bacteroides sp., enterococci	**Outpatient rx-mild diverticulitis, drained perirectal abscess:** (TMP/SMX-DS bid) or (CIP 500 mg bid) All po x7-10 d.	AM/CL 500/125 mg tid po x7-10 d. metro 500 mg q6h. All	Multiple regimens effective. Must "cover" both Gm-neg. aerobic and Gm-neg. anaerobic bacteria. **Drugs active vs aerobic Gm-neg. bacilli:** clinda, metro. **Drugs active only vs aerobic Gm-neg. bacilli:** APAG, P Ceph 2/3/4, aztreonam, AP Pen, CIP, TMP/SMX. **Drugs active vs both aerobic/anaerobic Gm-neg. bacteria:** cefotetan, cefoxitin, cefmetazole, TC/CL, PIP/TZ, AM/SB, ertapenem, IMP, MER, gati, moxi, & trova. **NOTE:** Ertapenem less active vs P. aeruginosa/Acinetobacter sp. than IMP or MER.
		Mild-moderate disease—Inpatient—Parenteral Rx: (e.g., focal peri-appendiceal peritonitis, peri-diverticular abscess, endomyometritis) **AM/SB** 3 gm IV q6h **or** **PIP/TZ** 3.375 gm IV q6h **or** or 4.5 gm IV q8h **or** **TC/CL** 3.1 gm IV q6h **or** **ertapenem** 1.0 gm IV qd	**Cefoxitin** 2 gm IV q6h **or** **cefotetan** 2 gm IV q12h **or** (CIP 400 mg IV q12h + metro 500 mg IV q6h)	Concomitant surgical management important, esp. with moderate-severe disease. Role of enterococci remains debatable. Probably pathogenic in infections of biliary tract. Probably need drugs active vs enterococci in pts with valvular heart disease.
		Severe life-threatening disease, ICU patient: **IMP** 500 mg IV q6h **or** **MER** 1 gm IV q8h	Trova 300 mg IV qd, then 200 mg qd **or** [AMP 2 gm IV q6h + metro 500 mg IV q6h + APAG (see Table 9C, page 70)] **OR** AMP² + metro + CIP 400 mg IV q12h	
GENITAL TRACT: Mixture of empiric & specific treatment. Divided by sex of the patient. See Guidelines for Dx of Sexually Transmitted Diseases, *MMWR 51(RR-6)*, 2002				
Both Women & Men:				
Chancroid	H. ducreyi	**Ceftriaxone** 250 mg IM single dose **OR** azithro 1.0 gm po single dose.	**CIP** 500 mg bid po x3 d. OR **erythro base** 500 mg qid po x7 d.	In HIV + pts, failures reported with single dose azithro (CID 21:409, 1995; IDCP 4:67, 1995). Ref: CID 28(Suppl. 1):S14, 1999
Chlamydia, et al. non-gonococcal or post-gonococcal urethritis/cervicitis. NOTE: assume concomitant N. gonorrhoeae, see treatment options above. For conjunctivitis, see *Coryneha, page 8*	Chlamydia 50%, Mycoplasma hominis. Other known etiologies (10-15%): Ureaplasma, Trichomonas, herpes simplex virus, Mycoplasma genitalium	(Doxy 100 mg bid po x7 d.) or (azithro 1.0 gm po single dose). Evaluate & tx sex partner. **In pregnancy: erythro base** 500 mg po qid x7 d. OR amox 500 mg po tid x7 d.	(Erythro base 500 mg qid po x7 d.) or (ofox 300 mg po bid x7 d.) or (levo 500 mg qd x7 d.) In pregnancy: azithro 1.0 gm po x1 Doxy & ofox contraindicated	Diagnosis: PCR/LCR of voided urine (male or female) sensitive and specific; if not available, culture or antigen detection. Doxy and FQ not recommended in pregnancy. Clarithro active in vitro vs C. trachomatis, but not FDA-approved for STDs. For recurrent or persistent disease: either metro 2.0 gm po x1 + either erythro base 500 mg po qid x7 d. or erythro ethylsuccinate 800 mg po qid x7 d. Ref: Sex Trans Dis 26(Suppl.):S4, 1999.
Recurrent/persistent urethritis	Occult trichomonas, tetracycline-resistant U. urealyticum	**Metro** 2.0 gm po x1 + **erythro base** 500 mg po qid x7 d.	**Erythro ethylsuccinate** 800 mg po qid x7 d.	Evaluate & treat sex partners.
Gonorrhea [*MMWR 51(RR-6)*, 2002] **Conjunctivitis (adult)**	N. gonorrhoeae	**Ceftriaxone** 1 gm IM or IV x1 + lavage with saline x1		

NOTE: All dosage recommendations are for adults (unless otherwise indicated) and assume normal renal function

TABLE 1 (14)

ANATOMIC SITE/DIAGNOSIS/ MODIFYING CIRCUMSTANCES	ETIOLOGIES (usual)	SUGGESTED REGIMENS* PRIMARY	ALTERNATIVE†	ADJUNCT DIAGNOSTIC OR THERAPEUTIC MEASURES AND COMMENTS
GENITAL TRACT/Both Women & Men/Gonorrhea [MMWR 51(RR-6), 2002] (continued)				
Disseminated gonococcal infection (DGI, dermatitis arthritis syndrome)	N. gonorrhoeae	(Ceftriaxone 1.0 gm IV q d) or (cefotaxime 1.0 gm q8h IV) or (ceftizoxime 1.0 gm q8h IV)—see Comment	Spectinomycin 2.0 gm q12h IM OR (CIP 400 mg IV q12h or oflox 400 mg IV q12h or levo 250 mg IV q12h)—see Comment	Continue IM or IV regimen for 24 hrs after symptoms ↓; reliable pts may be discharged 24 hrs after resolve to complete 7 days in with ceftime 400 mg po bid or CIP 500 mg po bid or oflox 400 mg po bid or levo 500 mg po bid x7 d. R/O meningitis/endocarditis. Treat presumptively for concomitant C. trachomatis.
Endocarditis/Meningitis	N. gonorrhoeae	Ceftriaxone 1-2 gm IV q12h		
Pharyngitis	N. gonorrhoeae	Ceftriaxone 125 mg IM x1	CIP 500 mg po x1	If chlamydia not ruled out: Azithro 1 gm po x1 or doxy 100 mg po bid x7 d
Urethritis, cervicitis, proctitis (uncomplicated) For prostatitis, see page 17	N. gonorrhoeae (50% of pts with urethritis, cervicitis have concomitant C. trachomatis—**treat for both**). Dx by amplification (PCR/LCR) of DNA in voided urine.	(Ceftriaxone 125 mg IM x1) or (cefixime 400 mg po x1) or (CIP 500 mg po x1) or (oflox 400 mg po x1) or (levo 250 mg po x1) or (gati 400 mg po x1) **PLUS** (Azithro 1 gm po x1) or (doxy 100 mg po 2x/d x7 days) — Evaluate and rx sex partner. Due to ↑ resistance, do not use a quinolone to treat gonorrhea that may have been acquired in Hawaii, Asia, or other Pacific areas.	Spectinomycin 2 gm IM x1. Other single-dose cephalosporins: ceftizoxime 500 mg IM, cefotaxime 500 mg IM, cefoxitin 2 gm IM + probenecid 1 gm po. Other single-dose oral quinolones: lome 400 mg, gati 400 mg, norflox 800 mg. Azithro 1 gm po x1 effective for chlamydia but need 2 gm for GC; not recommended for GC due to GI side-effects and expense.	**Treat for both GC and C. trachomatis.** Screen for syphilis. Other alternatives for GC:
Granuloma inguinale (Donovanosis)	Calymmatobacterium granulomatis	Doxy 100 mg bid po x3 wks OR TMP/SMX-DS 2x/d x3 wks	Erythro 0.5 gm po x21 d OR CIP 750 mg po bid x3 wks OR azithro 1.0 gm po q wk x3 wks	Clinical response usually seen in 1 week. Rx until all lesions healed, may take 4 weeks. Treatment failure & recurrences seen with doxy and TMP/SMX. Report of efficacy with F/Q and chloro. Ref. CID 25,24, 1997.
Herpes simplex virus	See Table 14, page 106			
Lymphogranuloma venereum	Chlamydia trachomatis, serovars L1, L2, L3.	Doxy 100 mg bid po x21 d	Erythro 0.5 gm po x21 d	Dx based on serology; biopsy contraindicated because sinus tracts develop. Rectal LGV may require re-treatment.
Phthirus pubis (pubic lice, "crabs") & scabies	[Phthirus pubis & Sarcoptes scabiei]	See Table 12, page 97		
Syphilis [MMWR 51(RR-6), 2002] Early: primary, secondary, or latent <1 year	T. pallidum	Benzathine pen G 2.4 mU IM x1	(Doxy 100 mg po x14 d) or (tetracycline 500 mg po qid x14 d) or (ceftriaxone 1 gm IV/IM daily x8-10 d). Follow-up mandatory.	Every effort should be made to document penicillin allergy before choosing alternative (good general ref. NEJM 326:1060, 1992). All pts with early or congenital syphilis should have quantitative VDRL at 3, 6, 12 & 24 months. If pt had 1° or 2° VDRL should ↓ 2 tubes at 6 months. 3 tubes 12 months, & 4 tubes 24 months. Early latent: 2 tubes ↓ at 12 months. With 1°, 50% will be RPR seronegative at 2 months, 24% neg 1 TA/ABS at 2–3 yrs [AJM 114:1.005, 1991]. Re-treat if (1) clinical signs persist or recur, (2) a sustained 4-fold ↑ titer over initial, (3) an initially high titer fails to decrease to <1:8 at 1 year. Ref. on syphilis serology: JDCP 5:351, 1996
More than 1 yr's duration (latent of indeterminate duration, cardiovascular, late benign)		Benzathine pen G 2.4 mU IM q week x3 = 7.2 mU total	Doxy 100 mg bid po x28 d OR tetracycline 500 mg po qid x28 d	No published data on efficacy of alternatives. The value of routine lumbar puncture in asymptomatic late syphilis is being questioned in the U.S., i.e., no LP in all patients who are asymptomatic recommendation, AMM 145:465, 1986. Indications for LP (CDC): neurologic symptoms, treatment failure, serum non-treponemal titer ≥1:32, other evidence of active syphilis (aortitis, gumma, iritis), non-penicillin rx, + HIV test.
Neurosyphilis—Very difficult to treat. Includes ocular (retrobulbar neuritis) syphilis.		Pen G 3-4 mU q4h IV x10-14 d OR AMP 4.0 gm q4h x10-14 d	(Procaine pen G 2.4 mU IM + probenecid 0.5 gm po qid) x10-14 d—See Comment	Ceftriaxone 2.0 gm po (IV or IM) x14 d. 23% failure rate reported during study. For pts with penicillin allergy: either desensitize to penicillin or obtain infectious diseases consultation. Serologic criteria for rx: 4-fold or greater ↓ in VDRL titer over 6–12 mos. CID 28 [Suppl. 1]:S21, 1999.

(Footnotes and abbreviations on page 45)

NOTE: All dosage recommendations are for adults (unless otherwise indicated) and assume normal renal function

TABLE 1 (15)

ANATOMIC SITE/DIAGNOSIS/ MODIFYING CIRCUMSTANCES	ETIOLOGIES (usual)	SUGGESTED REGIMENS* PRIMARY	ALTERNATIVE†	ADJUNCT DIAGNOSTIC OR THERAPEUTIC MEASURES AND COMMENTS
GENITAL TRACT/Both Women & Men/Syphilis (continued)				
HIV Infection (AIDS) (See SANFORD GUIDE TO HIV/AIDS THERAPY for details)	T. pallidum	Adding 10 d. of **amox** + **probene- cid** to **pen G** did not change effi- cacy in 1° & 2° syphilis (NEJM 337: 307, 1997)	For neurosyphilis, recommendations vary; some use **pen G** 2.4 mU as an alternative agent.	Clinical presentations, serology & response to rx may be atypical (AJM 99:55, 1995). Higher doses & longer periods of rx may be required. Repeat VDRL titer (RPR) at 3, 6, 12, 24 months. Reinfection with T. pallidum not uncommon. Erythro should not be used as an alternative agent. Re-treat if needed (AJM 93:481, 1992): see Syphilis, above, for indications.
Pregnancy and syphilis	Same as for non-pregnant, some recommend 2ⁿᵈ dose (2.4 mU) **benzathine pen G** 1 wk after initial dose esp. in 3ʳᵈ trimester or with 2° syphilis.		Skin test for penicillin allergy. Desensitize if necessary.	Monthly quantitative VDRL or equivalent. Doxy, tetracycline contraindicated. Erythro not recommended because of high risk of failure to cure fetus.
Congenital syphilis	T. pallidum	**Aqueous crystalline pen G** 50,000 u/kg/dose IV/IM q8-12h, x10-14 d.	**Procaine pen G** 50,000 U/kg IM qd IM for 10 d. OR **pen G** 50,000 u/kg/dose IV x10-14 d.	Another alternative: Ceftriaxone <30 days old. 75 mg/kg IV/M qd or >30 days old 100 mg/kg IV/IM qd. Treat 10-14 d. If symptomatic, ophthalmologic exam indicated. If more than 1 day of rx missed, restart entire course. **Need serologic follow-up!**
Warts, anogenital	See Table 14, page 109			
Women:				
Amnionitis, septic abortion	Bacteroides, esp. Prevotella bivius, Group B, A strepto- cocci. Enterobacteriaceae; C. trachomatis	[(**Cefoxitin** or **TC/CL** or **IMP** or **MER** or **PIP/TZ**)] OR [**AM/SB** or (**APAG** or **P Ceph 3**)] OR [**Clinda** + (**APAG** or **P Ceph 3**)] *Dosage: see footnote⁹*		D&C of uterus. In septic abortion, Clostridium perfringens may cause fulminant intravascular hemolysis. In postpartum patients with enigmatic fever and/or pul- monary emboli, **consider septic pelvic vein thrombophlebitis** (see Vascular, septic pelvic vein thrombophlebitis, page 44). After discharge, doxy or continue clinda. NOTE: IV clinda effective for C. trachomatis, no data on IV clinda (CID 19:720, 1994).
Cervicitis, mucopurulent	N. gonorrhoeae C. trachomatis trachomatis	Treat for gonorrhoeae, page 15 Treat for non-gonococcal urethritis, page 14		Criteria for dx: yellow or green pus on cervical swab., >10 WBC/oil field. Gram stain of cervical exudate >5 PMNs per oil field. If in doubt, send swab or urine for culture. EIA or ligase chain reaction (LCR) and n. for both.
Endomyometritis/septic pelvic phlebitis				
Early postpartum (1ˢᵗ 48 hrs) (usually after C-section)	Bacteroides, esp. Prevotella bivius, Group B, A strepto- cocci. Enterobacteria- ceae; C. trachomatis	[(**Cefoxitin** or **TC/CL** or **ertapenem** or **IMP** or **MER** or **AM/SB** or **PIP/TZ**) + **doxy**] OR [**Clinda** + (**APAG** or **P Ceph 3**)] OR **trova** *Dosage: see footnote⁹*		See Comments under Amnionitis, septic abortion
Late postpartum (48 hrs to 6 wks)	Chlamydia trachomatis, M. hominis	**Doxy** 100 mg q12h IV or po x14 d.		Tetracyclines not recommended in nursing mothers; discontinue nursing. M. hominis sensitive to tetra, clinda, not erythro (CID 17:S292, 1993)
Pelvic inflammatory disease (PID): salpingitis, tubo-ovarian abscess				
Outpatient rx: limit to pts with temp <38°C, WBC <11,000/mm³, minimal evi- dence of peritonitis, active bowel sounds & able to tolerate oral nourishment	N. gonorrhoeae, chlamydia, bacteroides, Enterobacteria- ceae, streptococci	**Outpatient rx:** [(Ofloxᵃ 400 mg po qd) + (**metro** 500 mg po qid x14 d.)] OR [(**ceftriaxone** 250 mg IM or (**cefoxitin** 2.0 gm IM or IV x1) + (**doxy** 100 mg po bid x14d.) ± **metro** 500 mg po bid x14 d.]	**Inpatient regimens:** [(**Cefotetan** 2.0 gm IV q12h or **cefoxitin** 2 gm IV q6h) + (**doxy** 100 mg IV/po q12h)] OR [(**Clinda** 900 mg IV q8h) + (**gentamicin** 2 mg/kg loading dose, then 1.5 mg/kg q8h or 5.0 mg/kg q24h)]	**Alternative parenteral regimens:** 1. (Oflox 400 mg IV q12h or levo 500 mg IV qd) + **metro** 500 mg IV q8h + doxy. 2. AM/SB 3 gm IV q6h + doxy 100 mg IV/po q12h + levo Remember: Evaluate and treat sex partner

---

*¹ **P Ceph 2** (**cefotetan** 2.0 gm q8-8h IV, **cefotan** 2.0 gm q12h IV, **cefuroxime** 750 mg q8h IV); **TC/CL** 3.1 gm q6h IV; **AM/SB** 3.0 gm q6h IV; **PIP/TZ** 3.375 gm q6h or 4.5 gm q8h IV; **doxy** 100 mg q12h IV or po; **clinda** 450-900 mg q8h IV; **APAG** (**gentamicin**, see Table 9C, page 71); **P Ceph 3** (**cefotaxime** 2.0 gm q8h IV, **ceftriaxone** 2.0 gm qd IV); **ertapenem** 1.0 gm qd IV; **IMP** 0.5 gm q6h IV; **MER** 1.0 gm q8h IV; **azithro** 500 mg IV qd; **trova** 300 mg IV qd. **trova** 300 mg IV/d. Then 200 mg po 1x/d. in hospital only. NOTE: All dosage recommendations are for adults (unless otherwise indicated) and assume normal renal function*

(Footnotes and abbreviations on page 45)

TABLE 1 (16)

ANATOMIC SITE/DIAGNOSIS/ MODIFYING CIRCUMSTANCES	ETIOLOGIES (usual)	SUGGESTED REGIMENS[*] PRIMARY	ALTERNATIVE[5]	ADJUNCT DIAGNOSTIC OR THERAPEUTIC MEASURES AND COMMENTS
GENITAL TRACT, Women (continued)				
Vaginitis—MMWR 51(RR-6), 2002				
Candidiasis Pruritus, thick cheesy discharge, pH <4.5 See Table 10	Candida albicans 80–90%. C. glabrata, C. tropicalis increasing—they are less susceptible to azoles	**Oral azoles:** **Fluconazole** 150 mg po po bid x1 day or **Itraconazole** 200 mg po bid x1 day	**Intravaginal azoles:** variety of strengths—from 1 dose to 7-14 d. Many available (all end in –azole): butocon, clotrim, micon, tiocon, tercon (doses: Table TOA, Sanford Guide)	Nystatin vag. tabs x14 d. less effective. Other rx for azole-resistant strains: gentian violet, boric acid. For recurrent candidiasis (4 or more episodes/yr), 6 mos. suppression with fluconazole 150 mg po q week or itraconazole 100 mg po qd or clotrimazole 100 mg vag. suppositories 500 mg q week.
Trichomoniasis Copious foamy discharge, pH >4.5 Treat sexual partners—see Comment	Trichomonas vaginalis	**Metro** 2.0 gm as single dose or 500 mg po bid x7 d. In pregnancy, defer rx until after 1st trimester.	For rx failure: Re-treat with metro 500 mg po bid x7 d. If 2nd failure: metro 2.0 gm po qd x3–5 d. If still fails, suggest ID consultation and/or contact CDC: 770-488-4115 or www.cdc.gov/std.	**Treat male sexual partners (2.0 gm metronidazole as single dose).** Another option if metro-resistant: **Tinidazole** 500 mg po bid x1 d (not approved for this indication). **Metro 2.0 gm po x1 not as effective as 5–7 day course** (JAMA 260:52, 1992). Metro extended release tabs 750 mg po qd x7 d. available: no published data. **Pregnancy:** Rx same as non-pregnancy, except avoid clindamycin cream (↑ risk premature birth).
Bacterial vaginosis Malodorous vaginal discharge, pH >4.5	Polymicrobic: associated with Gardnerella vaginalis, bacteroides non-fragilis, mobiluncus, peptococcus, Mycoplasma hominis	**Metro** 0.5 gm po bid x7 d. or **metro vaginal gel** (1 applicator intravaginally 1x/d x5 d. (avoid in 1st trimester pregnancy)	**Clinda** 0.3 gm po bid x7 d. or **metro** 2.0 gm po x1 or **clinda vaginal cream** 5 gm intravaginally hs x7 d. or **clinda ovules** 100 mg intravaginally hs x3 d.	Fix of male sex partner not indicated unless balanitis present. **Metro 2.0 gm po x1** not as effective as 5–7 day course (JAMA 260:52, 1992). Ref: CID 33:1341, 2001.
Men:				
Balanitis	Candida 40%, Group B strep, gardnerella	**Oral azoles** as for vaginitis		Occurs in ¼ of male partners of women infected with candida. Exclude circinate balanitis (Reiter's syndrome). Plasma cell balanitis (non-infectious) responds to hydrocortisone cream.
Epididymo-orchitis				
Age <35 years	N. gonorrhoeae, Chlamydia trachomatis	**Ceftriaxone** 250 mg IM x1 + **doxy** 100 mg po bid x10 d.		Also: bedrest, scrotal elevation, and analgesics.
Age >35 years or homosexual men (insertive partners in anal intercourse)	Enterobacteriaceae (coliforms)	**Oflox** 300 mg bid po or **oflox** 300 mg bid po or 400 mg bid po or **(oflox** 300 mg bid po) x10–14 d.	**AM/SB, P Ceph 3, TC/CL, PIP/TZ** (Dosage: see footnote page 16)	Midstream pyuria and scrotal pain and edema. Also: bedrest, scrotal elevation, and analgesics.
Prostatitis—Review: AJM 106:327, 1999				
Acute <35 years of age	N. gonorrhoeae, C. trachomatis	**Oflox** 400 mg po x1 then 300 mg po bid x10 d. or **cef-triaxone** 250 mg IM x1 then **doxy** 100 mg bid x10 d.		Oflox effective vs gonococci & C. trachomatis and penetrates prostate. In AIDS pts. prostate may be focus of Cryptococcus neoformans.
≥35 years of age	Enterobacteriaceae (coliforms)	**FQ** (Dosage: see Epididymo-orchitis, ≥35 yrs, above) or **TMP/SMX** 1 tablet po bid x10–14 d.		Treat as acute urinary infection, 14 days (not single dose regimen). Some authorities recommend 3-4 weeks (J AAFP 4:325, 1991).
Chronic bacterial	Enterobacteriaceae 80%, enterococcus 15%, P. aeruginosa	**FQ:** **CIP** 500 mg po bid x4 wks or **oflox** 300 mg po bid x4 wks—see Comment	**TMP/SMX-DS** 1 tab po bid x1–3 mos.	With rx failures consider infected prostatic calculi.

[*] 1 applicator contains 5.0 gm of gel with 37.5 mg metronidazole

(Footnotes and abbreviations on page 45)   NOTE: All dosage recommendations are for adults (unless otherwise indicated) and assume normal/renal function

TABLE 1 (17)

ANATOMIC SITE/DIAGNOSIS/ MODIFYING CIRCUMSTANCES	ETIOLOGIES (usual)	SUGGESTED REGIMENS* PRIMARY	ALTERNATIVE[1]	ADJUNCT DIAGNOSTIC OR THERAPEUTIC MEASURES & COMMENTS
GENITAL TRACT, Men/Prostatitis (continued)				
Chronic prostatitis/chronic pain syndrome (New NIH classification, *JAMA 282:236, 1999*)	The most common prostatitis syndrome. Etiology is unknown; molecular probe data suggest infectious etiology (*Clin Micro Rev 11: 604, 1998*).	α-adrenergic blocking agents are controversial (*AIM 133:367, 2000*).		Pt has sx of prostatitis but negative cultures and no cells in prostatic secretions. Rev. *JAC 46:157, 2000.*
HAND *(Bites: See Skin)*				
Paronychia				
Nail biting, manicuring	Staph. aureus, anaerobes	**Clinda** 300 mg qid po	**Erythro** 500 mg qid po	Onset usually 2–5 days after trauma. No lymphangitis.
Contact with oral mucosa- dentists, anesthesiologists, wrestlers	Herpes simplex (Whitlow)	**Acyclovir** 400 mg tid po x10 days	**Famciclovir or valacy- clovir** should work, see *Comment*	Gram stain and routine culture negative. Famciclovir/valacyclovir doses used for primary genital herpes, see *Table 14, page 106*
Dishwasher (prolonged water immersion)	Candida sp.	**Clotrimazole** (topical)		Avoid submersion of hands in water as much as possible
HEART				
Atherosclerotic coronary artery disease	Chlamydia pneumoniae—under study	— Summary of current data in published symposium: *JID 181(Suppl.3):S393–S586, 2000.*		
Infective endocarditis—Native valve—empirical rx awaiting cultures	NOTE: Diagnostic criteria include evidence of endocarditis on echocardiography (transthoracic or transesophageal); evidence of valvular vegetations. Review: *NEJM 345:1318, 2001.*			
Valvular or congenital heart disease including mitral valve prolapse but no modifying circumstances. *See Table 15 for prophylaxis*	Viridans strep 30–40%, "other" strep 15–25%, entero- cocci 5–18%, staphylo- cocci 20–35%	[**Pen G** 20 mU q4h IV, con- tinuous or div. q4h] PLUS (**AMP** 12 g/day IV, continuous or div. q4h) + (**nafcillin** OR **oxacillin** 2.0 gm q4h IV) + **gentamicin** 1.0 mg/kg q8h IV, not once daily dos- ing]	**Vanco** 15 mg/kg[2] q12h IV (not to exceed 2 gm q24h unless serum levels moni- tored) + **gentamicin** 1.0 mg/kg q8h IM or IV	If patient not acutely ill and not in heart failure, we prefer to wait for blood culture results. If initial 3 blood cultures neg. after 24–48 hrs, obtain 2–3 more blood cultures before empiric rx started. Nafcillin/oxacillin + gentamicin may not be adequate coverage of enterococci, hence addition of penicillin G pending cultures. When blood cultures + modify regimen from empiric rx to specific based on organism, in vitro susceptibilities. Clinical experience.
Infective endocarditis—Native valve—culture positive (Consensus opinion on treatment by organism: *JAMA 274:1706, 1995/Review: NEJM 345:1318, 2001*)				
S. viridans, S. bovis, strep	S. viridans, S. bovis	[**Pen G** 12–18 mU/d IV, con- tinuous or q4h] **x4 wks** OR [(**Pen G** 12–18 mU/d IV, con- tinuous or q4h) PLUS (**gentamicin** 1 mg/ kg q8h IV) **x2 wks**]		Also effective: (ceftriaxone 2.0 gm qd IV + (netilmicin[AUS] 4 mg/kg qd) x2 wks (*CID 21: 1406, 1995*). Target gent peak levels ~3 μg/ml, trough <1 μg/ml. If very obese pt, recommend consultation for dosage adjustment. Infuse vanco over ≥1 hr to avoid "red man" syndrome. S. bovis suggests occult bowel pathology. Once daily gentamicin may not be as effective; more data needed.
S. viridans, S. bovis with peni- cillin G MIC ≤0.1 μg/ml	S. viridans, S. bovis	[**Pen G** 12–18 mU/d IV (con- tinuous or q4h) **x4 wks**] OR [**ceftriaxone** 2.0 gm qd IV **x4 wks**]	**Vanco** 30 mg/kg/d IV in 2 div. doses to max. 2 gm/d unless serum levels docu- mented **x4 wks**	Can use ceftriaxone for pen G in pt whose allergy that is not IgE-mediated (e.g., anaphy- laxis). Alternatively, can use vanco. (See Comment above on gent and vanco)
S. viridans, S. bovis with peni- cillin G MIC >0.1 to <0.5 μg/ml nutritionally variant strep	S. viridans, S. bovis nutritionally variant strep, tolerant strep	[**Pen G** 18 mU/d IV (con- tinuous or q4h) **x4 wks**] PLUS **gentamicin** 1 mg/ kg q8h IV **x2 wks**		Also cefazolin for pen G in pt with allergy that is not IgE-mediated. Penicillin-gentamicin synergism theoretically may be advantageous in this group.

---

[1] Assumes estimated creatinine clearance ≥80 ml/min, see *Table 17.*
[2] Tolerant streptococci = MBC 32-fold greater than MIC
(Footnotes and abbreviations on page 45)
NOTE: All dosage recommendations are for adults (unless otherwise indicated) and assume normal renal function

TABLE 1 (18)

ANATOMIC SITE/DIAGNOSIS/ MODIFYING CIRCUMSTANCES	ETIOLOGIES (usual)	SUGGESTED REGIMENS*		ADJUNCT DIAGNOSTIC OR THERAPEUTIC MEASURES AND COMMENTS
		PRIMARY	ALTERNATIVE†	
HEART/Infective endocarditis—Native valve—culture positive (continued)				
For S. viridans or S. bovis with pen G MIC ≤ 0.1 and entero-coccus susceptible to AMP/pen G, vanco, gentamicin suggested	"Susceptible" entero-cocci, S. bovis, nutritionally variant streptococci	(Pen) 18-30 mu/24h continuous rx or q4h x4-6 wks PLUS genta-micin 1-1.5 mg/kg q8h IV x4-6 wks) OR (AMP 12 gm/d IV continuous or q4h x4-6 wks) gent and as above	Vanco 30 mg/kg/d IV in 2 div. doses to max. of 2 gm/d not to exceed meas-ured PLUS gentamicin 1.5 mg/kg q8h IV x4-6 wks	4 wks of rx if symptoms <3 mos.; 6 wks of rx if symptoms >3 mos. Vanco for pen-allergic pts; do not use cephalosporins. Do not give gent once-daily for enterococcal endocarditis. Target gent levels: peak 3-4 μg/ml, trough <1 μg/ml. Vanco target serum levels: peak 20-50 μg/ml, trough 5-12 μg/ml. NOTE: Because of ↑ frequency of resistance (see below), all enterococci causing endocarditis should have in vitro tests for susceptibility to penicillin, β-lactamase production, gent susceptibility, vanco & high-level resistance to aminoglycosides. 10-25% E. faecalis and 45-50% E. faecium resistant to high gent levels. May be sensitive to streptomycin, check MIC. (Scand J Inf Dis 29:628, 1997).
Enterococci, high-level aminoglycoside resistance MIC streptomycin >2000 μg/ml, MIC gentamicin >500-2000 μg/ml, no resistance to penicillin		Pen G or AMP IV as above x4-12 wks		Case report of success with combination of AMP, IMP, and vanco (Scand J Int Dis 29:628, 1997).
Enterococci, penicillin resistance β-lactamase production test is positive and β-lactamase resistance		AM/SB 3.0 gm q6h IV PLUS gentamicin 1-1.5 mg/kg q8h IV x4-6 wks	Vanco 30 mg/kg/d IV in 2 div. doses (check levels if >2 gm) x4-6 wks	β-lactamase not detected by MIC tests with standard inocula. Detection requires testing with the chromogenic cephalosporin nitrocefin. Once-daily gentamicin rx not efficacious in animal model of E. faecalis endocarditis (JAC 39:519, 1997). Review of aminoglycoside dosage regimens, JAC 49:422, 2002.
Enterococci, intrinsic pen G/AMP resistance (β-lactamase test neg, pen G MIC >16 μg/ml; no gentami-cin resistance)		Vanco 30 mg/kg/d IV in 2 div. doses PLUS gent 1-1.5 mg/kg q8h IV x4-6 wks		Desired vanco serum levels: peak 30-50 μg/ml, trough 5-12 μg/ml
Enterococci, vanco-resistant, usually E. faecium Pen/AMP resistant + high-level gent/strep resistant + vanco resistant, usually vanco-resistant E. faecium		No reliable effective rx. Can try quinupristin/ dalfopristin (Synercid) or linezolid—see Comment, footnote, and Table 5.	Synercid active against E. faecium, not E. faecalis. Teicoplanin is not available in U.S.	Synercid activity limited to E. faecium and is usually bacteriostatic, therefore expect relapse rate. Dose: 7.5 mg/kg IV (via central line, q8h) synercid, also bacteriostatic. Dose: 600 mg 2x/d. IV or po.
Coronavirus endocarditis			Teicoplanin active against enterococci. Teicoplanin is not available in U.S.	Avoid cephalosporins in pts with immediate allergic reaction to penicillin; in allergic pt, vanco may be as effective as oxacillin. No definitive data, pro or con, on once-daily gentamicin for S. aureus endocarditis. At present, favor q8h dosing x3-5 d.
Staphylococcal endocarditis Aortic and/or mitral valve infection	Staph. aureus, methicillin-sensitive	Nafcillin (oxacillin) 2.0 gm q4h IV x4-6 wks PLUS gentamicin 1.0 mg/kg q8h IV x3-5 d]	Cefazolin 2.0 gm q8h IV x4-6 wks PLUS gentami-cin 1.0 mg/kg q8h IV x3-5 d] OR Vanco 30 mg/kg/d IV in 2 div. doses (check levels if >2 gm) x4-6 wks	↑ recognition of IV catheter-associated S. aureus endocarditis. May need TEE to detect endocarditis. 23% of S. aureus bacteremia in association with IV catheter had endocarditis (CID 115:106 & 115, 1999). If TEE neg., only need 2 wks of therapy in this setting.
Tricuspid valve infection (usually IVDUs): MSSA	Staph. aureus, methicillin-sensitive	Nafcillin (oxacillin) 2 gm q4h IV PLUS gentami-cin 1 mg/kg q8h IV x2 wks	If penicillin allergy: Not clear, may not have failure rate with Cefazolin IV without gentamicin (AnIM 125:969, 1996). Can try longer duration x4-6 wks OR Vanco 30 mg/kg/d IV in 2 div. doses (check levels if >2 gm) x4-6 wks	2-week regimen not recommended if metastatic infection (e.g., osteo) or left-sided endocarditis. Cloxacillin IV without gentamicin 89% successful (AnIM 125:969, 1996). 2 reports of success with 4-week oral regimen: CIP 750 mg bid + RIF 300 mg bid. Less than 10% pts had MRSA (Ln 2:1071, 1989; AJM 101:68, 1996).
Methicillin resistance (MRSA)	Staph. aureus, methicillin-resistant	Vanco 30 mg/kg/d IV in 2 div. doses (check levels if >2 gm) x4-6 wks	Fails if resistant to vanco, can try quinu/dalfo or linezolid	For MRSA, no difference in duration of bacteremia or fever between pts rx with vanco or vanco + RIF (AnIM 115:674, 1991).

Three interesting (recent reports): (1) Successful rx of vanco-resistant E. faecium prosthetic valve endocarditis with Synercid without change in MIC (CID 25:163, 1997); (2) resistance to Synercid emerged during treatment of E. faecium bacteremia (CID 24:90, 1997); and (3) super-infection with E. faecalis occurred during Synercid rx of E. faecium

† **Quinupristin/dalfopristin (Synercid):** 7.5 mg/kg IV (via central line) q8h. **Linezolid** 600 mg IV or po q12h.

(Footnotes and abbreviations on page 45) NOTE: All dosage recommendations are for adults (unless otherwise indicated) and assume normal renal function

TABLE 1 (19)

ANATOMIC SITE/DIAGNOSIS/ MODIFYING CIRCUMSTANCES	ETIOLOGIES (usual)	SUGGESTED REGIMENS*		ADJUNCT DIAGNOSTIC OR THERAPEUTIC MEASURES AND COMMENTS
		PRIMARY	ALTERNATIVE[§]	
HEART: Infective endocarditis—Native valve–culture positive (continued)				
Slow-growing fastidious Gm-neg. bacilli	**HACEK group** (see Comments) [Mayo Clin Proc 72: 532, 1997]	Ceftriaxone 2.0 gm qd IV x4 wks	AMP 12 gm qd IV or div. q4h) x4 wks + gentamicin 1.0 mg/kg q8h IV or IM x4 wks	HACEK (acronym for Hemophilus parainfluenzae, H. aphrophilus, Actinobacillus, Cardiobacterium, Eikenella, Kingella). H. aphrophilus resistant to vanco, clinda and methicillin. Penicillinase-positive HACEK organisms should be susceptible to AM/SB + gentamicin. For hemophilus, see CID 24:1087, 1997
	B. henselae, B. quintana	**Bacteremia & NO endocarditis:** (Doxy 100 mg po bid) or (erythro 500 mg po qid) or (azithro 500 mg po qd)– all for 4–6 wks	**For endocarditis:** As for endocarditis + either gentamicin or ceftriaxone in 1st 2–3 wks. Rx 4–6 wks. May require valve replacement.	Dx: Microimmunofluorescence antibody titer ≥1:1600; blood cultures only occ. positive. Surgery: Without surgery, 1/3 cured, surgery + anti-infectives, 81% cure. B. quintana transmitted by body lice among homeless; asymptomatic colonization of RBCs described [Ln 360:226, 2002].
Infective endocarditis—culture negative				
Fever, valvular disease and ECHO vegetations ± emboli and neg. cultures	T. whipplei, Q fever, psittacosis, brucellosis, bartonella (see above)	Emphasis on dx on diagnosis. See specific organism for treatment regimens.		For Q fever, doxycycline 100 mg po bid + hydroxychloroquine 200 mg po tid x18 mos See CID 33:1347, 2001. 4 pts with afebrile culture-neg. endocarditis had T. whipplei identified by PCR of resected heart valves [AnIM 131:112 & 144, 1999]. Review Whipple's endocarditis: CID 33:1309, 2001
Infective endocarditis—Prosthetic valve—empiric therapy (cultures pending)				
Early (< 2 months post-op)	S. epidermidis, S. aureus. Rarely, Enterobacteriaceae, diphtheroids, fungi.	**Vanco** 15 mg/kg q12h IV + **gentamicin** 1.0 mg/kg q8h IV + **RIF** 600 mg daily		Early surgical consultation advised. Watch for evidence of heart failure.
Late (≥ 2 months post-op)	S. epidermidis, S. viridans, enterococci, S. aureus			
Infective endocarditis—Prosthetic valve–culture-positive				
Staph. epidermidis	Staph. aureus	(**Vanco** 15 mg/kg q12h IV + **RIF** 300 mg q8h po) x6 wks + **gentamicin** 1.0 mg/kg IV or IM q8h **x14 d.**		If S. epidermidis is susceptible to nafcillin/oxacillin (not common), then substitute nafcillin (or oxacillin) for vanco.
		Methicillin sensitive: (**Nafcillin** 2.0 gm q4h IV + **RIF** 300 mg q8h po) x6 wks + **gentamicin** 1.0 mg/kg q8h IV **x14 d.**		
	Staph. aureus	Methicillin resistant: (**Vanco** 1.0 gm q12h IV + **RIF** 300 mg q8h po) x6 wks + **gentamicin** 1.0 mg/kg q8h IV **x14 d.**		
	Strep. viridans, enterococci	See infective endocarditis, native valve, culture positive, pages 18, 19		
	Enterobacteriaceae or P. aeruginosa	**Aminoglycoside** (tobra if P. aeruginosa) + **AP Pen** or **P Ceph 3** AP or **P Ceph 4**		In theory, could substitute CIP for APAG, but no clinical data.
	Candida, aspergillus	**Ampho B** ± an **azole**, e.g. fluconazole (Table 10, page 73)		High mortality. Valve replacement plus antifungal therapy standard therapy but some success with antifungal therapy alone [CID 22:262, 1996].
Pericarditis, purulent	Staph. aureus, Strep. pneumoniae, Group A strep, Enterobacteriaceae	(**Nafcillin** or **oxacillin**) + **APAG** (dosage, see footnotes)	**IMP** or **TC/CL** or **PIP/TZ** or **AM/SB** or **MER** or **CFP** (see footnote)	Drainage required if signs of tamponade. If MRSA suspected, use vanco 1.0 gm q12h IV.
Rheumatic fever with carditis Ref.: CID 33:806, 2001 For acute rheumatic fever, see page 41; reactive arthritis below	Post-infectious sequelae of Group A strep infection (usually pharyngitis)	Diuretics, ASA, and usually prednisone 2 mg/kg po		Clinical features: Carditis, polyarthritis, chorea, subcutaneous nodules, erythema marginatum. For Jones criteria: Circulation 87:302, 1993. Prophylaxis: see page 41

[§] **APAG** (see Table 9C, page 71), **IMP** 0.5 gm q6h IV, **MER** 1.0 gm q8h IV, **nafcillin** or **oxacillin** 2.0 gm q4h IV, **TC/CL** 3.1 gm q4h IV, **PIP/TZ** 3.375 gm q6h or 4.5 gm q8h IV, **AM/SB** 3.0 gm q6h IV, **P Ceph 1** (**cephalothin** 2.0 gm q4h IV or **cefazolin** 2.0 gm q8h IV), **CIP** 750 mg bid po or 400 mg q12h IV, **RIF** 600 mg qid po, **aztreonam** 2.0 gm q8h IV, **CFP** 2.0 gm IV q12h

Footnotes and abbreviations on page 45

NOTE: All dosage recommendations are for adults (unless otherwise indicated) and assume normal renal function

TABLE 1 (20)

ANATOMIC SITE/DIAGNOSIS/ MODIFYING CIRCUMSTANCES	ETIOLOGIES (usual)	SUGGESTED REGIMENS* PRIMARY	ALTERNATIVE†	ADJUNCT DIAGNOSTIC OR THERAPEUTIC MEASURES AND COMMENTS
JOINT—Also see Lyme Disease, page 39				
Reactive arthritis				
Reiter's syndrome (See Comment for definition)	Occurs wks after infection with C. trachomatis, Campylobacter jejuni, Yersinia enterocolitica, Shigella, Salmonella sp.	Only treatment is non-steroidal anti-inflammatory drugs		Definition: Urethritis, conjunctivitis, arthritis, and sometimes uveitis and rash. Arthritis: asymmetrical oligoarthritis of ankles, knees, feet, sacroiliitis. Rash: palms and soles—keratoderma blennorrhagica; circinate balanitis of glans penis. HLA-B27 positive predisposes to Reiter's.
Poststreptococcal reactive arthritis (See Rheumatic fever, above)	Immunologic reaction after strep pharyngitis: (1) arthritis onset in 10 (2) lasts months, (3) unresponsive to ASA	Treat strep pharyngitis and then NSAIDs (prednisone needed in some pts)		A reactive arthritis after a β-hemolytic strep infection in absence of sufficient Jones criteria for acute rheumatic fever. Ref: Mayo Clin Proc 75:144, 2000.
Septic arthritis: Treatment requires both adequate drainage of purulent joint fluid and appropriate antimicrobial therapy. There is no need to inject antimicrobials into joints. Empiric therapy after collection of blood and joint fluid for culture; review Gram stain of joint fluid. For full differential, see Table 16/197, 1998.				
Infants <3 months (neonate)	Staph. aureus, Enterobacteriaceae, Group B strep, N. gonorrhoeae	Nafcillin (or oxacillin) + P Ceph 3 at dosage, see Table 16, page 126	Nafcillin (or oxacillin) + APAG (If MRSA prevalent, vanco in place of nafcillin/ oxacillin)	Blood cultures frequently positive. Adjacent bone involved in 2/3 pts. Group B strep and gonococcal most common community-acquired etiologies.
Children (3 months–14 years)	Staph. aureus 27%, S. pyogenes & S. pneumo 14%, H. influenzae 3%, Gm-neg bacilli 6%, other (GC, N. meningitidis) 14%, unknown 36%	(Nafcillin or oxacillin) + P Ceph 3	Vanco + P Ceph 3 See Table 16 for dosage	Marked ↓ in H. influenzae since use of conjugate vaccine. NOTE: Septic arthritis due to salmonella has no association with sickle cell disease, unlike salmonella osteomyelitis. Duration of treatment varies with specific microbial etiology.
Adults (review Gram stain): See page 39 for Lyme Disease				
Acute monoarticular				
Sexually active	N. gonorrhoeae (see page 15), S. aureus, streptococci, rarely aerobic Gm-neg bacilli	**Gram stain negative:** Ceftriaxone 1.0 gm qd IV or cefotaxime 1.0 gm q8h IV or ceftizoxime 1.0 gm q8h IV	If Gram stain shows Gm+ cocci in clusters, nafcillin (or oxacillin) 2.0 gm q4h IV	For rx comments, see Disseminated GC, page 15
Not sexually active	S. aureus, streptococci, Gm-neg. bacilli	**All empiric choices guided by Gram stain** Nafcillin/oxacillin + P Ceph 3 For treatment duration, see Table 3 For dosage, see footnote page 23	Nafcillin/oxacillin + CIP See Tables 2, 10 & 11	Differential includes gout and chondrocalcinosis (pseudogout). Look for crystals in joint fluid. Levo has appropriate in vitro spectra and should work, but no clinical data. NOTE: Substitute vanco for nafcillin/oxacillin if MRSA suspected or proven. For bites, see page 35
Chronic monoarticular	Brucella, nocardia, mycobacteria, fungi			
Polyarticular, usually acute	Gonococci, B. burgdorferi, acute rheumatic fever, viruses, e.g., hepatitis B, rubella vaccine, parvo B19	Gonococcemia: Gram stain usually negative for GC. If sexually active, culture urethra, cervix, anal canal, throat, blood, joint fluid, and treat: ceftriaxone 1.0 gm IV daily		If GC, usually associated petechiae and/or pustular skin lesions and tenosynovitis. Consider Lyme disease (if exposure areas known to harbor infected ticks. See page 39 Expanded differential includes gout, pseudogout, reactive arthritis (HLA-B27 pos)
Prosthetic joint, postoperative or infection post intra-articular injection [CID 33(Suppl.2):S94, 2001]	MSSE/MRSE 40%, MSSA/MRSA 20%, Enterobacteriaceae, Pseudomonas sp.	**Culture first!** Isolation/rx susceptibility of etiologic organisms essential.		**For infections after intra-articular injections,** arthroscopy for culture, washout, and treat specifically for 14 days. **Management of infected prosthetic joint** remains variable. Most infections at bone-prosthesis interface or osteomyelitis. 2 strategies: open debridement, prosthesis retention, 6 wks antibiotics vs 2-stage exchange arthroplasty with 6 wks antibiotics (see CID 32:419–430, 2001; CID 33(Suppl.2):S94, 2001).
Empiric rx, no culture data		Vanco + CIP (or aztreonam or APAG or CFP) for dosage, see footnote page 23	CIP 750 mg bid po + RIF 900 mg x1/d, po) or (ofloxacin 400 mg bid po + RIF 900 mg x1/d, po)	

(Footnotes and abbreviations on page 45)   *NOTE: All dosage recommendations are for adults (unless otherwise indicated) and assume normal renal function*

TABLE 1 (21)

ANATOMIC SITE/DIAGNOSIS/ MODIFYING CIRCUMSTANCES	ETIOLOGIES (usual)	SUGGESTED REGIMENS*		ADJUNCT DIAGNOSTIC OR THERAPEUTIC MEASURES AND COMMENTS
		PRIMARY	ALTERNATIVE§	
JOINT/Prosthetic joint, postoperative or infection post intra-articular injection (continued)				
Culture results known; specific rx	[MRSA/MRSE or MSSA/ MSSE]: **CIP/RIF suscep- tible**	[FQ + RIF] in above dosage	Oxacillin 2.0 gm q4h IV + RIF 300 mg x1/d po	Data on staph species infection of stable implants treated by debridement and prolonged oral antimicrobials: (1) po RIF + oflox x3–9 mos, 74% success (AAC 36:1214, 1993); (2) initial IV drug (vanco, then oxacillin or vanco, then po) CIP + RIF x3 mos. (hip) or 6 mos. (knee). Cure in 100% (JAMA 279:1537 & 1575, 1998); (3) po TMP/SMX (20 mg/kg/d of TMP) successful in 2/3 pts with staph species (AAC 42:3086, 1998). Most S. aureus are sensitive to RIF; most MRSA and roughly ½ of MSSE are resistant to Cip/oflox.
	[MRSA/MRSE or MSSA/ MSSE]: **CIP resistant**	Vanco + RIF (if sensitive) Another alternative: **Linezolid + RIF** (no published studies)		
Septic bursitis	Staph. >80%, M. tuberculosis (rare), M. marinum (rare)	Nafcillin or oxacillin 2 gm IV q4h or dicloxacillin 500 mg po qid	Cefazolin 2 gm IV q8h or vanco 1 gm IV q12h or CIP 750 mg q12h (or RIF 300 mg bid po) Other doses, see footnote page 23	Initially aspirate daily and treat for a minimum of 2–3 weeks. If recurrence, surgical excision of bursa—should not be necessary often if treated for 3 weeks + Ref. Semin Arth & Rheum 24:391, 1995.
KIDNEY, BLADDER AND PROSTATE [For review, see CID 29:745, 1999 & AJM 113(Suppl 1A):1S, 2002]				
Acute uncomplicated urinary tract infection (cystis-urethritis) [NOTE: Routine urine culture not necessary; self-rx works (Arth 135:9, 2001)]				
Dipstick: positive leucocyte esterase or hemoglobin for positive Gram stain on urine	Enterobacteriaceae (E. coli), Staph. saprophyticus, enterococcus	If local E. coli resistant to TMP/SMX <20%, then TMP/SMX-DS bid x3 d; if resistance >20%, then FQ po x3 d: CIP 250 mg bid or CIP-ER 500 mg qd, gati 400 mg or 400 mg qd, levo 250 mg qd, oflox 200 mg bid	TMP/SMX-DS 1 DS tab (160 mg TMP) bid po x3 d. Other option: O Ceph, NF, doxy, TMP or AM/CL. Usual dura- tion of rx is 3 d, for dosage, see footnote*	7-day rx recommended in pregnancy (discontinue or do not use sulfonamides (TMP/SMX) near term (2 weeks before EDC) because of potential ↑ in kernicterus). If failure on 3-day course, culture and rx 2 weeks. O In sexually active young women, risk of symptomatic UTI assoc. with recent intercourse. use of diaphragm/spermicide, and hx of recurrent UTIs (NEJM 335:468, 1996). Single dose fosfomycin 3.0 gm po x1 less effective vs E. coli than multi-dose TMP/SMX or FQ (Med Lett 39:66, 1997).
Risk factors for STD. Dipstick: positive leucocyte esterase or hemoglobin, neg. Gram stain.	C. trachomatis	Doxy 100 mg po x7 d.	Azithro 1.0 gm single dose	Pelvic exam for vaginitis & herpes simplex; urine LCR/PCR for GC and C. trachomatis.
Recurrent (3 or more episodes/ year) in young women	Any of the above bacteria	Eradicate infection, then TMP/SMX long term	TMP/SMX-DS, 2 tabs, 320/1600 mg) at symptom onset. Another alternative: 1 DS tablet TMP/SMX post-coitus.	A cost-effective alternative to continuous prophylaxis is self-administered single-dose rx
Child: ≤5 yrs old and grade 3–4 reflux	Coliforms	TMP/SMX (2 mg TMP/10 mg SMX)/kg po qd (or nitrofurantoin 2 mg/kg po qd)		Treat as for uncomplicated UTI. Evaluation for potentially correctable urologic factors—see Comment.
Recurrent UTI in postmenopausal women See CID 30:152, 2000	E. coli & other Enterobac- teriaceae, enterococci. S. saprophyticus			Definition of recurrent UTI. Reinfection vs. relapse. (1) 3 culture + symptomatic UTIs in 1 year or 2 UTIs in 6 months. Urologic factors: (1) cystocele, (2) incontinence, (3) ↑ residual urine volume (≥50 ml). In postmenopausal women, use of vaginal estrogen cream↓ frequency of urinary tract infections.

¹ O Ceph listed in Table 9B, page 66; nitrofurantoin 100 mg po qid; doxy 100 mg po bid; TMP 100 mg po bid; AM/CL 875/125 mg po bid.
NOTE: Dosage recommendations are for adults (unless otherwise indicated) and assume normal renal function
(Footnotes and abbreviations on page 45)   NOTE: All dosage recommendations are for adults (unless otherwise indicated) and assume normal renal function

TABLE 1 (22)

ANATOMIC SITE/DIAGNOSIS/ MODIFYING CIRCUMSTANCES	ETIOLOGIES (usual)	SUGGESTED REGIMENS*		ADJUNCT DIAGNOSTIC OR THERAPEUTIC MEASURES AND COMMENTS
		PRIMARY	ALTERNATIVE†	
KIDNEY, BLADDER AND PROSTATE (continued)				
Acute uncomplicated pyelonephritis (usually women 18–40 yrs., temperature >102°F, definite costovertebral tenderness) [NOTE: Culture of urine and blood indicated prior to therapy. Report of hemolytic uremic syndrome as result of toxin-producing E. coli UTI (NEJM 335:635, 1996)]				
Moderately ill (outpatient)	Enterobacteriaceae (most likely E. coli), enterococci	An **FQ** po x7 d: **CIP** 500 mg bid, **gati** 400 mg qd, or **oflox** 400 mg qd	**AM/CL**, **O Ceph**, or **TMP/SMX-DS**. Treat for 14 days.	In randomized double-blind trial, bacteriologic and clinical success higher for 7 days of CIP than for 14 days of TMP/SMX. Failures correlated with TMP/SMX in vitro resistance (JAMA 283:1583, 2000).
	Note: In hospital, can use **oflox** 400 mg qd IV. (When able to take po, and urine may allow identification of Gm-neg. bacilli vs Gm+ cocci).			Since CIP worked with 7-d. rx, suspect other FQs effective with 7-d. rx. Do not use moxi or trova due to low urine concentrations.
Hospitalized	E. coli most common, enterococci 2° in frequency	**FQ** (IV) or [**AMP** + **gent**: or **amikin**] or **P Ceph 3** or **AP Pen** Treat for 14 d.	**TC/CL** or **AM/SB** or **PIP/TZ** or **ertapenem**. Treat for 14 d.	Treat IV until afebrile 24–48 hrs, then complete 2-wk course with oral drugs (as Moderately ill, above). If no clinical improvement in 3 days, we recommend imaging. On CT if single focal mass-like lesion avg. response requires 6 d. If lesions diffuse avg. response 13 d. (AJM 93:289, 1992). **If pt hypotensive, prompt imaging (Echo or CT) is recommended to ensure absence of obstructive uropathy.**
		Dosages in footnotes² Do not use P Ceph 3 for suspect or proven enterococcal infection		NOTE: P Ceph 3 & ertapenem not active vs enterococci
		For dosages, see footnote 2 page 23		
Complicated UTI/catheters Obstruction, reflux, azotemia, transplant, Foley catheter-related	Enterobacteriaceae, P. aeruginosa, enterococci	[**AMP** + **gent**] or **PIP/TZ** or **TC/CL** or **IMP** or **MER** x2–3 wks	**FQ CIP gati. levo. oflox** x2–3 wks	Rule out obstruction. Often able to switch to oral quinolone or TMP/SMX in a few days. Watch out for enterococci and P. aeruginosa—not all listed drugs have predictable activity.
		For dosages, see footnote 2 page 23		
Asymptomatic bacteriuria				
Screen high-risk children		Base regimen on C&S, not empirical		Diagnosis requires ≥10⁵ CFU/ml urine of same bacterial species in 2 specimens obtained 3–7 days apart.
Pregnancy	Aerobic Gm-neg. bacilli & Staph. hemolyticus	Screen monthly. If positive, rx 3 d. with **amox, NF, O Ceph, TMP/SMX**, or **TMP/SMX** alone		Screen monthly for recurrence. Some authorities treat continuously until delivery (stop TMP/SMX 2 wks before EDC). ↑ resistance of E. coli to TMP/SMX.
Before and after invasive uro-logic intervention, e.g., Foley catheter	Aerobic Gm-neg. bacilli	Obtain urine culture and then rx 3 d. with **TMP/SMX DS**, bid		In one study, single dose 2-TMP/SMX DS 80% effective (AnIM 114:713, 1991). Use of silver-alloy Foley catheter may ↓ risk of clinically significant bacteriuria (AJM 105:236, 1998; AnIM 160:3294, 2000).
Neurogenic bladder		No rx in asymptomatic; intermittent catheterization if possible		Ref.: AJM 113(1A):67S, 2002.
Asymptomatic, advanced age: male or female		No rx indicated unless in conjunction with surgery to correct obstructive uropathy.		Chronic pyelo with abnormal inflammatory response. See CID 29:444, 1999
Malacoplakia	E. coli	Bethanechol chloride + [**CIP** or **TMP/SMX**]	**Vanco**	
Perinephric abscess				
Associated with staphylococcal bacteremia	Staph. aureus	**Nafcillin/oxacillin** or **P Ceph 1** (Dosage, page 20)		Drainage, surgical or image-guided aspiration
Associated with pyelonephritis	Enterobacteriaceae	See pyelonephritis, complicated UTI, above		Drainage, surgical or image-guided aspiration
Prostatitis		See prostatitis, page 17		

¹ **AM/CL** (amoxicillin/clavulanate) 875/125 mg q12h or 500/125 mg tid po. **aztreonam** 2.0 gm IV q8h. **FQ (IV) CIP** 400 mg bid. **gati** 400 mg qd. **levo** (250 mg qd for mild uncomplicated disease, 500 mg q24h IV for life-threatening infections; **ceftriaxone** 1.0–2.0 gm IV q24h). **cefoxitin** 2.0 gm IV q8h. **P Ceph 3 (ceftazidime** 1.0 gm q8h IV or 2.0 gm q8h IV for uncomplicated infections; **ceftriaxone** (see Table 9C, page 71), **AP Pen (PIP** 3.0 gm q6h IV, **AM/SB** 3.0 gm q6h IV, **TC/CL** 3.1 gm q6h IV, **PIP/TZ** 3.375 gm q6h or 4.5 gm q8h IV, **gentamicin** (see Table 10D, page 79). 2.0 gm tid IV (use 2.0 gm under age 40)). **AP Pen (PIP** 3.0 gm q6h IV, **AM/SB** 3.0 gm q6h IV, **P Ceph 4 (CFP** 2.0 gm q12h IV). **ertapenem** 1.0 gm qd IV, **IMP** 0.5 gm q6h IV, **MER** 1.0 gm q8h IV. **Nafcillin** or **oxacillin** 2.0 gm q4h IV. For **oral cephalosporin** dosages, see Table 9B, page 66. **Dicloxacillin** 500 mg po qid. **Metronidazole** 500 mg po qid. **Vanco** 1.0 gm IV q12h. (max. 4 gm/day) and assume normal renal function
(Footnotes continued on page 45) *NOTE: All dosage recommendations are for adults (unless otherwise indicated) and assume normal renal function*

TABLE 1 (23)

ANATOMIC SITE/DIAGNOSIS/ MODIFYING CIRCUMSTANCES	ETIOLOGIES* (usual)	SUGGESTED REGIMENS*		ADJUNCT DIAGNOSTIC OR THERAPEUTIC MEASURES AND COMMENTS
		PRIMARY	ALTERNATIVE‡	
LIVER (for spontaneous bacterial peritonitis, see page 31)				
Cholangitis	Enterobacteriaceae bacteroides, enterococci, Entermoeba histolytica, Yersinia enterocolitica (rare)	See Gallbladder, page 10		
Hepatic abscess		Metro − (P Ceph 3 or ciprofloxacin or TC/CL or PIP/TZ or AM/SB or FQ) AMP + APAG + metro	Metro (for amoeba) + either IMP or MER (Dosage, see footnote page 23)	Serological tests for amebiasis should be done on all patients; if neg, surgical drainage or percutaneous aspiration indicated in pyogenic abscess. ½ have identifiable GI source. If amoeba serology positive, treat with metro alone without surgery. Metro included for E. histolytica & bacteroides.
		Azithro—see page 30		Hemochromatosis associated with Yersinia enterocolitica liver abscess (CID 18:938, 1994); regimens listed are effective for yersinia
Cat-scratch disease (CSD)	Bartonella henselae			Ref. on hepatosplenic CSD: CID 28:778, 1999
Leptospirosis	Leptospirosis, see page 40			
Peliosis hepatis	Bartonella henselae and B. quintana	See page 38 and the SANFORD GUIDE TO HIV/AIDS THERAPY		
Viral hepatitis	Hepatitis A, B, C, D, E, G	See Table 14		
LUNG/Bronchi				
Bronchiolitis/wheezy bronchitis (expiratory wheezing) Respiratory syncytial Infants/children (≤ age 5)	**Respiratory syncytial virus** (RSV) 50%, parainfluenza 25%, other viruses 20%	Antibiotics not useful, mainstay of rx is oxygen. Ribavirin no benefit (AJRCCM 160:829, 1999). Ribavirin aerosol plus RSV-immune globulin products available for prevention: RSV-immune globulin and a humanized monoclonal antibody, palivizumab. See Table 14, page 109		RSV most important. Rapid dx with antigen detection methods. Ribavirin: No data on IV ribavirin but little enthusiasm. Emphasis now on vaccine development. Reviews: PIDJ 17:1123, 2000; Red Book of Peds 2000 25th Ed., pp. 483–488
Bronchitis				
Infants/children (≤ age 5)	< Age 2: Adenovirus; age 2–5 virus, parainfluenza 3 virus	Respiratory syncytial		Antibiotics indicated only with associated sinusitis or heavy growth on throat culture for S. pneumo., Group A strep, H. influenzae or no improvement in 1 week. Otherwise rx is symptomatic.
Adolescents and adults with acute tracheobronchitis (Acute bronchitis) Ref.: AnIM 162:256, 2002; AnIM 134:521, 2001	≤ Age 2: M. pneumoniae 5%; C. pneumoniae 5%. See Persistent cough, below	Antibiotics not indicated. Antitussive ± inhaled bronchodilators		Purulent sputum alone not an indication for antibiotic rx. Azithro was no better than low-dose vitamin C in a controlled trial (Ln 359:1648, 2002). Expect cough to last 2 weeks. If fever/rigors, get chest x-ray.
Persistent cough (>14 d.), afebrile during community outbreak: Pertussis (whooping cough) Reports indicate 10–20% adults with cough > 14 d. have pertussis (CID 32:1691, 2001)	Bordetella pertussis & occ. Bordetella parapertussis. Also consider asthma, gastroesophageal reflux, post-nasal drip.	**Peds doses: Erythro** estolate po 40 mg/kg/d div q6–12h x14 d OR **TMP/SMX** po 8 mg/kg/d div q12h x14 d	**Adult doses: Erythro** estolate 500 mg po qid x14 d OR **TMP/SMX-DS** 1 tab po bid x14 d OR **clarithro** 500 mg po bid or 1.0 gm ER qd x7 d	3 stages of illness: catarrhal (1–2 wks), paroxysmal coughing (2–4 wks), and convalescence (1–2 wks). Erythro may abort or eliminate pertussis in catarrhal stage; erythro does not shorten paroxysmal stage. **Rx** aimed at decreasing spread by eradicating nasopharyngeal carriage. Two antibiotic prophylaxis reported in infants under 6 wks of age given erythro (MMWR 48:1117, 1999).
Prophylaxis of household contacts		**Erythromycin—Children:** 50 mg/kg/d po in 4 doses x14 d. **Alternative: clarithro** 7.5 mg/kg po bid x14 d. See footnote	**Adults:** 500 mg po qid. See footnote	Recommended by Am. Acad. Ped. Red Book 2000 for all household or close contacts; community-wide prophylaxis not recommended.

---

[1] Peds doses: (azithro 10–12 mg/kg/d po) or (clarithro 7.5 mg/kg po bid) x5–7 d.

[2] Compliance with erythro poor due to nausea/vomiting, clarithro costs more but compliance should be better.

(Footnotes and abbreviations on page 45)

NOTE: All dosage recommendations are for adults (unless otherwise indicated) and assume normal renal function

TABLE 1 (24)

ANATOMIC SITE/DIAGNOSIS/ MODIFYING CIRCUMSTANCES	ETIOLOGIES (usual)	SUGGESTED REGIMENS*		ADJUNCT DIAGNOSTIC OR THERAPEUTIC MEASURES AND COMMENTS
		PRIMARY	ALTERNATIVE[1]	
LUNG/Bronchi/Bronchitis *(continued)*				
Acute bacterial exacerbation of chronic bronchitis (AECB), adults (almost always smokers with COPD) Refs.: AnIM 134:595 & 600, 2001; NEJM 346:988, 2002; AnIM 162:256, 2002	Viruses 20–50%, C. pneu-moniae 5%, M. pneumoniae <1%, role of S. pneumo, H. influenzae & M. catarrhalis controversial. Tobacco use, air pollution contribute.	**Severe AECB** = ↑ dyspnea, ↑ sputum viscosity/purulence, ↑ sputum volume. For severe ABECB: (1) consider chest x-ray, esp. if febrile &/or low O_2 sat, (2) inhaled anticholinergic bronchodilator; (3) oral corticosteroid. Taper over 2 wks; (4) D/C tobacco use; (5) non-invasive positive-pressure ventilation. **Role of antimicrobial rx debated even for severe disease. For mild or moderate disease, no antimicrobial treatment** or maybe amox, doxy, TMP/SMX, or O Ceph. **For severe disease,** AM/CL, azithro/ clarithro, or O Ceph or telithro or FQs with enhanced activity vs drug-resistant S. pneumo (gati, levo, or moxifloxacin) *Drugs & doses in footnote. Duration varies with drug: range 5–10 d.*		
Pneumonia: Birth to 1 month	Viruses: CMV, rubella, H. simplex **Bacteria:** Group S strep, listeria, coliforms, S. aureus, P. aeruginosa **Other:** Chlamydia trachomatis, syphilis	**AMP + gentamicin ± cefotaxime** Add **vanco** if MRSA a concern. For chlamydia rx, **erythro** 12.5 mg/kg po or IV qid x14 d		Blood cultures indicated. Consider C. trachomatis if afebrile pneumonia, staccato cough. IgM > 1:8; rx with erythro or sulfisoxazole
CONSIDER TUBERCULOSIS IN ALL PATIENTS; ISOLATE ALL SUSPECT PATIENTS				
Age 1–3 months *(Adapted from NEJM 346:429, 2002)* Pneumonitis syndrome. Usually afebrile	C. trachomatis, RSV, parainfluenza virus 3, Bordetella, S. pneumoniae, S. aureus (rare)	**Outpatient: po erythro** 10 mg/kg q6h **or po azithro** 10 mg/kg x1, then 5 mg/kg x4 d. For RSV, see bronchiolitis, page 24	**Inpatient: If afebrile erythro** 10 mg/kg IV q6h or **azithro** 2.5 mg/kg IV q12h (see Comment). **If febrile,** add **cefotaxime** 200 mg/kg/d. div q8h	Pneumonitis syndrome: cough, tachypnea, dyspnea, diffuse infiltrates, afebrile. Usually requires hospital care. Reports of hypertrophic pyloric stenosis after erythro under age 6 wks; not sure about azithro. If lobar pneumonia, give AMP 200–300 mg/kg/d iv div for S. pneumoniae.
Age 4 months–5 years For RSV, see bronchiolitis, page 24 & Table 14 Ref.: NEJM 346:429, 2002	RSV, other resp. viruses, S. pneumo, H. flu, myco-plasma, S. aureus (rare), M. tbc	**Outpatient: Amox** 100 mg/kg/d div q8h **Inpatient (not ICU):** No antibiotic if viral or trivial. **AMP** 200 mg/kg/d div q6h	**Inpatient (ICU): Cefotaxime** 200 mg/kg/d div q8h	Common "other" viruses: rhinovirus, influenza, parainfluenza, adenovirus *(PIDJ 19:293, 2000).* Often of mild to moderate severity. S. pneumo, non-type B H. flu in 4–20%. Treat x10–14 d. NOTE: High frequency of resistance of DRSP to cefotaxime. See footnote 1, page 24, footnote 1 page 26, and Table 5, page 55, for rx of drug-resistant S. pneumo.

[1] **TMP/SMX** 1 double-strength tab (160 mg TMP) po, **doxy** 100 mg bid po, **amox** 500 mg bid po, **AM/CL** 875/125 mg bid po, adult dose of **O Ceph** [**cefaclor** 500 mg tid po or 500 mg CD (extended release) q12h po, **cefdinir** 300 mg q12h po or 600 mg q24h po, **cefixime** 400 mg qd po, **cefpodoxime proxetil** 200 mg q12h po, **cefprozil** 500 mg q12h po, **cefditoren** 400 mg q12h po, **ceftibuten** 400 mg qd po or **cefuroxime axetil** 250 or 500 mg q12h po, **cefdinir** 300 mg q12h po or 600 mg q24h po], **azithro** 500 mg po x1, then 250 mg/d po x4 d or 500 mg po x3 d, **clarithro** 500 mg q12h po or **clarithro ER** 1000 mg q24h po, **levo** 500 mg qd po, **CIP** 750 mg q12h po, **oflox** 400 mg q12h po, **gati** 400 mg qd po, or **gati** 400 mg qd po, or **levo** 500 mg qd po, **gati** 400 mg qd po, or **moxi** 400 mg qd po. **Ketolide: Telithromycin** 800 mg po qd x5 d.
NOTE: CIP and ceftibuten have relatively poor in vitro activity vs S. pneumo. *NOTE: All dosage recommendations are for adults (unless otherwise indicated) and assume normal renal function*
(Footnotes and abbreviations on page 45)

TABLE 1 (25)

ANATOMIC SITE/DIAGNOSIS/ MODIFYING CIRCUMSTANCES	ETIOLOGIES (usual)	SUGGESTED REGIMENS*		ADJUNCT DIAGNOSTIC OR THERAPEUTIC MEASURES AND COMMENTS
		PRIMARY	ALTERNATIVE†	
LUNG/Bronchi/Bronchitis *(continued)*				
Age 5 years–15 years, Non-hospitalized NEJM 346:429, 2002	Mycoplasma, Chlamydia pneumoniae, S. pneumoniae, M. pneumoniae, Mycobacterium tuberculosis	**(Clarithro** 500 mg po bid (if or 1 gm ER qd; Peds dose: 7.5 mg/kg q12h) **OR** (**azithro** 0.5 gm po x1 (then 0.25 gm/d; Peds dose: 10 mg/kg/d, max. of 500 mg po, then 5 mg/ kg/d, max. 250 mg) **See Comment regarding macrolide resistance**	**Doxy** 100 mg po bid (if >8 yrs old) **or erythro** 500 mg po 4/d. (Peds dose: 10 mg/kg po q6h)	It otherwise healthy and if not concomitant with or post-influenza, S. pneumoniae uncommon in this subset; suspect S. pneumo if sudden onset and large amount of purulent sputum, which might raise suspicion of penicillin (macrolide)-resistant S. pneumo in pts >5 yrs old (JAMA 286:1857, 2001). Mycoplasma PCR/viral culture usually not done for outpatients. **Mycoplasma requires 2–3 wks of rx; C. pneumoniae up to 6 wks.** (Ln Int Dis 1:334, 2001).
Hospitalized	S. pneumoniae, viruses, mycoplasma	**Ceftriaxone** 50 mg/kg/d iV (to max. 2 gm/d) + **azithro** 10 mg/kg/d up to 500 mg po q12h	**Alternatives are a problem in children:** No doxy under age 8, no FQs under age 18. For S. pneumo, vanco. Linezolid reported efficacious in children. MIC ≥2 μg/ml, see *Table 5, page 55* for options; e.g., vanco. (PIDJ 20:489, 2001).	
Presumed viral pneumonia in adults: cough, no sputum, dyspnea/hypoxia, interstitial infiltrates. Also see *Table 14, page 108.* Rapid diagnostic tests available.	Influenza (Dec.–Mar. in U.S.) parainfluenza, adenovirus, RSV, hantavirus.	**For influenza A or B: zan-amivir** 10 mg inhaled bid x5 d. **or oseltamivir** 75 mg po bid x5 d. Start within 48 hrs of symptom onset.	**For influenza A: riman-tadine** 100 mg po 2x/d or **amantadine** 100 mg po 2x/d	**Zanamivir & oseltamivir** shortened course and ↓ complications of influenza A & B (Ln 355:1877 & 1872, 1999); also efficacious in prevention (JAMA 282:31 & 75, 1999.) Amantadine/rimantadine shorten course of influenza bronchitis if started early; presumably same benefit in pneumonia; renal excretion: adjust dose for est. CrCl <90 ml/min—*see Table 17.*
Adults (over age 18)—Guidelines for community-acquired pneumonia AnIM 160:1399, 2000 (CDC); CID 31:347, 2000 (IDSA); CID 31-383, 2000 (Canadian); AJRCCM 163:1730, 2001 (ATS)				
Community-acquired; non-Smokers: S. pneumo, H. influenzae, Moracella cata-hospitalized rhalis, Post-viral bronchitis: (esp. S. pneumo, H. influenzae). Chlamydia pneumoniae, viral. Rarely: S. pneumo, anaerobes, coliforms. Alcoholic stupor: S. aureus. Epidemic Legionnaires: Birds: Psittacosis. Rabbits: Tularemia. Parturient livestock or cats: Coxiella burnetii (Q fever, assoc. hepatitis (Med 79: 109, 2000)). Airway obstruction:		**Azithro** 0.5 gm po x1, then 0.25 gm/d. **OR clarithro** 500 mg po bid **or clarithro** (see Comment)	**FQ** with enhanced activity vs S. pneumo (see footnote¹) **OR** & **O Ceph 2** (see footnote²) (CID 34:556 & 565; AnIM 160:1399). **OR AM/CL** (Augmentin XR) 2000/125 po bid **OR doxy** 100 mg po bid or **telithro** 800 mg po qd x7–10 d.	2000 (IDSA); CID 31-383, 2000 (Canadian); AJRCCM 163:1730, 2001 (ATS) Empiric drug selection based on uncertainty due to ↑ prevalence of DRSP (DRSP [CID 34/Suppl.1]:S4, 2002]. No drug is foolproof; e.g. reports of rare failures with macrolides (CID 35:556 & 565, 2002; DMID 43:163, 2002) and FQ (AnIM 138:612, 2003). Regardless of treatment regimens, if pt fails to respond, consider presence of a resistant organism. **AM/CL** and **O Ceph 2** not active vs legionella, mycoplasma, chlamydia. **Amoxicillin** alone not used due to susceptibility to β-lactamases from H. influenzae & Moraxella. Retrospective review suggests outcomes better with dual therapy—need prospective confirmation (AnIM 161:1837, 2001).
		Rx duration varies; usually rx until afebrile 3–5 d. Duration of rx can range from 7–14 d.		

TABLE 1 (26)

ANATOMIC SITE/DIAGNOSIS/ MODIFYING CIRCUMSTANCES	ETIOLOGIES (usual)	SUGGESTED REGIMENS* PRIMARY	ALTERNATIVE§	ADJUNCT DIAGNOSTIC OR THERAPEUTIC MEASURES AND COMMENTS
LUNG/Bronchi, Pneumonia/Adults (continued) **Community-acquired, hospitalized-adults, 15–52)** NOTE: Severe S. pneumo in post-splenectomy, myeloma, lymphoma, CA pts & other immuno-compromised. For level of specific bacteria results, see below & Table 2, page 48	(continued) (See previous page)	**In Intensive Care: (P Ceph 3¹ IV + erythro 15–20 mg/kg/ IV q6h or azithro 500 mg IV once daily)** (If pt enhanced activity vs S. pneumo, see footnote 1 page 26) *(Dosage in footnote)*	**In Intensive Care: (P Ceph 3¹ IV + (erythro 15-20 mg/kg/ IV q6h or azithro 500 mg IV once daily) OR (P Ceph 3¹ IV + FQ with enhanced activity vs S. pneumo, see footnote 1 page 26)** *(Dosage in footnote)*	**Dx:** Sputum Gram stain and culture. Blood cultures. Urine legionella antigen. Pleural fluid if present. AFB smear/culture if indicated. Pneumococcal urine antigen pos. in 50% children with asymptomatic carriage (PIDJ 20:78, 2001), hence of limited value. **Rx:** Need to know local prevalence of drug-resistant S. pneumo. If **high-level** resistant—i.e., MIC ≥ 4—failures (rare) documented. With macrolide-resistance & unclear etiology, **start Rx with enhanced activity FQ (see footnote 1 page 26) pending culture results.** For Legionnaire's: Azithro IV requires less diluent than erythro; many prefer an FQ. Levo superior to macrolide in ICU (Activity vs DRSP & legionella). Editors see no need for empiric combination of P Ceph 3 + FQ as in ATS & IDSA Guidelines.
Hospital-acquired: NOT mechanical ventilation. NOT neutropenic NOTE: Suggested regimens do not address specific resistant pathogens. Check results & Table 2, page 48	**Post-CVA aspiration:** S. pneumo, anaerobes. **Water colonization:** Legionella. **Organ failure:** Coliforms, S. pneumo, S. aureus. **Airway obstruction:** Anaerobes. **Steroids:** Yeast, PCP (see AIDS)	**To cover coliforms, S. pneumo & anaerobes:** IMP (0.5 gm IV q6h) OR MER (1 gm IV q8h) OR (AP Pen + APAG) or (P Ceph 3 AP + APAG) = (TC/CL or PIP/TZ) + (CIP or levo) OR (P Ceph 4¹ ± clinda) See Comment	**To include DRSP & coli-forms/anaerobes: (trova 300 mg IV x1, then 200 mg IV q24h) or, if suspect legionella: gati, levo, moxi, or trova IV alone or in combination to primary rx regimen.** See Comment	**Dx of ventilator-associated pneumonia:** Fever & lung infiltrates often not pneumonia (Chest 108:221, 1994). Quantitative cultures helpful: bronchoalveolar lavage (>10⁵/ml pos.) or protect. spec. brush (>10³/ml pos.). Ref: AJRCCM 165:867, 2002. **Treatment:** Drugs active vs non-resistant S. pneumo—vanco, gati, levo, trova, & perhaps IMP & clinda (in U.S.). If no other option possible, linezolid is active. Review on use of quinolones for Legionnaire's disease. AnIM 129:328, 1998. Also, if macrolide selected for Legionnaire's, prefer azithro IV than erythro, no need for lessen diluent volume. **Prevention:** If possible, keep head of bed elevated 30° or more. Remove N-G tubes as soon as possible. If avoidable, continuous subglotic suctioning. Limit stress ulcer prophylaxis. Ref: NEJM 340:627, 1999.
Hospital- or community-acquired, neutropenic pt (<500 neutrophils/mm³)	Any of organisms listed under community-acquired & nosocomial-acquired, plus fungi (aspergillus, Candida sp.)	See footnotes below & on pages 16, 23 & 25 See Hospital-acquired, immediately above & Vanco not listed in initial empiric rx unless high suspicion of resistant-S. pneumo. Add vanco if immediate access of drug-resistant S. pneumo is a possibility. If clinical, wait until febrile after 3 days or high clinical likelihood See Comment		See consensus document on management of febrile neutropenic pt: CID 25:551. Failures due to drug-resistant S. pneumo. AnIM 158:868, 1998
Adults—Selected specific rx drug culture results (sputum, blood, pleural fluid, etc.) **Gram-negative**		See footnotes below & on pages 16, 23 & 25 See Table 2, page 48		
Burkholderia (Pseudomonas) pseudomallei (etiology of melioidosis)		**Severe (Rx Table 2, page 63)** ceftazidime 2 gm IV q6h or (IMP 1 gm IV q6h or MER 1 gm IV q8h) x2 wks, then TMP/SMX-DS po bid x6 months	**Also see Table 2, page 48** Can also use **TMP/SMX** azithro/clarithro, doxy	Resistant to TMP/SMX in Thailand. Can also use ceftaz; IMP in lieu of ceftaz or IMP. Mortality with ceftaz: 35–40%. Relapse rate 4–16% Ref for AM/CL 875/125 po bid x6 months
Haemophilus influenzae β-lactamase negative β-lactamase positive		**AMP IV, amox po, TMP/SMX, azithro/clarithro, doxy AM/CL, O Ceph 2/3, FQ, azithro/clarithro, telithro²**		Ref for AM/CL. Trans N Soc Trop Med Hyg 89:546, 1995. 25–35% strains β-lactamase positive to both TMP/SMX and doxy See Table 98, page 63 for dosages
Legionella species Hospitalized/immunocompromised		**(azithro IV or levo IV or trova IV or (erythro IV ± (RIF)) See Table 98, page 63 for dosages**		Active FQs: trova, peflox Xd levo, moxi, gati. Refs: AnIM 129:328, 1998; JAC 43:747, 1999. Best legionella website: www.legionella.org
Moraxella catarrhalis 93% β-lactamase positive		**AM/CL, O Ceph 2/3, macrolide²telithro², FQ, TMP/SMX, Doxy**		O Ceph another option. See Table 98, page 63 for dosages

<hr>

*¹ P Ceph 3 (cefotaxime dose ranges from 2.0 gm q8h IV for severe infection to 2.0 gm q4h IV for life-threatening infection. ceftriaxone 1.0 gm qd IV standard. However, unpublished data suggest possible superiority with 2.0 gm qd IV. Dosing of oral cephalosporins as in Strep. pneumo & other Gram-positive infections in urine. **P Ceph 3 AP** (ceftazidime 2.0 gm q8h IV, **P Ceph 4** (CFP 2.0 gm q12h IV) **cefpirome 2.0 gm q12h IV. TC/CL** 3.1 gm q4-6h IV, **(TC/CL)** 3.1 gm q4h IV + **tobra** 5 mg/kg IV once daily). If no P. aeruginosa, **PIP/TZ** can be 3.375 gm q6h or 4.5 gm q8h IV, **PIP/TZ** 3.375 gm q4h + **tobra** 5 mg/kg once daily) and assume normal renal function

² **Telithro²** = telithromycin 800 mg po qd

³ **Macrolide** = azithromycin, clarithromycin, dirithromycin, and erythromycin
(Footnotes and abbreviations on page 45)
NOTE: All dosage recommendations are for adults (unless otherwise indicated) and assume normal renal function

TABLE 1 (27)

ANATOMIC SITE/DIAGNOSIS/ MODIFYING CIRCUMSTANCES	ETIOLOGIES (usual)	SUGGESTED REGIMENS* PRIMARY	ALTERNATIVE³	ADJUNCT DIAGNOSTIC OR THERAPEUTIC MEASURES AND COMMENTS
LUNG/Bronchi, Pneumonia/Adults, when culture results available (continued)				
Strep. pneumoniae	Penicillin-susceptible Penicillin-resistant, high level	**AMP** IV, **amox** po, **macrolide²**, **pen G** IV,³ **doxy**, **O Ceph** 2, **P Ceph** 2/3, (telithro 800 mg po qd). See Table 98, page 63 for other dosages. **FQs** with enhanced activity: **gati, levo, moxi, trova** (IV); **P Ceph** 3 (if susceptible); high-dose IV **AMP** (**vanco** IV ± **RIF**)—see Table 5, page 55 for more data. If all options not possible or (e.g., allergy), **linezolid** active 600 mg IV or po q12h.		
LUNG—Other				
Anthrax	Bacillus anthracis			

Inhalation (applies to oro-pharyngeal & gastrointestinal forms): **Treatment** (Cutaneous: See Page 34)
Refs.: JAMA 287:2236, 2002 & MMWR 50:909, 2001
Also see Table 1B, page 46
	To report possible bioterrorism event:
	770-488-7100
		Adults (including pregnancy): CIP 400 mg IV (q12h) or (**doxy** 100 mg IV q12h) **plus (clindamycin** 900 mg IV q8h and/or **RIF** 300 mg IV q12h). Switch to po when pts stable; CIP to 500 mg po bid, clinda to 450 mg po bid & RIF 300 mg po bid; treat x60 days.	**Children:** CIP 10–15 mg/kg IV q12h) or (**Doxy**: >8 y/o & >45 kg: 100 mg IV q12h; >8 y/o & ≤45 kg: 2.2 mg/kg IV q12h; ≤8 y/o: 2.2 mg/kg IV q12h) **plus clindamycin** 7.5 mg/kg q8h
			and/or RIF 20 mg/kg (max. 600 mg) IV q12h.
			treat x60 d. See Table 16, page 126 for oral dosage.
				1. Clinda may block toxin production
				2. Rifampin penetrates CSF & intracellular sites.
				3. If isolate shown penicillin-susceptible:
				  a. **Adults: Pen G** 4 mU IV q4h
				  b. **Children: Pen G** <12 y/o: 50,000 U/kg IV q6h; >12 y/o: 4 mU IV q4h alone.
				4. Constitutive & inducible β-lactamases—do not use pen or amp alone.
				5. Do not use cephalosporins or TMP/SMX.
				6. Erythro, azithro actively borderline, clarithro active.
				7. No person-to-person spread.

Post-exposure prophylaxis	info: www.bt.cdc.gov	**Adults (including pregnancy):** CIP 500 mg po bid x60 d. **Children:** CIP 20–30 mg/kg/d div q12h x60 d.	**Adults (including pregnancy): Doxy** 100 mg po bid x60 d. **Children** (see Comment): **Doxy** >8 y/o & >45 kg: 100 mg po bid; >8 y/o & ≤45 kg: 2.2 mg/kg po bid; ≤8 y/o: 2.2 mg/kg po bid. All for 60 days.	1. Once organism shows suscept. to penicillin, switch to amoxicillin 80 mg/kg/d div q8h (max. 500 mg q8h); pregnant pt to amoxicillin 500 mg po tid. 2. Do not use cephalosporins or TMP/SMX. 3. Other FQs (gati, levo, moxi) & clarithro should work but no clinical experience.
Aspiration pneumonia & lung abscess: NEJM 88:409, 1995)	Bacteroides sp. (~15% B. fragilis), Prevotella sp. Peptostreptococci, Fusobacterium sp. S. milleri group, nocardia (pts taking steroids)	**Clinda** 450–900 mg q8h IV or **Cefoxitin** 2.0 gm q8h IV or **P Ceph** 2/3, see Table 10, Table 10, page 77	**Cefoxitin** 2.0 gm q8h IV or **TC-CL** 3.1 gm q6h IV or **PIP/TZ** 3.375 gm q6h IV or 4.5 gm q8h IV. **Historically (pen G** HD) has been effective.	Bronchoscopy to r/o neoplasm if pt fails to clear or recurs. Metro not as effective in treating lung abscess (Clin Infect Dis 16:S248, 1993). A recent review questioned the etiologic role of anaerobic bacteria, the editors respectfully disagree (NEJM 344:665, 2001).
Chronic pneumonia with fever, night sweats and weight loss	M. tuberculosis, coccidio-mycosis, histoplasmosis	See Tables 10, 11		HIV+, foreign-born, alcoholism, contact with TB, travel into developing countries
Cystic fibrosis: NEJM 335:179, 1996	S. aureus early in disease; P. aeruginosa later in disease	For **P. aeruginosa** (**Tobra** 3 mg/kg q8h IV + **ticarcillin** or **PIP** 100 mg/kg IV) or (**tobra** 3 mg/kg q8h IV) + (**ceftaz** 50 mg/kg q8h IV)—see footnotes⁴	For S. aureus: (1) MSSA oxacillin/nafcillin 2.0 gm IV q4h (Peds data, Table 16). (2) MRSA—vanco 1.0 gm q12h & check serum levels	Monitor serum levels of aminoglycosides due to altered kinetics and drug accumu-lation in CF cells (JAC 41:215, 1998). Consensus report on FQs in pediatrics lists P. aeruginosa exacerbation in CF as an indication (PIDJ 14:1, 1995).
Acute exacerbation of pulmonary symptoms 1. Parenteral administration of antibiotics x14–21 d. + intensified airway clearance of secretions		Once-daily tobra under study. AAC 44:869, 2000. **SubRVAC** 10.0 mg/kg IV or q8h po	**Chloro** 15–26 mg/kg IV or q8h po	For chronic suppression of P. aeruginosa, inhaled tobra led to modest ↑ in FEV, & bacterial density. May not work if P. aeruginosa resistant to tobra. Dose (page >6 yrs): 300 mg with designated inhaler bid x28 days, no treatment x28 d, then repeat cycle (NEJM 340:23, 1999; Chest 120:1073, 2001). No major resistance so far (JID 179:1190, 1999).
Suppressive therapy for use of inhaled tobra for chronic suppression of P. aeruginosa Bronchiectasis ref.: NEJM 346:1383, 2002	Burkholderia (Pseudomo-nas) cepacia	For other alternatives, see Table 2		1. B. cepacia is a major pathogen. Patients develop progressive respiratory failure, 62% mortality in 1 yr (AAC 43:213, 1999). 2. Patients with B. cepacia should be isolated from other CF patients. **NOTE:** 3- & 4-drug combinations under study in refractory pts.

¹ **Macrolide** = azithromycin, clarithromycin, dirithromycin, and erythromycin

² **IV Pen G dosage:** (Blood cultures neg., 1 mU IV q4h; blood cultures pos. & no meningitis: 2 mU IV q4h; Another option is continuous infusion (CI) 3 mU loading dose & then CI of 10–12 mU over 12 hrs

³ Other options: (Tobra + aztreonam 50 mg/kg q8h IV); (IMP 15–25 mg/kg q8h IV + tobra); (CIP IV/po + ceftaz IV—see comment on FQs in Cystic fibrosis and ref.: PIDJ 16:572, 1997).
NOTE: All dosage recommendations are for adults (unless otherwise indicated) and assume normal renal function
(Footnotes and abbreviations on page 45)

TABLE 1 (28)

ANATOMIC SITE/DIAGNOSIS/ MODIFYING CIRCUMSTANCES	ETIOLOGIES (usual)	SUGGESTED REGIMENS* PRIMARY	ALTERNATIVE†	ADJUNCT DIAGNOSTIC OR THERAPEUTIC MEASURES AND COMMENTS
LUNG/Other Refs: CID 22:747, 1996; COID 11:163, 1998. Pleural effusion review: NEJM 346: 1971, 2002				
Empyema	Pneumonia, neonatal, peds 25	See Pneumonia, age 1 month–5 years, page 25		Drainage indicated
Child <5 yrs to Adult—Diagnostic thoracentesis, chest tube for empyemas				
Infants/children (1 month–5 yrs)	Staph. aureus, Strep. pneumoniae, H. influenzae	See Pneumonia, age 1 month–5 years, page 25		Drainage indicated
Acute, usually parapneumonic	Strep. pneumoniae, Group A strep	Cefotaxime or ceftriaxone (Dosage: see footnote 2, page 27)	Vanco	
Subacute/chronic	Staph. aureus	Naficillin or oxacillin	TMP/SMX or AM/SB	Randomized trial showed benefit of intrapleural streptokinase (250,000 units in 20 ml saline with 2-hr dwell qd x3 days) (Thorax 52:416, 1997). Urokinase 100,000 IU/d x3 d, effective in double-blind study (AJRCCM 159:37, 1999).
	H. influenzae	P Ceph 3		Gram-pos. cocci in clusters
	Anaerobic strep, Strep. milleri, Bacteroides sp, Enterobacteriaceae, M. tuberculosis	Clinda 450–600 mg q8h IV + P Ceph 3	Cefoxitin or IMP or TC/CL or PIP/TZ or AM/SB (Dosage: see footnote 1 page 27)	Pleomorphic Gm-neg. bacilli. ↑ resistance to TMP/SMX. If organisms not seen, treat as subacute. Drainage. R/O tuberculosis or tumor. Pleural biopsy with culture for mycobacteria and histology if TBc suspected (CID 22:747, 1996).
Human immunodeficiency virus infection (HIV+)				
CD4 T-lymphocytes <200/ mcl or clinical AIDS	Pneumocystis carinii most likely, also M. tbc, fungi, Kaposi's sarcoma, & lymphoma NOTE: AIDS pts may develop pneumonia due to bacterial or other pathogens—see next box below	Rx listed here is for *severe* pneumonia; see Table 12, page 63 for non-severe pneumonia. **Prednisone 1st (see Comment), then:** TMP/SMX IV· 15 mg/kg/d of trim component (TMP component) div q6h-q8h (TMP component) × 21 days	**Prednisone 1st (see Comment), then:** TMP/SMX or AM/SB Could use gatl, levo, moxi, or trova IV as alternative (see Comment) primaquine 30 mg (qd po base) + clinda 600 mg (q6h IV) or (450 mg po q8h), total of 21 days nate 4 mg/kg/d IV) x21 d See Comment	Diagnostic procedure of choice is sputum induction. (If negative, bronchoscopy). Pts with PCP & pO2 <200 (A-a ≥35) should be on anti-PCP prophylaxis for life. **Prednisone 40 mg bid po x5 d, then 40 mg qd po x5 d then 20 mg qd po x11 d is indicated with PCP (pO2 <70 mmHg), should be given at initiation of anti-PCP rx; don't wait until pt's condition deteriorates** (Table 12, page 63). If PCP studies negative, consider bacterial pneumonia, TBc, cocci, histo, crypto, Kaposi's sarcoma or lymphoma. **NOTE: Pentamidine not active vs bacterial pathogens. NOTE: Pneumocystis resistant to TMP/SMX, albeit rare, does exist.** Examination of sputum shows Gm-neg. bacilli, options include P Ceph 3 AP, TC/CL, PIP/TZ, IMP or MER FQs: Levo 500 mg po/IV qd; trova 200 mg IV qd; gatl 400 mg qd V/po qd; moxi 400 mg po/IV qd
CD4 T-lymphocytes normal Acute onset, purulent sputum ± pulmonary infiltrates ± pleuritic pain. **Isolate pt until TBc excluded. Adults**	Strep. pneumoniae, H. influenzae, aerobic Gm-neg. bacilli (including P. aeruginosa), Legionella rare, M. tbc	As for HIV+ adults with pneumonia. If diagnosis is LIP, rx with steroids		In children with AIDS: LIP responsible for 1/3 of pulmonary complications, usually > 1 yr of age vs PCP, which is seen at < 1 yr of age. Clinically: clubbing, hepatosplenomegaly, salivary glands enlarged (take up gallium), lymphocytosis.
As above: Children	Same as adult with HIV + lymphoid interstitial pneumonia (LIP)			
LYMPH NODES (approaches below apply to lymphadenitis without an obvious primary source)				
Lymphadenitis, acute				
Generalized	EBV, early HIV infection, syphilis, toxoplasma, tularemia, Lyme disease, sarcoid, lymphoma, systemic lupus erythematosus, and Kikuchi-Fujimoto disease. Complete history and physical examination followed by appropriate serological tests. Treat specific agent(s).			
Regional				
Cervical—see cat-scratch disease (CSD), page 30	CSD (B. henselae), Grp A strep, Staph. aureus, anaerobes, M TBc (scrofula), M. avium, M. scrofulaceum, M. malmoense, toxo, tularemia.	History & physical exam directs evaluation. If nodes fluctuant, aspirate and base rx on Gram & acid-fast stains. Review of mycobacterial etiology: CID 20:954, 1995. Kikuchi-Fujimoto disease causes fever and benign self-limited adenopathy: the etiology is unknown (AJM 171:401, 1995).
Inguinal				
Sexually transmitted	HSV, chancroid, syphilis, LGV	Treatment depends on specific dx		
Not sexually transmitted	GAS, SA, tularemia, CSD	Treatment depends on specific dx, geography, hx of insect bites, distal lesions may help. See cervical adenopathy Comment		
Axillary	GAS, SA, CSD, tularemia, Y. pestis, sporotrichosis	See cervical adenopathy Comment		

(Footnotes and abbreviations on page 45)   NOTE: All dosage recommendations are for adults (unless otherwise indicated) and assume normal renal function

TABLE 1 (29)

ANATOMIC SITE/DIAGNOSIS/ MODIFYING CIRCUMSTANCES	ETIOLOGIES (usual)	SUGGESTED REGIMENS* PRIMARY	SUGGESTED REGIMENS* ALTERNATIVE†	ADJUNCT DIAGNOSTIC OR THERAPEUTIC MEASURES AND COMMENTS
LYMPH NODES/lymphadenitis, Acute/Regional (continued)				
Extremity, with associated nodular lymphangitis (For full description: AnIM 118:883, 1993)	Sporotrichosis, leishmania, Nocardia brasiliensis, Mycobacterium marinum, Mycobacterium chelonae, tularemia	Treatment varies with specific etiology		A distinctive form of lymphangitis characterized by subcutaneous swellings along inflamed lymphatic channels. Primary site of skin invasion usually present; regional adenopathy present.
Cat-scratch disease— immunocompetent patient Axillary/epitrochlear nodes 46%, neck 26%, inguinal 17%	Bartonella henselae Review: IDC No. Amer 12: 137, 1998	**Azithro dosage—Adults** (>45.5 kg): 500 mg po x1, then 250 mg/d x4 d. **Children** (<45.5 kg): liquid azithro 10 mg/kg x1, then 5 mg/kg/d x4 d. Rx is controversial—see Comment	No rx: resolves in 2–4 mos. Needle aspiration relieves pain in suppurative nodes Avoid I&D.	**Clinical:** Approx. 10% nodes suppurate. Atypical presentation in <5% pts, i.e. lung nodules, liver/spleen lesions, Parinaud's oculoglandular syndrome, CNS manifestations in 2% of pts (encephalitis, peripheral neuropathy, retinitis). **Dx:** Cat exposure. Positive IFA serology. Rarely need biopsy. **Rx:** Only 1 prospective randomized blinded study. used azithro with ↑ rapidity of resolution of enlarged lymph nodes (PIDJ 17:447, 1998)
MOUTH				
Odontogenic infection, including Ludwig's angina Can result in more serious parapharyngeal space infection (see page 33)	Oral microflora incl infec- tion polymicrobial	**Clinda** 300–450 mg q6h po or 600 mg IV q6–8h	**(AM/CL** 875/125 mg bid or 500/125 mg tid po) or **cefotetan** 2 gm IV q12h	Surgical drainage and removal of necrotic tissue essential. β-lactamase producing organisms are ↑ in frequency. Ref. Canadi Dental Assn J 64:508, 1998 Other parenteral alternatives: AM/SB, PIP/TZ, or TC/CL
Buccal cellulitis Children <5 y.o.	H. influenzae	**Cefuroxime** or **P Ceph 3** Dosage: see Table 16, page 126	**AM/CL** or **TMP/SMX**	With Hib immunization, invasive H. influenzae infections have ↓ by 95%. Now occurring in infants prior to immunization.
Herpetic stomatitis	Herpes simplex virus 1 & 2	See Table 14		
Aphthous stomatitis, recurrent; HIV-neg.	Etiology unknown	Topical steroids (Kenalog in Orabase) may ± pain and swelling; if AIDS, see SANFORD GUIDE TO HIV/AIDS THERAPY.		
MUSCLE				
"Gas gangrene" Traumatic or non-traumatic wound Can be spontaneous without trauma (CID 28:159, 1999)	Cl. perfringens, other histo- toxic Clostridium sp.	**(Clinda** 900 mg q8h IV) + **(pen G** 24 mU IV/d div. q4–6h IV)	**Ceftriaxone** 2.0 gm q12h IV or **(erythro** 1 gm q6h IV (not by bolus)	Surgical debridement primary rx. Hyperbaric oxygen adjunctive efficacy debated, 1998. Follow exercise injury, rare but focus in temperate zones (IDCP 7:265, 1998). Follow exercise injury, see Necrotizing fasciitis. Now seen in HIV/AIDS (Ln 348:1741, 1997). Add clinda or metro if anaerobes suspected/proven (IDCP 8:252, 1999)
Pyomyositis	Staph. aureus, Group A strep, rarely Gm-neg bacilli, variety of anaerobic organisms	**(Nafcillin** or **oxacillin** 2.0 gm IV q4h) or **Cefazolin** 2.0 gm q8h IV)	**Vanco** 1.0 gm q12h IV	Has been common in tropics, rare but occurs in temperate zones (IDCP 7:265, 1998). Follow exercise injury, see Necrotizing fasciitis. Now seen in HIV/AIDS (Ln 348:1741, 1997). Add clinda or metro if anaerobes suspected/proven (IDCP 8:252, 1999)
PANCREAS: Review—NEJM 340:1412, 1999				
Acute alcoholic (without necrosis) (idiopathic) pancreatitis	Not bacterial	None		1–9% become infected (see Comment). Prospective studies show no advantage to initial AMP (Ln 346:652, 1995). Observe for pancreatic abscesses or necrosis which require rx.
Pancreatic abscess, infected pseudocyst, infected necrosis	Enterobacteriaceae, entero- cocci, S. aureus, S. epider- midis, anaerobes, candida	For necrotizing pancreatitis (dose in footnote1 page 31) and continue 1–4 weeks (SGO 176: 480, 1993; ArSurg 132:487, 1997)	(see Comment), start **IMP**	For dx of pancreatic necrosis: contrast-enhanced CT. Accuracy >90% if >30% glandular necrosis. If infection uncertain, do CT-guided fine-needle aspiration (sens. 96%, spec. 99%).
PAROTID GLAND				
"Hot" tender parotid swelling	S. aureus, oral flora, & aerobic Gm-neg. bacilli (rare), mumps, rarely enteroviruses/	**Nafcillin** or **oxacillin** IV q4h (see above)		Predisposing factors: stone(s) in Stensen's duct, dehydration. Rx depends on ID of specific etiologic organism.
"Cold" non-tender parotid swelling	Granulomatous disease (e.g. mycobacteria, fungi, sarcoidosis, Sjögren's syn- drome), drugs (iodides, etc.), diabetes, cirrhosis, tumors			History/lab results may narrow differential, may need biopsy for dx.

(Footnotes and abbreviations on page 45)   NOTE: All dosage recommendations are for adults (unless otherwise indicated) and assume normal renal function

TABLE 1 (30)

ANATOMIC SITE/DIAGNOSIS/ MODIFYING CIRCUMSTANCES	ETIOLOGIES (usual)	SUGGESTED REGIMENS* PRIMARY	ALTERNATIVE†	ADJUNCT DIAGNOSTIC OR THERAPEUTIC MEASURES AND COMMENTS
PERITONEUM/PERITONITIS: Reference—CID 24:1035, 1997 **Primary (spontaneous bacterial peritonitis, SBP)** Rev.: CID 27:669, 1998 ESBL ref.: CID 28:683, 1999 Microbiology: CID 33:1513, 2001	Enterobacteriaceae 63%, S. pneumo 15%, enterococci 6–10%, anaerobes <1%.	**[Cefotaxime** 2.0 gm q8h IV (if life-threatening, q4h) or **TC/CL** or **PIP/TZ** or **AM/SB**] OR **[ceftriaxone** 2.0 gm IV q24h] If blood culture pos. & suspect E. coli/klebsiella problem (ESBL+) then: [IMP or MER] or [FQ: CIP, levo, trova, gati, moxi] (Dosage in footnote)		One-year risk of SBP in pts with ascites and cirrhosis as high as 29% (Gastro 104: 1133, 1993). 30–40% of pts have neg. cultures of blood and ascitic fluid. Neg. culture if blood & ascitic fluid inoculated into blood culture bottles. Duration of rx unclear. Suggest 2 wks if blood culture pos. One report suggests repeat paracentesis after 48 hrs of cefotaxime. If PMNs <250/mm³ and ascitic fluid bacteria, (stop) at 5 days of rx (AJM 97:169, 1994. Hepato 5:457, 1985). IV antibiotics × 5 days & IV albumin 1.5 gm/kg at dx & 1 gm/kg day 3 ↓ frequency of renal impairment (p 0.002) & ↓ hospital mortality (p 0.01) (NEJM 341:403, 1999). Ref. for CIP:
Prevention of SBP Cirrhosis & ascites		**TMP/SMX-DS** 1 tab po 5 d./wk. or **CIP** 750 mg po q wk.	**TMP/SMX** ↓ peritonitis or spontaneous bacteremia from 27% to 3% (AnIM 122:595, 1995).	
Cirrhosis & UGI bleeding			**CIP** 500 mg po bid × 7 d. (Ref. Gastroenterol 93:962, 1986)	
Secondary (bowel perforation, ruptured appendix, ruptured diverticuli) Ref.: NEJM 338:1521, 1998	Enterobacteriaceae, Bacteroides sp, enterococcus, P. aeruginosa (3–15%)	**Mild-moderate disease—Inpatient—parenteral rx:** (e.g. focal periappendiceal peritonitis, abscess, endomyometritis) **AM/SB** 3 gm IV q6h or **cefoxitin** 2 gm IV q8h or **PIP/TZ** 3.375 gm IV q6h or **cefotetan** 2 gm IV q12h or or 4.5 gm IV q8h, OR [CIP 400 mg IV q12h) + **TC/CL** 3.1 gm IV q6h, OR metro 500 mg IV q6h **ertapenem** 1 gm IV q24h **Severe life-threatening disease—ICU patient:** **IMP** 500 mg IV Trova 300 mg IV then 200 mg q6h or **MER** 1 gm IV qd OR [AMP 2 gm IV q6h + metro q8h or 1.0 gm 500 mg IV q6h + APAG] + metro IV q6h q8h OR [(AMP + metro + CIP 400 mg q12h)]		Multiple regimens effective. Must "cover" both Gm-neg. aerobic & Gm-neg. anaerobic bacteria. **Drugs active only vs anaerobic Gm-neg. bacilli:** clinda, metro. **Drugs active only vs aerobic Gm-neg. bacilli:** APAG, P Ceph 2/3/4, aztreonam, AP Pen, FQ, TMP/SMX. **Drugs active vs both aerobic/anaerobic Gm-neg. bacteria:** cefoxitin, cefotetan, cefmetazole, TC/CL, PIP/TZ, AM/SB, IMP, MER, & trova. **NOTE:** Ertapenem less active vs P. aeruginosa/Acinetobacter species than IMP or MER. **Concomitant surgical management important.** If rx has been ill for >24–48 hrs and there is absence of ongoing fecal contamination, aerobic/anaerobic culture of peritoneal exudate/abscess of help in guiding specific therapy. With large number of effective drugs, less need for aminoglycosides. With severe penicillin allergy, can "cover" Gm-neg. aerobes with CIP or aztreonam. Remember IMP/MER are β-lactams.
Associated with chronic ambulatory peritoneal dialysis (defined as >100 WBC/μL, >50% PMNs)	Staph. aureus (most common), Staph. epidermidis, aeruginosa 7%, Gm-neg. bacilli 11%, sterile 20%, M. fortuitum (rare)	If of moderate severity, can rx by adding thru IV to dialysis fluid—see Table 7? for dosage. Reasonable empiric combinations: vanco + P Ceph 3 or vanco + APAG (if severely ill, rx with same drugs IV (adjust dosage for renal failure, Table 17) & via addition to dialysis fluid Excellent ref.: Perit Dialysis Int 13:14, 1993		For diagnosis, concentrate several hundred ml of removed dialysis fluid by centrifugation. Gram stain concentrate and then inject into aerobic/anaerobic blood culture bottles. A positive Gram stain will guide initial therapy. If culture shows Staph. epidermidis, good chance of "saving" dialysis catheter. If multiple Gm-neg. bacilli cultured, consider bowel perforation and catheter removal.

† Parenteral IV therapy for peritonitis: **TC/CL** 3.1 gm IV q6h, **PIP/TZ** 3.375 gm IV q6h, **AM/SB** 3.0 gm IV q6h, **IMP** 0.5 gm q6h, **MER** 1.0 gm q8h, **FQ** [**CIP** 400 mg q12h; **oflox** 400 mg q12h; **levo** 500 mg qd; **trova** 300 mg qd; **gati** 400 mg qd, **moxi** 400 mg qd], **AMP** 1.0 gm q6h, **APAG** (see Table 7?), **AMP/SB** 3.0 gm q6h, **cefmetazole** 2.0 gm q6–12h, **P Ceph 3** [**cefotaxime** 2.0 gm q4–8h, **ceftizoxime** 2 gm qd, **ceftriaxone** 2.0 gm q24h], **P Ceph 4** (**CFP** 2.0 gm q12h), **cefpirome** 2.0 gm q12h, **clinda** 450–900 mg q8h, **metro** 1.0 gm loading then 0.5 gm q6h or 1.0 gm q12h, **aztreonam** 2.0 gm q8h, (metro 1 gm loading then 0.5 gm q6h) NOTE: All dosage recommendations are for adults (unless otherwise indicated) and assume normal renal function

(Footnotes and abbreviations on page 46)

TABLE 1 (31)

ANATOMIC SITE/DIAGNOSIS/ MODIFYING CIRCUMSTANCES	ETIOLOGIES (usual)	SUGGESTED REGIMENS* PRIMARY	ALTERNATIVE†	ADJUNCT DIAGNOSTIC OR THERAPEUTIC MEASURES AND COMMENTS
PHARYNGITIS Pharyngitis—Reviews: NEJM 344:205, 2001; AnIM 134:506 & 509, 2001. Overuse of antibiotics in adults: JAMA 286:118, 2001; Guideline for Group A strep: CID 35:113, 2002.				
Exudative or diffuse erythema *For relationship to acute rheumatic fever, see footnote†* Rheumatic fever ref.: Ln 349:935, 1997	(Group A,C,G strep, viral, infectious mononucleosis, HHV-6, (CID 26:1479, 1998), haemophilicum, Mycoplasma pneumoniae)	**Pen V** po x10 d. or **O Ceph benzathine pen** IM x1	**Erythro** x10 d. or **O Ceph 2** x4–6 d. or **clinda** or **azithro** x5 d., **clarithro** x10 d. or **azithro** x10 d.	**If Group A strep:** shortens duration/severity of symptoms and ↓ risk of rheumatic fever. Rapid strep test >95% specific; sensitivity varies (60–100%) **Groups C & G cause pharyngitis but not a risk for post-strep rheumatic fever.** To prevent rheumatic fever, eradicate Group A strep. Requires 10 d. of pen V po; 4–6 d. of po P Ceph 2, 5 d. of po azithro, 10 d. of clarithro. In controlled trial, better eradication rate with 10 d. azithro (91%) than 5 d. azithro (82%)(CID 32:1798,2001)
	Gonococci	**Ceftriaxone** 125 mg IM x1 + (**azithro** or **doxy**) (see Comment)	(**CIP** 500 mg po x1) or (**gati** 400 mg po x1) or (**oflox** 400 mg po x1) + (**azithro** or **doxy**) (see Comment)	Because of risk of concomitant genital C. trachomatis, add either azithro 1.0 gm po x1) or (doxy 100 mg po 2x/d x7 d.)
Asymptomatic post-rx carrier	Group A strep	**No rx required**		Routine post-rx throat culture not advised.
Multiple repeated culture-positive episodes (CID 25:574, 1997)	Group A strep	**Clinda** or **AM/CL** po	Parenteral **benzathine pen G** + **RIF** (see Comment) *Dosages in footnote[3]*	Small % of pts have recurrent culture-pos. Group A strep with symptomatic pharyngitis. Hard to tell if true Group A strep infection or active viral infection in carrier of Group A strep. Addition of RIF may help: 20 mg/kg/d x4 d. to max. of 300 mg bid po (J Ped 106:481 & 876, 1985).
Vesicular, ulcerative Whitish plaques; HIV+; (thrush)	Candida albicans [see Table 10, page 73]		Antibacterial agents not indicated, but for HSV-	
	Coxsackie A9, B1-5, ECHO (multiple types). Enterovirus 71. Herpes simplex 1,2	Antibiotics not indicated	1,2, **acyclovir** 400 mg tid x4 d.	
Membranous	C. diphtheriae	**Antitoxin + erythro** 20-25 mg/kg (up to 2 gm) IV q12h x7–14 d. or **Pen G** 25,000-50,000 U/kg/d x5 d. then po **VK** 50 mg/kg/d x5 d.	**Clinda** 600 mg q8h IV	Diphtheria occurs in immunized individuals. Antibiotics may ↓ toxin production (J...35:271, 1998). Penicillin superior to erythro in randomized trial (CID 27:845, 1998).
Vincent's angina (anaerobes/spirochetes)		**Pen G** 4 mU q4h IV	**Clinda** 600 mg q8h IV	May be complicated by F. necrophorum bacteremia; see jugular vein phlebitis (Lemierre's), below.
Epiglottitis (IDCP 6:500, 1997) Children	H. influenzae (rare), S. pyogenes, S. pneumoniae, S. aureus	**Peds dosage: Cefotaxime** 50 mg/kg q8h IV or **ceftriaxone** 50 mg/kg q24h IV or **cefuroxime** 50 mg/kg q8h IV	**Peds dosage: AM/SB** 100–200 mg/kg/d div q6h or **TMP/SMX** 8–12 mg TMP comp./kg/d div q12h	Have tracheostomy set "at bedside." Chloro is effective, but potentially less toxic alternative agents available. Review (adults): JAMA 272:1358, 1994.
Adults	Group A strep, H. influenzae (rare)	**Adult dosage:** See footnote[3]	**Adult dosage: AM/SB** 3.0 gm IV q6h; **TC/CL** 3.1 gm IV q4-6h; **TMP/SMX** 8–10 mg/kg/d (based on TMP component) div q6h, q8h, or q12h.	

---

[1] Primary rationale for treatment is eradication of Group A strep (GAS) and prevention of acute rheumatic fever (ARF). Benzathine penicillin G has been shown in clinical trials to ↓ rate of ARF from 2.8 to 0.2%. This was associated with clearance of GAS on pharyngeal cultures. Subsequent studies have been based on cultures, not actual prevention of ARF. Treatment ↓ duration of symptoms.

[2] Treatment at Group A strep: **All po unless otherwise indicated. PEDIATRIC DOSAGE: Benzathine penicillin** 25,000 u/kg IM to max. 1.2 mU; **Pen V** 25–50 mg/kg/d div q8h x10 d; **AM/CL** 45 mg/kg/d div q12h x10 d; **erythro estolate** 20 mg/kg/d div bid x10 d. or **ethylsuccinate** 40 mg/kg/d div bid x10 d; **cefprozil** 7.5 mg/kg/d div q12h x10 d; **clinda** 20-30 mg/kg/d div q8h x10 d; **cefpodoxime** 10 mg/kg/d div q12h x5–10 d; **cefdinir** 14 mg/kg/d div q12-24h x10 d; **clarithro** 15 mg/kg/d div q12h x10 d; **azithro** 12 mg/kg x1 d. then 6 mg/kg/d x4 d.
ADULT DOSAGE: Benzathine penicillin 1.2 mU IM x1; **Pen V** 500 mg (or 250 mg qid) x10 d; **erythro, dosage varies**—with erythro base 500 mg qid x10 d.; **cefuroxime axetil** 250 mg bid x4 d, **cefpodoxime proxetil** 100 mg bid x4 d, **cefdinir** 300 mg q12h x5–10 d. or 600 mg qd x10 d; **cefprozil** 500 mg qd x10 d. **NOTE: All O Ceph 2 drugs** approved for 10 d. rx of strep. pharyngitis; increasing number of studies show efficacy of 4-6 d.: **clarithro** 250 mg bid x10 d., **dirithromycin** 500 mg x1 and then 250 mg daily x4 d.

[3] **Cefuroxime** 0.75–1.5 gm IV q8h; **cefotaxime** 2.0 gm IV qd; **ceftriaxone** 2.0 gm IV q24h; **cefotaxime** 2.0 gm IV q-8h IV. **AM/SB** 3.0 gm IV q6h; **TC/CL** 3.1 gm IV q4-6h; **TMP/SMX** 8–10 mg/kg/d (based on TMP component) div q6h, q8h, or q12h. *NOTE: All dosage recommendations are for adults (unless otherwise indicated) and assume normal renal function*

(Footnotes and abbreviations on page 45)

TABLE 1 (32)

ANATOMIC SITE/DIAGNOSIS/ MODIFYING CIRCUMSTANCES	ETIOLOGIES (usual)	SUGGESTED REGIMENS* PRIMARY	SUGGESTED REGIMENS* ALTERNATIVE§	ADJUNCT DIAGNOSTIC OR THERAPEUTIC MEASURES AND COMMENTS
PHARYNX (continued)				
Parapharyngeal space infection. Poor dental hygiene, dental extractions, foreign bodies (e.g. toothpicks, fish bones)	Spaces include: sublingual, submandibular, submaxillary (Ludwig's) angina, used loosely for these), lateral pharyngeal, retropharyngeal, prevertebral. Polymicrobic: Strep. sp., anaerobes, Eikenella corrodens	Pen G 24 mU iv q4-6h IV + metro 1.0 gm load and then 0.5 gm q6h IV	Clinda 600-900 mg q8h IV	Critical is maintenance of airway (73 intubation, MRI guide needle aspiration, surgical drainage if pus. CT to identify abscess; if present, surgical drainage. (Dosage see footnote 2 page 31) Metro may be given 1.0 gm q12h IV
Jugular vein septic phlebitis (Lemierre's) (CID 31:524, 2000)	Fusobacterium necrophorum in vast majority	Pen G¹ 24 mU iv q4-6h IV or cont. infusion or div. q4-6h¹	Clinda 600-900 mg q8h IV	Usual rx includes external drainage of lateral pharyngeal space. Emboli, pulmonary and systemic common. Erosion into carotid artery can occur.
Laryngitis (hoarseness)/tracheitis	Viral (90%)	Not indicated		
SINUSES, PARANASAL				
Sinusitis, acute; current terminology: acute rhinosinusitis. Obstruction of sinus ostia, viral infection, allergens	Strep. pneumoniae 31%, H. influenzae 21%, M. catarrhalis 2%, Group A strep 2%, anaerobes 6%, viruses 15%, Staph. aureus 4% By CT scans, sinus mucosa inflamed in 87% of viral URIs; only 2% develop bacterial rhinosinusitis	Reserve antibiotic rx for pts given decongestants and analgesics for 7 d. who have (1) maxillary/facial pain & (2) purulent nasal discharge; if severe illness (pain, fever), treat sooner—usually requires hospitalization. For mild/mod. disease: Antibiotics in prior month and/or DRSP prevalence >30%?? NO: Amox or AM/CL-ER or cefdinir or cefpodoxime or cefuroxime axetil or telithro Treat x10 days. Adult and pediatric doses, footnote¹ and footnote 2 page 7 (Otitis)	**For pts with penicillin/cephalosporin allergy, esp. severe IgE-mediated allergy, e.g. hives, anaphylaxis; treatment options: clarithro, azithro, telithro, TMP/SMX, doxy & FQs if under age 18. Dosages in footnote 2 page 32.** YES: AM/CL-ER (adults) or FQ (adults). For pen. allergy, see Comment. Use AM/CL susp. in peds.	Rx goals. (1) Resolve infection, (2) prevent complications of bacterial disease, e.g. bacteremia, meningitis, brain abscess, (3) avoid chronic sinus disease, (4) avoid unnecessary antibiotic rx. High rate of spontaneous resolution. In areas with prevalence of DRSP >30%, and recent prior antibiotic use, consider increasing amoxicillin dose to 3–3.5 gm/d. use extra amox. do not increase AM/CL beyond standard dosage. Usual rx 10 days, results of 3 & 10. d. of TMP/SMX, the same (JAMA 273:1015, 1995). Watch for pts with fever & facial erythema: ?risk of S. aureus infection, requires IV nafacillin/oxacillin (if antistaphylococcal penicillin, penicillinase-resistant). Pts aged 1-18 yrs. No difference in multiple measures of efficacy (Pediatrics 107:619, 2001).
Clinical failure after 3 days	As above; consider diagnostic tap/aspirate	Mild/Mod. Disease: AM/CL-ER OR (cefpodoxime, cefurox-ime or cefdinir) Treat 10 days. Adult doses in footnote 2 page 32 &	Severe Disease: Gati, levo, moxi	Pts aged 1-18 yrs randomized to placebo, amox, or AM/CL for 14 d. No difference in multiple measures of efficacy (Pediatrics 107:619, 2001).
Diabetes mellitus with acute ketoacidosis; neutropenia; deferoxamine rx	Rhizopus sp. (mucor); aspergillus	See Table 10, page 77. Ref: NEJM 337:254, 1997		

¹ Penicillin may be given in divided doses q4-6h or by continuous infusion

¹ **Pediatric doses for sinusitis (all oral):** Amoxicillin high dose 90 mg/kg/div div q12h, **clarithro** 15 mg/kg/d div q12h, **cefpodoxime** 10 mg/kg/d div. q12h, **cefprozil** 30 mg/kg/d div q12h, **AM/CL-ES** (extra strength) pediatric susp.: 90 mg/kg component/kg/div div q12h, **azithro** 10 mg/kg x1 then 5 mg/kg/day, **TMP/SMX** 8-12 mg TMP/40-60 mg SMX/kg/d div q12h, **cefuroxime axetil** 30 mg/kg/d div q12h, **cefdinir** 14 mg/kg/d q24h or once daily or divided bid, **TMP/SMX** 8-12

² **Adult doses for sinusitis (all oral):** **AM/CL** (Augmentin XR) 2000/125 mg bid, **amox** 500 mg tid, **clarithro** 500 mg bid or **clarithro ext. release** 1.0 gm od, **doxy** 100 mg bid, **FQs (gati)** 400 mg od, **levo** 500 mg od, **moxi** 400 mg qd.), **O Ceph** (**cefdinir** 300 mg q12h or 600 mg qd, **cefpodoxime** 200 mg q12h bid, **cefuroxime** 250-500 mg bid), **TMP/SMX** 1 double-strength (TMP 160 mg) bid, **telithro** 800 mg qd.

(Footnotes and abbreviations on page 45) NOTE: All dosage recommendations are for adults (unless otherwise indicated) and assume normal renal function

TABLE 1 (33)

ANATOMIC SITE/DIAGNOSIS/ MODIFYING CIRCUMSTANCES	ETIOLOGIES (usual)	SUGGESTED REGIMENS* — PRIMARY	SUGGESTED REGIMENS* — ALTERNATIVE§	ADJUNCT DIAGNOSTIC OR THERAPEUTIC MEASURES AND COMMENTS
SINUSITIS, PARANASAL/Sinusitis, Acute				
Hospitalized + nasotracheal or nasogastric intubation	Gm-neg. bacilli 47% (pseudomonas, acinetobacter, E. coli common), Gm+ (S. aureus) 35%, yeasts 18%. Polymicrobial in 80%	Remove nasotracheal tube and if fever persists, recommend sinus aspiration for C/S prior to empiric rx. **IMP** 0.5 gm q6h IV or **ceftaz** + **vanco** IV or (**CFP** 2.0 gm q12h IV)		After 7 d. of nasotracheal or gastric tubes, 95% have x-ray "sinusitis" (fluid in sinuses), but on transnasal puncture only 38% culture + [AJRCCM 150:776, 1994]. For pts requiring mechanical ventilation for ≥1 wk. bacterial sinusitis occurs in <10% [CID 27:851, 1998]. May need fluconazole if yeasts on Gram stain of aspirate. Review: CID 25:1441, 1997. Epidemiology: CID 27:463, 1998
Sinusitis, chronic	Prevotella anaerobic strep, & fusobacterium—common anaerobes. Strep sp., hemophilus, P. aeruginosa, S. aureus, & moraxella—aerobes [CID 35:428, 2002]	Antibiotics usually not effective	Otolaryngology consultation. If acute exacerbation, rx as acute	Pathogenesis unclear and may be polyclactoral complex & maybe due to osteomeatal complex obstruction; allergy ± polyps, occult immunodeficiency, and/or odontogenic disease (periodontitis in maxillary teeth).
SKIN				
Acne vulgaris [NEJM 336:1156, 1997; Ln 351:1871, 1998; Med Lett 44:52, 2002]				
Comedonal acne, blackheads, "whiteheads," earliest form, no inflammation	Excessive sebum production & gland obstruction. No Propionibacterium acnes	Topical **tretinoin** (cream 0.025 or 0.05%) or (gel 0.01 or 0.025%) Once-daily	All once-daily. Topical **adapalene** 0.1% gel OR **azelaic acid** 20% cream OR **tazarotene** 0.1% cream, gel	Goal is prevention. ↓ number of new comedones and create an environment unfavorable to P. acnes. Adapalene causes less irritation than tretinoin. Azelaic acid as topically less potent but less irritating than retinoids.
Mild inflammatory acne: small papules or pustules	Proliferation of P. acnes and abnormal desquamation of follicular cells	Topical **erythro** 3%, & **benzoyl peroxide** 5% bid	Can substitute **clinda** 1% gel for erythro	Topical metro has anti-inflammatory activity but P. acnes not susceptible
Inflammatory acne: comedones, papules & pustules. Less common: deep nodules (cysts)	Progression of above events	(Topical **erythro** 3% + **benzoyl peroxide** 5% bid) & oral antibiotic	Oral drugs: (**doxy** 100 mg bid) or (**minocycline** 50 mg bid) or (**tetracycline** 500 mg bid) or erythro, TMP/SMX, clinda	Systemic **isotretinoin** reserved for pts with severe widespread nodular cystic lesions that fail oral antibiotic rx: 4–5 mo. course of 0.1–1.0 mg/kg/day. Aggressive, violent behavior reported. Tetracyclines stain developing teeth. Doxy can cause photosensitivity. Minocycline side-effects: urticaria, vertigo, pigment deposition in skin or oral mucosa.
Acne rosacea	? skin mite Demodex folliculorum	**Metro** (topical), cream or gel	**Doxy** 100 mg bid po	Metro efficacious in randomized double-blind, placebo-controlled trial [Cutis 61:44, 1998]
Anthrax, cutaneous, inhalation (pulmonary, mediastinal) **To report bioterrorism event: 770-488-7100;** For info: www.bt.cdc.gov Refs: JAMA 281:1735, 1999; & MMWR 50:909, 2001	B. anthracis. See Lung, page 28, and Table 1B, page 46	**Adults (including pregnancy):** CIP 400 mg IV q12h or **doxy** 100 mg IV q12h. **Children:** CIP 20-30 mg/kg/d div q12h to max. 1 gm/d.) x60 d.	**Adults (including pregnancy): Doxy** 100 mg po bid x60 d. **Children: Doxy** >8 yo & >45 kg: 100 mg po bid; >8 yo & <45 kg: 2.2 mg/kg po bid; ≤8 yo: 2.2 mg/kg po bid. All for 60 days.	1. If penicillin susceptible, then: **Adults: Amox** 500 mg po q8h x60 d. **Children: Amox** 80 mg/kg/d div. q8h (max. 500 mg q8h) 2. Usual treatment of cutaneous anthrax is 7–10 d.; 60 d. in setting of bioterrorism with presumed aerosol exposure 3. Other FQs (gati, levo, moxi) should work based on in vitro susceptibility data
Bacillary angiomatosis: For other Bartonella infections, see Cat-scratch disease lymphadenitis, page 30, and Bartonella, page 38	Bartonella henselae and quintana	In immunocompromised (HIV-1, bone marrow transplant) patients Also see SANFORD GUIDE TO HIV/AIDS THERAPY	**Clarithro** 500 mg bid po or **azithro** 500 mg qd po or **CIP** 500–750 mg bid po (see Comment)	**Erythro** 500 mg qid po or **doxy** 100 mg bid po	In immunocompromised pts with severe disease, doxy 100 mg po/IV bid + RIF 300 mg po bid reported effective [IDC No. Amer 12:37, 1998; Adv PID 11:1, 1996]

(Footnotes and abbreviations on page 45)

NOTE: All dosage recommendations are for adults (unless otherwise indicated) and assume normal renal function

TABLE 1 (34)

ANATOMIC SITE/DIAGNOSIS/ MODIFYING CIRCUMSTANCES	ETIOLOGIES (usual)	SUGGESTED REGIMENS*		ADJUNCT DIAGNOSTIC OR THERAPEUTIC MEASURES AND COMMENTS
		PRIMARY	ALTERNATIVE§	
SKIN (continued)				
Bite: Prophylaxis within 12 hrs of bite or empirical rx of established infection. Ref. CID 14 633, 1992; remember tetanus prophylaxis—see Table 20.				
Bat, raccoon, skunk		AM/CL 875/125 mg po bid or 500/125 mg tid po		In Americas, antirabies rx indicated, rabies immune globulin + vaccine. (See Table 20C, page 135)
Cat (Ref. NEJM 340 85 & 138, 1999) Cat-scratch disease: page 30	**Pasteurella multocida.** Staph. aureus	AM/CL 875/125 mg po bid or 500/125 mg tid po	Cefuroxime axetil 0.5 gm q12h po or doxy 100 mg po. Do not use cephalexin	Pts may become infected. P. multocida resistant to dicloxacillin, cephalexin, clinda and erythro (most sensitive to azithro but no clinical data) P. multocida infection develops within 24 hrs. Observe for osteomyelitis. If culture +, for only P. multocida, can switch to pen G IV or pen VK po.
Catfish sting	Toxins	See Comments		Presents as immediate pain, erythema and edema. Resembles strep cellulitis. May become secondarily infected. AM/CL is reasonable choice for prophylaxis
Dog (Ref. NEJM 340 85 & 138, 1999)	P. multocida, S. aureus, Bacteroides sp., Fusobacterium sp., EF-4, Capnocytophaga	AM/CL 875/125 mg bid or 500/125 mg tid po	Clinda 300 mg q8h po + FQ (adults) or clinda + TMP SMX (children)	Only 5% dog bites become infected. (Arch EM 23 535, 1994). Consider antirabies rx, rabies immune globulin + vaccine (Table 20C). May transmit blastomycosis. Capnocytophaga in splenectomized pts may cause local eschar, sepsis with DIC. P. multocida resistant to dicloxacillin, cephalexin, clinda and erythro; sensitive to FQs in vitro (AAC 43 1475, 1999).
Human	Viridans strep 100%, Staph epidermidis 53%, corynebacterium 41%, Staph. aureus 29%, eikenella 15%, bacteroides 82%, peptostrep 26%	**Early** (not yet infected): AM/CL 875/125 mg bid po x5 **Later:** Signs of infection (usually in 3–24 hrs) (AM/SB) 1.5 gm q6h IV or cefoxitin 2.0 gm q8h IV) or (TC/CL 3.1 gm q6h IV) or (PIP/TZ (3.375 gm q6h or 4.5 gm q8h IV)	**Pen allergy: Clinda** + (either cipro or TMP/SMX). P Ceph 3 or TC/CL or AM/SB or IMP	Cleaning, irrigation and debridement most important. For clenched fist injuries, x-rays should be obtained. Bites inflicted by hospitalized pts, consider aerobic Gm-neg. bacilli. Eikenella resistant to clinda, nafcillin/oxacillin, metro and to Ceph 1 and erythro; susceptible to FQs and TMP/SMX. For in vitro susceptibility to FQs and macrolides JAC 41 391, 1998
Pig (swine)	Polymicrobic: Gm+ cocci, Gm-neg. bacilli, anaerobes, Pasteurella sp.	AM/CL 875/125 mg bid po		Information limited but infection is common and serious (Ln 348 888, 1996).
Primate, non-human	Herpesvirus simiae	Acyclovir. See Table 14B, page 110		
Rat	Spirillum minus & Streptobacillus moniliformis	AM/CL 875/125 mg bid po		CID 20 421, 1995
Snake pit viper (Ref. NEJM 347 347, 2002)	Pseudomonas sp., Enterobacteriaceae, staph. epidermidis, Clostridium sp.	AM/CL 875/125 mg bid po	Doxy	Antirabies rx not indicated.
Spider				
Widow (Latrodectus)	Not infectious	None		May be confused with "acute abdomen." Diazepam or calcium gluconate helpful to control pain, muscle spasm. Tetanus prophylaxis.
Brown recluse (Loxosceles) (not west of Nebraska)	Not infectious	Dapsone 50 mg qd po (see Comments)	Systemic antibiotics and drainage Primary therapy is antivenom. Penicillin generally used but would not be effective vs organisms isolated. Ceftriaxone should be more effective.	Most pts do well without systemic rx. Dapsone followed by excision at 6 weeks (AnSurg 202 659, 1985) reported effective. Screen for G6PD deficiency. Caution: dapsone inhibits PMNs
Boils—Furunculosis				
Acute episode	Staph. aureus	Not effective: hot packs and drainage		Incision and drainage. Systemic antibiotics do not shorten course of a boil. (See Skin, furunculosis, page 36)
Prevention of recurrences (goal is to eliminate nasal carriage of Staph. aureus)	Staph aureus-MSSA For control of MRSA, see below	Mupirocin nasal (2%, apply small amount intranasally bid x5 d.)	RIF 600 mg po x10 d or (diclox 500 mg qid po x10 d or TMP/SMX 1 DS tab (TMP 160 mg) po) x10 d.	Mupirocin intranasal effective vs S. aureus including MRSA (JAC 19 1, 1987). RIF + cloxacillin also effective (AnIM 114 101, 1991). Subset of pts with impaired neutrophil function responded to vitamin C, 1 gm/d. (JID 140 1140, 1996)
Hidradenitis suppurativa	Lesions secondarily infected aureus, Enterobacteriaceae, pseudomonas, anaerobes	Aspirate base rx on culture		Acute rx: clinda or keflex or cloxa, plugging of apocrine glands of axillary and/or inguinal areas. Many pts ultimately require surgical excision.

(Footnotes and abbreviations on page 45)

NOTE: All dosage recommendations are for adults (unless otherwise indicated) and assume normal renal function

TABLE 1 (35)

ANATOMIC SITE/DIAGNOSIS/ MODIFYING CIRCUMSTANCES	ETIOLOGIES (usual)	SUGGESTED REGIMENS* PRIMARY	ALTERNATIVE§	ADJUNCT DIAGNOSTIC OR THERAPEUTIC MEASURES AND COMMENTS
SKIN/Boils, recurrent—Furunculosis				
Methicillin-resistant S. aureus—colonization (continued)	MRSA	**Mupirocin** (2% to nares and wounds) bid x 1–2/ wks	(**Novobiocin** 250 mg po) + (**TMP/SMX** po) + **RIF**)	Mupirocin cleared 95% when applied to nares and wounds but resolves even if use is continued. Silver nitrate leaches electrolytes from wounds & stains ev- erything. Meticare inhibits cationic, anhydrate and can cause metabolic acidosis. (AJM 94:371, 1993; AAC 37:1334, 1993)
Burns				
Initial burn wound care (NEJM 335:1581, 1996)	Not infected	**Silver sulfadiazine** cream, 1% apply 1–2x/ day	0.5% silver nitrate solution or **mafenide acetate** cream. Apply 2x/day	Marrow-induced neutropenia can occur during 1st wk of sulfadiazine but resolves even if use is continued. Silver nitrate leaches electrolytes from wounds & stains every- thing. Mafenide inhibits carbonic anhydrase and can cause metabolic acidosis.
Burn wound sepsis	Strep. pyogenes, Enterobac- ter sp., S. aureus, S. epi- dermidis, E. faecalis, E. coli, P. aeruginosa. Fungi rare. Herpesvirus rare	**Vanco** 1.0 gm q12h IV + **PIP** 4.0 gm q4h IV (give ½ daily dose of **piperacillin** into subeschar tissues with surgical eschar removal within 12 hours)	**Vanco** 1.0 gm q12h IV + (load- ing dose then 7.5 mg/kg q4h IV + **PIP** 4.0 gm q4h IV)	Infection a/w serum antibiotics ↓ . Staph. aureus has become the most local- ized burn wound. If patient more than expected, consider toxic shock syndrome. Candida too seldom invade. Pneumonia has become the major infectious complication, most often staph. Other infectious complications include septic thrombophlebitis.
Cellulitis, erysipelas				
Extremities, not associated with venous catheter (see Comments) non-diabetic For diabetes, see below	Group A strep, occ. Group B, C, G; Staph. aureus (un- common but difficult to ex- clude)	**Pen G** 1–2 mU IV q6h or **Nafcillin** or **oxacillin** 2.0 gm q4h IV. If not severe, **dicloxacillin** 500 mg po qid or **cefazolin** 1.0 gm q8h IV	**Erythro*** or **P Ceph 1** or **AM/CL** or **azithro** or **clarithro** or **dirithro** or **moxi.** See footnote	"Spontaneous" erysipelas of leg in non-diabetic is usually due to strep. Gps A,B,C or G. Hence OK to start with IV pen G 1–2 mU q6h & observe for localized S. aureus infection. Look for tinea pedis with fissures, a common portal of entry; can often culture strep from between toes (CID 23:1162, 1996). For Rx of pts with lymphedema & recurrent erysipelas, see prophylaxis, Table 15. Other alternatives clinda, gati, levo, moxi
Facial, adult (erysipelas)	Group A strep, Staph. aureus	**Nafcillin** or **oxacillin** (Dosage, see erysipelas of extremity, above)	**Cefazolin** or **vanco** if not severe, **AM/CL**	**Choice of empiric therapy must have activity vs S. aureus**
Diabetes mellitus and erysipelas	Group A strep, Staph. aureus, Enterobacteriaceae, clostridia (rare)	Early mild: **P Ceph 2/3** or **MER** or **ertapenem** or **trova** IV (Dosage, see page 10. Diabetic foot)	**IMP** or **MER** or **ertapenem** or **trova** IV	Prompt surgical debridement indicated to rule out necrotizing fasciitis or to obtain cultures. If septic, consider x-ray of extremity to demonstrate gas. Prognosis depen- dent on blood supply; assess arteries. See Diabetic foot, page 10.
Erysipelas, recurrent 2° to congenital lymphedema (Milroy's disease)	S. pyogenes, Groups A, C, G	**Benzathine pen G** 1.2 mU IM q4 wks (of minimal benefit in reducing recurrences in pts with underlying predisposing conditions (CID 25:685, 1997)		Indicated only if pt is having frequent episodes of cellulitis. Pen V 250 mg po bid should be effective but never adequately tested in controlled trials. In pen-allergic pts: erythro 500 mg po qid or azithro 250 mg qd, or clarithro 500 mg qd.
Dandruff (seborrheic dermatitis)	Malassezia species	**Ketoconazole shampoo** 2% or **selenium sulfide** 2.5% (see page 6, chronic external otitis)		
Decubitus or venous stasis or arterial insufficiency ulcers; with sepsis	Polymicrobic: S. pyogenes (Gps A,C,G) enterococci, anaerobic strep, Enterobac- teriaceae, Pseudomonas sp., Bacteroides sp., Staph. aureus	**IMP** or **MER** or **TC/CL** or **PIP/TZ**	**P Ceph 1** (cefti, levo, or moxi) + **(clinda** or **metro)** Dosages, see footnotes pages 10, 16, 20, 42	Without sepsis or extensive cellulitis local care may be adequate. Debride as needed. Topical mafenide or silver sulfadiazine adjunctive. R/O underlying osteo- myelitis. In nursing home with MRSA, vanco required for Staph. aureus. May need wound coverage with skin graft or skin substitute. (JAMA 283:716, 2000)
Erythema multiforme	H. simplex type 1, mycoplasma, Strep. pyogenes, drugs (sulfonamides, phenytoin, penicillins)			**Rx: Acyclovir** if due to H. simplex
Erythema nodosum	Sarcoidosis, inflammatory bowel disease, M. tbc, coccidioidomycosis, yersinia, sulfonamides			**Rx: NSAIDs, glucocorticoids** if refractory
Erythrasma	Corynebacterium minutissimum	**Erythro** 250 mg po x14 d		Coral red fluorescence with Wood's lamp. Alt: 2% aqueous clinda topically
Folliculitis	Many etiologies: S. aureus, candida, P. aeruginosa, malassezia, demodex	See individual entities. See Whirlpool folliculitis, page 38		
Furunculosis with cellulitis and/or sepsis (See Boils, recurrent, page 35)	Staph. aureus	**Nafcillin** or **oxacillin** 2.0 gm q6h IV or **cefazolin** 1.0–2.0 gm q8h IV or **vanco** 1.0 gm q12h IV		Surgical drainage. Hexachlorophene soap. Suppression of nasal carriage of Staph. aureus

* Rapid increase of resistance to erythro and clinda reported from Italy (EID 2:339, 1996).
NOTE: All dosage recommendations are for adults (unless otherwise indicated) and assume normal renal function
(Footnotes and abbreviations on page 45)

TABLE 1 (36)

ANATOMIC SITE/DIAGNOSIS/ MODIFYING CIRCUMSTANCES	ETIOLOGIES (usual)	SUGGESTED REGIMENS* PRIMARY	ALTERNATIVE†	ADJUNCT DIAGNOSTIC OR THERAPEUTIC MEASURES AND COMMENTS
SKIN (continued)				
Hemorrhagic bullous lesions Hx of sea water-contaminated abrasion or eating raw seafood, shock	**Vibrio vulnificus, V. damsela**	**Ceftazidime** 2.0 gm q8h IV + **doxy** 100 mg bid (IV or po)	Either **cefotaxime** 2.0 gm q8h IV or **CIP** 750 mg bid (po or 400 mg IV)	¾ pts have chronic liver disease. Mortality 50% (NEJM 312:343, 1985) No controlled studies. In Taiwan, where a number of cases are seen, the impression exists that ceftazidime is superior to tetracyclines (CID 15:271, 1992). Why not both?
No hx of saltwater exposure	Staph or strep septic shock. clostridia	See Gas gangrene, page 30		
Herpes zoster (shingles) See Table 14				
Impetigo, echyma—usually children "Honey-crust" lesions (non-bullous)	**Group A strep impetigo;** crusted lesions can be Staph. aureus + strepto-cocci	Oral **dicloxacillin** or **cloxacillin**	**Mupirocin** ointment tid or **azithro** or **erythro** or **O Ceph 2**. For dosages, see Table 9B for adults and Table 16, page 129 for children	24% failure with pen VK (AJDC 144:1313, 1990). O Ceph 2 >90% cure (AAC 36:1614, 1992).
Bullous (if ruptured, thin "varnish-like" crust)	**Staph. aureus impetigo**	**Dicloxacillin** p.o. or **oxacillin** p.o or **O Ceph 1** (not cefixime)	**Mupirocin** ointment or **AM/CL** or **azithro** or **clarithro**. For dosages, see Table 9B	NOTE: Cefixime not active vs Staph. aureus.
Infected wound, extremity—Post-trauma (for bites, see above) Mild to moderate, uncomplicated	Polymicrobic: Staph. aureus, Group A & anaerobic strep, Enterobacteriaceae, Cl. perfringens, etc. In fresh water sp. Aeromonas sp.)	(for post-operative, see below) **AM/CL** 875/125 mg bid po or **O Ceph 1** (Dosage, page 10)	**erythro** or **clarithro** or **azithro** or **clinda** (Dosage, page 26) or **levo** 500 mg qd	Wound cleansing and debridement. Gram stain may enable rapid diagnosis of clostridia. **Antitetanus prophylaxis** (See Table 20C, page 135) If freshwater exposure, Pseudomonas and Aeromonas species possible—FQ recommended
Febrile with sepsis		**AM/SB** or **TC/CL** or **PIP/TZ** or **IMP** or **MER** or **ertapenem** (Dosage, page 16)	(**Nafcillin** or **oxacillin** 2.0 gm q4h IV) + **CIP** + **clinda** or **levo** 750 mg IV/po qd	NOTE: Ertapenem not active vs P. aeruginosa. If sea water, see hemorrhagic bullous lesions and Vibrio vulnificus. If sea water, see hemorrhagic bullous lesions. Trova 200 mg IV qd should not work for life-threatening severe infection. NOTE: None of listed regimens predictably effective for MRSA. Treatment duration varies with severity, from 5–10 days
Infected wound, post-operative Surgery not involving GI or female genital tract Without sepsis	Staph. aureus, Group A strep. Enterobacteriaceae	**O Ceph 1** or **AM/CL, TC/CL** or **PIP/TZ** or **AM/SB** (Dosage, see page 16)	**Dicloxacillin** po ± **FQ** po. **P Ceph 1/2/3** (Dosage, see page 16)	Gram stain exudate to guide treatment choice. Surgical drainage alone often adequate. Where MRSA prevalent, add vanco. In pts without sepsis after 72 hours, pt can be switched to oral therapy.
With sepsis	Above + Bacteroides sp. other anaerobes, entero-cocci, Group B, C strep. See Necrotizing fasciitis, below	**Cefoxitin** or **cefotetan** or **TC/CL** or **PIP/TZ** or **AM/SB MER**. **Trova** another option	**P Ceph 2/3** + **metro** or **ertapenem** or **IMP** or **MER** or **ertapenem** or **IMP** or	For all treatment options, see Peritonitis, page 31 Trova dose 300 mg IV qd, then 200 mg po qd.
Surgery involving GI tract (includes oropharynx, esophagus) or female genital tract. Meleney's synergistic gangrene. See Necrotizing fasciitis, below				
Necrotizing fasciitis ("flesh-eating bacteria") Post-surgery, trauma, strepto-coccal skin infections (see Muscle, gas gangrene, page 30, & Toxic shock, page 43	Streptococci, Grp A, C, G; Clostridia sp., polymicrobic, aerobic + anaerobic. Rarely, aerobic coliform alone	For treatment of clostridia, see Muscle, gas gangrene. For treatment of Fournier's gangrene. necrotizing fasciitis have a common pathophysiology. **All require prompt surgical debridement** as well as antibiotics. Dx of necrotizing fasciitis—make incision & probe. If no resistance to probing, dx = necrotizing fasciitis. If inexperienced, frozen section at biopsy (NEJM 310:1689, 1984). Need Gram stain/culture to determine if etiology is strep, clostridia or polymicrobial. Treatment: **Pen G ±** clinda for strep or clostridia, **IMP** or **MER** or polymicrobial		The terminology of polymicrobic wound infections is not precise. Meleney's synergistic gangrene, Fournier's gangrene,

---

* Good evidence that incidence of invasive Group A strep infection (necrotizing fasciitis) is increasing. Also risk of transmission in households and health care institutions (NEJM 335:547, 1996).
NOTE: All dosage recommendations are for adults (unless otherwise indicated) and assume normal renal function

(Footnotes and abbreviations on page 45)

TABLE 1 (37)

ANATOMIC SITE/DIAGNOSIS/ MODIFYING CIRCUMSTANCES	ETIOLOGIES (usual)	SUGGESTED REGIMENS*		ADJUNCT DIAGNOSTIC OR THERAPEUTIC MEASURES AND COMMENTS
		PRIMARY	ALTERNATIVE§	
SKIN (continued)				
Staphylococcal scalded skin syndrome Ref: *PIDJ 19:819, 2000*	Toxin-producing S. aureus	**Nafcillin** or **oxacillin** 2.0 gm IV q4h (children: 150 mg/kg/d div. q6h) x5–7 days		Toxin causes intraepidermal split and positive Nikolsky sign. Drugs cause epidermal/dermal split, **called toxic epidermal necrolysis**—more serious *(Ln 351: 1417, 1998)*. Biopsy differentiates.
Whirlpool (Hot Tub) folliculitis See *Folliculitis, page 36*	Pseudomonas aeruginosa	Usually self-limited; treatment not indicated		Decontaminate hot tub: drain and chlorinate. Also associated with exfoliative beauty aids (loofah sponges) *(J Clin Micro 37:480, 1999).*
SPLEEN				
Splenic abscess				
Endocarditis, bacteremia	Staph. aureus, streptococci	**Nafcillin** or **oxacillin** 2.0 gm IV q4h IV	**Vanco** 1.0 gm IV q12h IV	MRI imaging is diagnostic procedure of choice. Standard rx is splenectomy + antibiotics. Burkholderia (Pseudomonas) pseudomallei is common cause of splenic abscess in SE Asia.
Contiguous from intra-abdominal site	Polymicrobic	*Treat as Peritonitis, secondary, page 31*		
Immunocompromised	Candida sp.	**Amphotericin B** (Dosage, see *Table 10, page 74*)	**Fluconazole**	
SYSTEMIC FEBRILE SYNDROMES				
Spread by infected **TICK, FLEA, or LICE** *(CID 29:888, 1999)*	Epidemiologic history crucial.	**Babesiosis, Lyme disease,**	**& granulocytic Ehrlichiosis** have same reservoir & tick vector *(CID 33:676, 2001).*	
Babesiosis: see *CID 32:1117, 1996*	Etiol: B. microti et al. Vector: Usually Ixodes ticks. Host: White-footed mouse & others	[(**Atovaquone** 750 mg po q12h) + **azithro** 600 mg po day 1, then 250 mg/d] x7 d. *(NEJM 343:1454, 2000)* OR [**clinda** 1.2 gm bid IV or 600 mg tid po x7 d. + **quinine** 650 mg tid po x7 d. **Ped. dosage:** Clinda 20–40 mg/kg/d and quinine 25 mg/kg/d		Exposure endemic areas May to Sept. Can result from blood transfusion *(JAMA 281: 927, 1999).* Usually subclinical. Illness likely in asplenic pts, pts with Lyme disease, older pts, pts with HIV. Dx: Giemsa-stained blood smear, antibody test available, PCR under study. Rx: Exchange transfusions successful adjunct, used early, in severe disease.
Bartonella				
Asymptomatic bacteremia	B. quintana	**Doxy** 100 mg po q12h x15 d]		Found in homeless, esp. if lice/leg pain *(NEJM 340:184, 1999; CID 35:684, 2002).*
Cat-scratch disease	B. henselae	Azithro (in symptomatic only—see *page 30*)		
Bacillary angiomatosis; Peliosis hepatis—pts with AIDS	B. henselae, B. quintana	(**Erythro** 500 mg qid po or **doxy** 100 mg bid po) x8 wks	(**Clarithro** 500 mg bid or **clarithro ER** 1.0 gm qd po or **azithro** 250 mg qd po or **CIP** 500–750 mg bid po) x8 wks	If severe, consider combination of doxy 100 mg po/IV bid + RIF 300 mg po bid *(IDC No Amer 12:137, 1998; Adv PID 11:1, 1996).*
Endocarditis *(see page 20)*	B. henselae, B. quintana	No definitive rx regimen Others have used **FQ** or **RIF** or **macrolide**	aminoglycoside + surgery macrolide ± surgery	Hard to detect with automated blood culture systems. Need lysis-centrifugation and/or blind subculture onto chocolate agar at 7 & 14 days. Diagnosis often by antibody titer ≥1:1600.
Trench fever	B. quintana	**Doxy** 100 mg bid po		
Ehrlichiosis: CDC def. of confirmed case as one of (1) 4x IFA antibody, (2) detection of Ehrlichia DNA by PCR, (3) visible morulae in WBC, and IFA ≥1:64 *(MMWR 46(RR-10):1–55, 1997)*				
Human monocytic ehrlichi- osis (HME) *(IUKCP 7:252, 1998)*	Ehrlichia chaffeensis (Lone Star tick is vector)	**Doxy** 100 mg bid po x7–14 d	**Tetracycline** 500 mg qid po x7–14 d. No current recom- mendation for children or pregnancy.	Exposure endemic areas May to Sept. Distribution: 30 states: mostly SE of line from NJ to IL to Missouri to Texas. History of outdoor activity and tick exposure. April–Sept. Fever, rash (36%), leukopenia and thrombocytopenia. Blood smears no help. PCR for early dx.
Human granulocytic ehrlichiosis (HGE) *(CID 31:554, 2000)*	Anaplasma (Ehrlichia) phagocytophilia/E. equi–like agent (Ixodes tick is vector)	**Doxy** 100 mg po or IV x7–14 d	**Tetracycline** 500 mg 4x/d po x7–14 d. Not in children or pregnancy.	Upper Midwest, NE, West Coast & Europe. H₂O tick exposure. April–Sept. Febrile flu- like illness after outdoor activity. No rash. Leukopenia/thrombocytopenia common. Dx: Up to 80% have positive blood smear. Antibody test for confirmation. Doxy successful in pregnancy *(CID 27:213, 1998).* Chloro, newer FQs active in vitro.

* In endemic area (New York), high % of both adult ticks and nymphs were jointly infected with both HGE and B. burgdorferi *(NEJM 337:49, 1997).*
(Footnotes and abbreviations on page 45)   NOTE: All dosage recommendations are for adults (unless otherwise indicated) and assume normal renal function

TABLE 1 (38')

ANATOMIC SITE/DIAGNOSIS/ MODIFYING CIRCUMSTANCES	ETIOLOGIES (usual)	SUGGESTED REGIMENS*		ADJUNCT DIAGNOSTIC OR THERAPEUTIC MEASURES AND COMMENTS
		PRIMARY	ALTERNATIVE§	
SYSTEMIC FEBRILE SYNDROMES: Spread by infected TICK, FLEA, or LICE/Ehrlichiosis *(continued)*				
Human/dog granulocytic ehrlichiosis *(NEJM 341:148 & 195, 1999)*	*Ehrlichia ewingii*	Doxy 100 mg bid po or IV x7-14 d		Previously only recognized in dogs; human cases now documented. Inclusion in granulocytes.
Lyme disease NOTE: Think about concomitant tick-borne disease—babesiosis *(JAMA 275:1657, 1996)* or ehrlichiosis				
Tick bite; possible bodies acquired in endemic area	*Borrelia burgdorferi* Urine antigen test reported unreliable *(JAMA 110:217 & 236, 2001)*	**If endemic area** and engorged deer tick: **doxy** 200 mg po x1 with food	**If not endemic area,** not engorged, no. deer tick. No treatment	Prophylaxis study in endemic area; erythema migrans developed in 3% of the control group and 0.4% doxy group *(NEJM 345:79 & 133, 2001).*
Early (erythema migrans) (See Comments)	Terminology ref.: *AnIM 136:413, 2002*	**Doxy** 100 mg bid po, or **amoxicillin** 500 mg tid po or **cefuroxime axetil** 500 mg bid po or **erythro** 250 mg qid. All regimens for 14–21 d		High rate of clinical failure with azithro & erythro *(Drugs 57:157, 1999)* **Peds** (all for 14–21 d.): Amox 50 mg/kg/d in 3 div. doses or cefuroxime axetil 30 mg/kg/d in 2 div. doses or erythro 30 mg/kg/d in 3 div. doses.
	Lyme Disease National Surveillance Case Definition available at either *NEJM or JAMA*		See Comment for peds doses	Lesions usually homogenous—not target-like *(AnIM 136:423, 2002).*
Carditis: See Comment		**Ceftriaxone** 2.0 gm qd IV or **cefotaxime** 2.0 gm q4h IV or **pen G** 24 mU qd IV) x14–21 d	**Doxy** (see Comments)100 mg bid po x14–21 d, or **amoxicillin** 500 mg tid po x14–21 d	First degree AV block: Oral regimen. High degree AV block: IV therapy—permanent pacemaker not necessary
Facial nerve paralysis (isolated finding, early)		(**Doxy** 100 mg bid po or **amoxicillin** 500 mg tid) x14–21 d		LP suggested to exclude neurologic disease. If LP neg., oral regimen OK. If abnormal or not done, suggest parenteral regimen
Meningitis, encephalitis. *For encephalopathy, see Comment*		**Ceftriaxone** 2.0 gm qd IV x14–28 d	**(Pen G** 20 mU qd in div. dose IV) or (**cefotaxime** 2.0 gm q8h IV) x14–28 d	Encephalopathy: memory difficulty, depression, somnolence or headache. CSF abnormalities. 89% had objective CSF abnormalities. 18/18 pts improved with ceftriaxone 2 gm/d x30 d. *(JID 180:377, 1999).*
Arthritis		**(Doxy** 100 mg bid po or **amoxicillin** 500 mg tid) po, both x30–60 d	**Ceftriaxone** 2 gm qd IV or **(cefotaxime** 2 gm q8h IV) x14–28 d	
Pregnant women		[Choice should not include doxy: **amoxicillin** 500 mg tid po x21 d]	**If pen. allergic: (azithro** 500 mg qd x7–10 d) or (**erythro** 500 mg qid po x14–21 d)	
Asymptomatic seropositivity and symptoms post-rx		None indicated		
Plague As biological weapon: *JAMA 283:2281, 2000, and Table 1B, page 46*	*Yersinia pestis* Reservoir: rat Vector: rat flea	**Gentamicin** 2.0 mg/kg IV loading dose then 1.7 mg/kg q8h IV or **streptomycin** 1.0 gm q12h IM or IV	**Doxy** 100 mg bid po or IV or (**chloro** 500 mg qid po or IV)	Reference IV: *streptomycin. CID 19:1150, 1994.* Septicemic form can occur with or without buboes. CDC reports 229 cases of plague in U.S. 1980–1994 *(MMWR 45(RR-14), 1996).* **CIP** effective in vitro + animal models *(JAC 41:301, 1998).* Plasmid-mediated resistance to aminoglycosides reported from Madagascar.
Relapsing fever *(CID 26:122, 1998).* Can be tick-borne or louse-borne	*Borrelia recurrentis* and other borrelia sp.	**Doxy** 100 mg bid po	**Erythro** 500 mg qid po	Jarisch-Herxheimer in most patients (occurs in ~2 hrs). Not prevented by prior steroids. **Dx: Examine peripheral blood smear during fever for spirochetes.**
Rickettsial diseases Spotted fevers (NOTE: Rickettsialpox not included) Rocky Mountain spotted fever (RMSF) *(CID 27:770, 1998).* NOTE: Can mimic ehrlichiosis. Pattern of rash important—see Comment	*R. rickettsii (Dermacentor ticks)*	**Doxy** 100 mg bid po or IV x7 d or for 2 days after temp. normal	**Chloro** 500 mg qid po x7 d, or for 2 days after temp. normal	Fever, rash (95%), petechiae 40–50%. Rash spreads from distal extremities to trunk. Dx: Immunohistology on skin biopsy; confirmation with antibody titers. Highest incidence in Mid-Atlantic states; also seen in Oklahoma, S. Dakota, Montana. NOTE: In early stages there are **no rash, no fever**, and **no tick exposure**; esp. in children many early deaths & empiric doxy reasonable *(MMWR 49: 888, 2000).*

(Footnotes and abbreviations on page 45)   NOTE: All dosage recommendations are for adults (unless otherwise indicated) and assume normal renal function

TABLE 1 (39)

ANATOMIC SITE/DIAGNOSIS/ MODIFYING CIRCUMSTANCES	ETIOLOGIES (usual)	SUGGESTED REGIMENS[§] PRIMARY	ALTERNATIVE[§]	ADJUNCT DIAGNOSTIC OR THERAPEUTIC MEASURES AND COMMENTS
SYSTEMIC FEBRILE SYNDROMES		**FLEA or LICE/Rickettsial diseases/Spotted fevers** (continued)		
Other spotted fevers, e.g.—6 species: R. conorii et al. Boutonneuse fever In sub-Saharan Africa, R. africae NEJM 344:1504, 2001	Spread by infected TICK.	**Doxy** 100 mg bid x7 d.	Cipro for RMSF Children <8 y.o. **azithro** or **clarithro** (see Comment)	Cipro 15 mg/kg/d in 2 div doses & azithro 10 mg/kg/d x1 for 3 days equally efficacious in children with Mediterranean spotted fever (CID 34:154, 2002).
Typhus group—Consider in returning travelers with fever Louse-borne		As for RMSF	As for RMSF	**Brill-Zinsser disease** (Ln 357:1198, 2001) is a relapse of remote past infection, e.g., WW II. Truncal rash spreads peripherally—opposite of RMSF. A winter disease.
Murine typhus (cat flea typhus, similar)	R. typhi (rat reservoir and flea vector)	As for RMSF	As for RMSF	Most U.S. cases south Texas and southern Calif. Flu-like illness. Rash in ~50%. Dx based on suspicion. Confirmed serologically.
Scrub typhus	O. tsutsugamushi (rodent reservoir, vector is larval stage of mites (chiggers)	As for RMSF. NOTE: Reports of doxy and chloro resistance from northern Thailand (Ln 348:86, 1996); **RIF** alone 450 mg bid x 7 d. reported effective (Ln 356:1057, 2000)		Limited to Far East (Asia, India). Cases imported into U.S. Evidence of chigger bite; flu-like illness. Rash like louse-borne typhus.
Tularemia, typhoidal type Ref: bioterrorism: see Table 1B, page 46, & JAMA 285:2763, 2001	Francisella tularensis. (Vector depends on geography, ticks, biting flies, mosquitoes identified)	**Gentamicin or tobra** 5 mg/kg/d div q8h IV x7–14 d.	Add **chloro** if evidence of meningitis. **CIP** reported effective in 12 children (PIDJ 19:449, 2000).	Typhoidal form in 5–30% pts. No lymphadenopathy. Diarrhea, pneumonia common. Dx: blood cultures. Antibody confirmation. A Jarisch-Herxheimer reaction may occur. Clinical failures with rx with P Ceph 3 (CID 17:976, 1993).
Trench fever (CID 10:131–?, 2000)	Bartonella quintana Vector: body louse	**Doxy** 100 mg bid x4–6 wks	**Azithro** 500 mg po qd x4–6 wks	For endocarditis, see page 20
Other Zoonotic Systemic Bacterial Febrile Illnesses: Obtain careful epidemiologic history				
Brucellosis—Reviews: CID 21:283, 1995; EID 3:213, 1997	Brucella sp.			
Adult or child >8 years	B. abortus—cattle B. suis—pigs B. melitensis—goats B. canis—dogs	[**Doxy** 100 mg bid po x6 wks + **gentamicin** x2–3 wks (see Table 10C, page 70)] or [**doxy** x6 wks + **streptomycin** 1 gm IM/d IM x2–3 wks] See Comment	[**Doxy** + **RIF** 600–900 mg qd po x6 wks] or [**TMP/SMX** 1 DS tab (160 mg TMP) po bid x6 wks + **gentamicin** x2 wks]	Doxy 100 mg bid po x6 wks + strep 1.0 gm qd IM x2 wks, relapse rate 6%. With doxy + RIF relapse rate 14%. Doxy + RIF may be less effective than doxy + SM in spondylitis (AnIM 119:25, 1992). CIP alone initially effective but relapse in 25% (AAC 34:150, 1992); however, oflox + RIF reported effective. Duration of rx unclear. For B. melitensis, gent for 7 d. + doxy for 45 d—fewer relapses than gent x7 d. + doxy for 30 d. (AAC 41:80, 1997). Usual recommendation is 6 wks of rx.
Child <8 years		**TMP/SMX** 5 mg/kg TMP po q12h po x4 wks + **gentamicin** 2 mg/kg q8h IV or IM x7–14 d.	**Doxy** 100 mg q12h IV or po x6 wks + **gentamicin** x2 wks	Longer rx for spondylitis—see CID 29:1440, 1999.
Leptospirosis (CID 21:1, 1995)	Leptospira—in urine of domestic livestock, dogs, small rodents	**Pen G** 20–24 mU qd IV div q4-6h	**Doxy** 100 mg q12h IV or po x7 d. or **AMP** 0.5–1.0 gm q6h IV	Illness varies. Two-stage mild anicteric illness to severe icteric disease (Weil's disease) with renal failure and myocarditis. Dx: Can culture first but slow and difficult. Sensitivity/specificity of rapid screening tests poor (J Clin Micro 40:1464, 2002).
Salmonella bacteremia (enteric fever most often caused by S. typhi)	Salmonella enteritidis—a variety of serotypes	**CIP** 400 mg q12h IV x14 d. or 750 mg/q12h IV bid (switch from IV to po when clinically possible)	**Ceftriaxone** 2.0 gm qd IV x7–14 d. (switch to po CIP when possible)	Usual exposure is contaminated poultry and eggs. Many others. Myriad of complications to consider, e.g., mycotic aneurysm (10% in adults over age 50. AJM 110:60, 2001), reactive arthritis, osteomyelitis, septic shock. Sporadic reports of resistance to CIP.
Miscellaneous Systemic Febrile Syndromes				
Kawasaki syndrome Unknown, syndrome of fever, lymphadenopathy, stomatitis, cervical adenitis, red hands/feet & coronary artery aneurysms (See Comment)		**IVIG** 2 gm/kg over 12 hrs PLUS **ASA** 80–100 mg/kg/d po div in 4 doses THEN **ASA** 3–5 mg/kg/d po 1x/d x6–8 wks	If still febrile after 1st dose of IVIG, give 2nd dose 2 gm/kg (PIDJ 17:1144, 1998)	IV gamma globulin (2.0 gm/kg over 10 hrs) in pts rx before 10th day of illness ↓ coronary artery aneurysms (NEJM 324:1633, 1991; CID 28:139, 1999). A current hypothesis: disease due to toxin production by staph or strep species (JID 179:1729, 1999; PIDJ 19:91, 2000). See Table 14B, page 112 for IVIG adverse effects and expense.

(Footnotes and abbreviations on page 45)   NOTE: All dosage recommendations are for adults (unless otherwise indicated) and assume normal renal function

TABLE 1 (40)

ANATOMIC SITE/DIAGNOSIS/ MODIFYING CIRCUMSTANCES	ETIOLOGIES (usual)	SUGGESTED REGIMENS* PRIMARY	ALTERNATIVE§	ADJUNCT DIAGNOSTIC OR THERAPEUTIC MEASURES AND COMMENTS
SYSTEMIC FEBRILE SYNDROMES/Miscellaneous Systemic Febrile Syndromes *(continued)*				
Rheumatic Fever, acute Ref: CID 33:806, 2001	Post–Group A strep, pharyngitis (not (Group B, C, or G).	(1) Symptom relief **ASA** 80–100 mg/kg/d in children; 4–8 gm/d in adults (2) Eradicate Group A strep: **Pen** x10 d. *(see Pharyngitis, page 32)* (3) Start prophylaxis: see below.		
Prophylaxis				
Primary prophylaxis	**Benzathine pen G** 1.2 mU IM *(see Pharyngitis)*	**Penicillin** for 10 days, prevents rheumatic fever even when started 7–9 days after onset of illness.		
Secondary prophylaxis (previous documented rheumatic fever)	**Benzathine pen G** 1.2 mU IM q3–4 wks		Alternative: **Penicillin V** 250 mg po bid or **sulfadiazine** (**sulfisoxazole**) 1.0 gm/d. po or **erythro** 250 mg po bid. Duration of 2° prophylaxis varies, with carditis continue 10 yrs or until age 25; without carditis continue 5 yrs or until age 18 (*AHA* 78:1082, *AJM* 78:401, 1993)	
Tumor necrosis factor (TNF) blockade for Crohn's disease, rheumatoid arthritis, or other	Drugs used: Etanercept (Enbrel), infliximab (Remicade)			Pts at increased risk of reactivation of latent tuberculosis	Suggest: TBc history, PPD ± chest x-ray prior to starting therapy.
Typhoidal syndrome (typhoid fever, enteric fever) (*JAMA* 278:847, 1997)	Salmonella typhi, S. paratyphi NOTE: 14% relapse rate with 5 d. of ceftriaxone (*AAC* 44:450, 2000)	**CIP** 500 mg bid po x10 d.) or (**ceftriaxone** 2.0 gm od IV x14 d.). If associated shock, give **dexamethasone** a few minutes before antibiotic. (*see Comment*)	**Azithro** 1 gm po day 1, then 500 mg po x6 d. (*AAC* 43:1441, 1999) or 1 gm po daily x5 d. (*AAC* 44:1855, 2000)	With shock or ↓ mental status, dexamethasone 3 mg/kg then 1 mg/kg q6h x8 doses ↓ mortality (*NEJM* 310:82, 1984). Look for other complications, e.g., osteo, septic arthritis, mycotic aneurysm (approx. 10% over age 50, *AJM* 110:62, 2001). Other rx options: Chloro 500 mg qid po or IV x14 d. or in children; cftox 15 mg/kg/d in 2 div. doses x2–3 d. (*AAC* 40:958, 1996) or ceftxime 10–15 mg/kg q12h po x8 d. (*JTP* 41:364, 1995). Sporadic reports of resistance to CIP.
Sepsis: Following assumes bacteremia is etiology, mimicked by viral, fungal, rickettsial infections and pancreatitis				
Neonatal—early onset —1 week old	Group B strep, E. coli, Klebsiella, enterobacter, Staph. aureus (uncommon), listeria	**AMP** 25 mg/kg q8h IV + **cefotaxime** 50 mg/kg q12h	**AMP + APAG** 2.5 mg/kg q12h IV or IM) or (**AMP + cefotaxime** 50 mg/kg q24h	Blood cultures are key but only 5–10% + Discontinue antibiotics after 72 hrs if cultures and course do not support diagnosis. In Spain, listeria predominates; in S. America, salmonella.
Neonatal—late onset 1–4 weeks old	As above + H. influenzae & S. epidermidis	**AMP** 25 mg/kg q6h IV + **cefotaxime** 50 mg/kg q8h) or (**AMP + ceftriaxone** 75 mg/kg q24h IV)	**AMP + APAG** 2.5 mg/kg q8h IV or IM	If Staph. aureus is common add nafcillin/oxacillin or vanco (if MRSA prevalence is high). Ref: PIDJ 16:768, 1997.
Child; not neutropenic	H. influenzae, Strep. pneumoniae, meningococci, Staph. aureus	**Cefotaxime** 50 mg/kg q6h IV or **ceftriaxone** 100 mg/kg q24h IV or **cefuroxime** 50 mg/kg q8h IV	**Nafcillin** or **oxacillin** + **cefotaxime** or **cefuroxime**	AM/SS and TC/CL not currently approved for children. In children who have received recommended course of conjugate Hib vaccine, invasive Hib disease has virtually disappeared, without an increase in other organisms (*PIDJ* 14:978, 1995; *EJCMID* 14:935, 1995). Meningococcemia mortality remains high (*Ln* 356:961, 2000).

(Footnotes and abbreviations on page 45)   *NOTE: All dosage recommendations are for adults (unless otherwise indicated) and assume normal renal function*

TABLE 1 (41)

ANATOMIC SITE/DIAGNOSIS/ MODIFYING CIRCUMSTANCES	ETIOLOGIES (usual)	SUGGESTED REGIMENS* PRIMARY	ALTERNATIVE§	ADJUNCT DIAGNOSTIC OR THERAPEUTIC MEASURES AND COMMENTS
SYSTEMIC FEBRILE SYNDROMES/Sepsis (continued)				
Adult, not neutropenic; Source unclear; life-threatening	Aerobic Gm-neg. bacilli, Gm-+ cocci; others	IMP or MER	APAG + one of: (P Ceph 3/4 or PIP/TZ or TC/CL). If suspect MRSA, add **vanco**. If suspect VRE, add **Q/D** or **linezolid**	Systemic inflammatory response syndrome (SIRS): 2 or more of the following: 1. Temperature >38°C or <36°C 2. Heart rate >90 beats/min. 3. Respiratory rate >20 breaths/min. 4. WBC >12,000/μL or <4000/μL or >10% bands. Sepsis: SIRS + a documented infection (+ culture). Severe sepsis: Sepsis + organ dysfunction hypotension or hypoperfusion abnormalities (lactic acidosis, oliguria, + mental status). Septic shock: Severe sepsis-induced hypotension (systolic BP <90 mmHg) not responsive to 500 ml IV fluid challenge + peripheral hypoperfusion (CCM 20:864, 1992; JAMA 273:117, 1995)
If asplenic	S. pneumo; H. influ; meningococci, Capnocytophaga (DF-2)	Cefotaxime or ceftriaxone (See Table 11B for prophylaxis)		
Suspect biliary source (see p. 10)	Enterococci + aerobic Gm-neg. bacilli	AM/SB, PIP/TZ or TC/CL	P Ceph 3 + metro	
Illicit use IV drugs	S. aureus	Nafcillin/oxacillin	Vanco	
Suspect intra-abdominal source	Mixture aerobic & anaerobic Gm-neg. bacilli [See secondary peritonitis, page 37]			
Suspect urinary source	Aerobic Gm-neg. bacilli & enterococci [See pyelonephritis, page 23]			
Neutropenic: Child or adult (absolute PMN count <500/mm³). Prophylaxis: **CID 34:730, 2002**				
Prophylaxis—afebrile				
Post-chemotherapy	Aerobic Gm-neg. bacilli, pneumocystis (PCP)	TMP/SMX-DS po bid—adults; 10 mg/kg/d div bid pd children	TMP/SMX or FQ works, not recommended 2° to ↑ bacterial resistance	TMP/SMX ↓ number of febrile episodes and prevents PCP. CIP also reported effective but no activity vs PCP. Problem is TMP/SMX- & FQ-resistant Gm-neg bacilli
Post-chemotherapy in children	↑ risk pneumocystis	TMP/SMX as above + (either acyclovir or ganciclovir) · fluconazole		Need TMP/SMX to prevent PCP. Hard to predict which leukemia/lymphoma/solid tumor pt at ↑ risk of PCP
Adult hematopoietic stem-cell transplant	↑ risk pneumocystis, herpes viruses, candida	TMP/SMX as above + (either acyclovir or ganciclovir) · fluconazole		Combined regimen justified by combined effect of neutropenia and immuno-suppression.
Empiric therapy—febrile (≥38.3°C x1 or ≥38°C for 2 hr)				
Low-risk adults (Def: low risk in Comment)	As above	CIP 750 mg po bid + AM/SB 875 mg bid		Treat as outpatients with 24/7 access to inpatient care if: no focal findings, no hypotension, no COPD, no dehydration, no fungal infection, age ~ <60 & >16. Neutropenic children with neg. blood cultures, safely switched to po cefixime 4 mg/kg q12h (CID 34:1469 & 1524, 2002; CID 31:1126, 2000; JAC 47:87, 2001).
High-risk adults and children	Aerobic Gm-neg. bacilli; ceph-resistant viridans strep, MRSA	**Monotherapy:** CFP or ceftaz or IMP or MER. Dosages: Footnote¹ and Table 10. Include empiric vanco if: suspect IV access infected; colonized with DRSP or MRSA blood culture pos for Gm-pos. cocci; pt hypotensive	**Combination therapy:** (Gent or tobra) + (TC/CL or PIP/TZ)	Increasing resistance of viridans streptococci to penicillins, cephalosporins & FQs. If severe IgE-mediated β-lactam allergy: No formal trials, but (APAG (or CIP) + aztreonam) ± vanco should work.
Persistent fever and neutropenia after 5 days of empiric antibacterial therapy—see CID 34:730, 2002	Candida species, aspergillus	Add either ampho B or voriconazole (NEJM 346:225, 2002)		

¹ **P Ceph 3** (cefotaxime 2.0 gm q8h IV; ceftizoxime 2.0 gm q8h IV; **ceftriaxone** 2.0 gm q24h IV; **ceftazidime** 3.0 gm q8h IV), **AP Pen** (piperacillin 3.0 gm q12h IV), **ticarcillin** 3.0 gm q4h IV, **TC/CL** 3.1 gm q4h IV, **PIP/TZ** 3.375 gm q4h IV, **AM/SB** 3.0 gm q6h IV, **APAG** (See Table 9C, page 71), **AMP** 3.0 gm q6h IV, **clinda** 900 mg q8h IV, **MER** 1.0 gm q8h IV, **IMP** 0.5 gm q6h IV, **Nafcillin** 1.0 gm q4h IV or **oxacillin** 2.0 gm q4h IV, **aztreonam** 2.0 gm q8h IV, **metro** 1.0 gm loading dose then 0.5 gm q6h IV, **vanco** 1.0 gm q12h IV, **P Ceph 3 AP** (ceftazidime 2.0 gm q8h IV), **P Ceph 4** CFP 2.0 gm q8h IV), **Q/D** = quinupristin/dalfopristin 7.5 mg/kg q8h IV, **linezolid** 600 mg q12h IV, neutropenic] IV, **cefpirome** 2.0 gm q12h IV, **CIP** 400 mg q12h IV, **ofloxa** 400 mg q12h IV, **levo** 500 mg qd, Q/D = quinupristin/dalfopristin 7.5 mg/kg q8h IV

² Not FDA-approved indication

NOTE: All dosage recommendations are for adults (unless otherwise indicated) and assume normal renal function

(Footnotes and abbreviations on page 45)

TABLE 1 (42)

ANATOMIC SITE/DIAGNOSIS/ MODIFYING CIRCUMSTANCES	ETIOLOGIES (usual)	SUGGESTED REGIMENS*		ADJUNCT DIAGNOSTIC OR THERAPEUTIC MEASURES AND COMMENTS
		PRIMARY	ALTERNATIVE†	
SYSTEMIC FEBRILE SYNDROMES (continued)				
Shock syndromes				
Septic shock	Bacteremia with aerobic Gm-neg. bacteria or Gm + cocci	**Proven therapy: (1)** Replete intravascular volume, **(2)** correct, if possible, disease that allowed bloodstream invasion; **(3)** appropriate empiric antimicrobial rx: see suggestions under life-threatening sepsis, above. **(4)** For recombinant activated **Protein C** (drotrecogin alfa) see Comment. **(5) Investigational but reasonable:** low-dose steroids if document relative adrenal insufficiency (see Comment for criteria). [Hydrocortisone 50 mg IV q8h + fludrocortisone (Florinef) 50 µg via NG once daily] x7 days. **(6)** Low-dose vasopressin reported effective for catecholamine-resistant septic shock (Ln 359:1209, 2002)		**Activ. Protein C. Drotrecogin (Xigris):** In a single prospective random double-blind study of 1690 pts. drotrecogin 24 µg/kg/hr x 96 hrs reduced mortality 6% from 31 to 25% in highly selected pts. shock with multi-organ failure, DIC, & low-risk of hemorrhage. **Major toxicity hemorrhage** (3.5% drotrecogin, 2% placebo) **Dose** 24 µg/kg/hr over 96 hrs by continuous IV infusion. Stop 2 hrs before & restart 12 hrs after surgery. Approx. **cost** of drug for 4-day course: $6800. **Low-dose steroids:** Based on one controlled random double-blind trial. Treat if ≤9 µg/dl response to 250 mg IV cosyntropin. 28-day mortality 63% placebo & 53% steroid group (JAMA 288:862 & 866, 2002).
Toxic shock syndrome, staphylococcal Colonization by toxin-producing Staph. aureus on: vagina (tampon-assoc.), surgical/traumatic wounds, & endometrial burns.	Staph. aureus (toxin-mediated)	**Nafcillin or oxacillin** 2.0 gm q4h IV	P Ceph 1 (**cefazolin** 1-2 gm q8h IV)	Nafcillin/oxacillin or cephalothin have no effect on initial syndrome, but ↓ recurrences. Seek occult abscess. TSS may occur with "clean" colonized post-op. wounds. Case fatality 5-15%. Consider eradication of carrier state (page 35). IVIG reasonable (see Streptococcal TSS)— dose 400 mg/kg (Curr Clin Top ID 16:1, 1996)
Toxic shock syndrome, streptococcal (Ref: JID 179[Suppl 2]:S366-374, 1999). NOTE: For necrotizing fasciitis without shock, see page 37.				
Associated with invasive disease, i.e., erysipelas, necrotizing fasciitis, secondary infection complicating (chicken-pox) (COID 7:423, 1994). Secondary cases TSS reported (NEJM 335:547 & 590, 1996; CID 27:150, 1998).	(Group A, B, C, & G Strep. pyogenes)	(**Pen G** 24 mU/d IV in div. doses) + (**clinda** 900 mg q8h IV) IVIG associated with ↑ 30-day survival in comparative study (CID 28:800, 1999); needs confirmation	**Erythro** 1.0 gm q6h IV or **clinda** 900 mg q8h IV [(**ceftriaxone** 2.0 gm q24h IV) + **clinda** 900 mg q8h IV] IVIG dose: 150 mg/kg/d x5 d.	Definition: Isolation of Group A strep., hypotension and ≥2 of: renal impairment, coagulopathy, liver involvement, ARDS, generalized rash, soft tissue necrosis (JAMA 269:390, 1993). Associated with invasive disease. **Surgery usually required.** Mortality with fasciitis 30-50%, myositis 80% even with early rx (CID 14:2, 1992). Clinda + toxin production ↓ use of NSAID may predispose to TSS. For discussion of possible reasons pen G may fail in fulminant S. pyogenes infections, see JID 167:1401, 1993.
Other Toxin-Mediated Syndromes—no fever unless complicated				
Botulinum (AnIM 129:221, 1998; CID 31:1018, 2000). As **biologic weapon:** JAMA 285:1069, 2001, and Table 1B, page 46)	C. botulinum	For all types. Follow vital capacity. If no ileus, purge GI tract	Trivalent (types A, B, E) equine serum antitoxin from State Health Dept. or CDC (see Comment)	**Equine antitoxin:** Obtain from State/Health Depts. or CDC (404-639-2206 M-F OR 404-639-2888 evenings/weekends). Skin test first & desensitize if necessary. One vial IV and one vial IM
Food-borne				**Antimicrobials:** May make infant botulism worse. Untested in wound botulism. When used, pen G 10-20 MU/d usual dose. Pen G possible if complications (pneumonia, UTI), avoid antimicrobials with assoc. neuromuscular blockade, i.e., aminoglycosides, tetracycline
Infant		Human botulism immunoglobulin (BIG) IV, single dose. Call 510-540-2646. Do not use equine antitoxin	No antibiotics; may lyse C. botulinum in gut and ↑ load of toxin	
Wound		Debridement & anaerobic cultures. Role of antibiotics untested.	Trivalent equine antitoxin (see Comment)	
Tetanus	C. tetani	**Pen G** 24 mU in div. dose or **doxy** 100 mg q12h IV	**Metro** 500 mg q6h or 1.0 gm q12h IV x7-10 d. (See Comment)	Primary rx is control of muscle spasms. Diazepam agent of choice. Morbidity less with metro than pen G (BMJ 291:648, 1985). Tetanus toxin and pen G both GABA antagonists (NEJM 332:812, 1995)

(Footnotes and abbreviations on page 45)   NOTE: All dosage recommendations are for adults (unless otherwise indicated) and assume normal renal function

(Footnotes and abbreviations on page 45)

TABLE 1 (43)

ANATOMIC SITE/DIAGNOSIS/ MODIFYING CIRCUMSTANCES	ETIOLOGIES (usual)	SUGGESTED REGIMENS*		ADJUNCT DIAGNOSTIC OR THERAPEUTIC MEASURES AND COMMENTS
		PRIMARY	ALTERNATIVE§	
VASCULAR Cavernous sinus thrombosis	Staph. aureus, Group A strep, H. influenzae, aspergillus/mucor/rhizopus	(Nafcillin or oxacillin 2.0 gm q4h IV) + P Ceph 3 **AP ceftazidime 2.0 gm IV** or **IMP** 0.5 gm q6h IV	Vanco for nafcillin/oxacillin 1.0 gm q12h IV or MER 1.0 gm q8h IV	CT or MRI scan for diagnosis. Heparin indicated (Ln 338:597, 1991). If patient diabetic with ketoacidosis or post-desferrioxamine rx or neutropenia, consider fungal: aspergillus, mucor, rhizopus, see Table 10A, pages 77 & 77. (General ref: Med 65:82, 1986)
IV line infection (see IDSA Guidelines: CID 32:1249, 2001) Heparin lock, midline catheter, non-tunneled central venous catheter (subclavian, internal jugular), peripherally inserted central catheter (PICC) Avoid femoral vein if possible. Risk of infection and thrombosis (JAMA 286:700, 2001)	Staph. epidermidis, Staph. aureus	Vanco 1.0 gm q12h IV. Comments re: rx and duration: (1) If S. aureus, remove catheter. Can use TEE result to determine if 2 or 4 wks of rx. (2) If S. epidermidis, can try to "save" catheter. 80% cure after 7–10 d. of rx. Catheter-hub/lumen: Infections may respond to "antibiotic lock" rx & allow salvage of catheter (JAC 48:597, 2001). Drug (vanco, gent, CIP) at 1–5 mg/ml mixed with 50–100 units heparin (or saline) in 2–5 ml volume, fill catheter when not in use. Continue 2 wks. For S. aureus, need full course of parenteral therapy.	Linezolid alternative—see Comments	Linezolid has predictable bacteriostatic activity vs most S. aureus and S. epidermidis. Authors prefer vanco in order of linezolid activity. If MRSA/MRSE and either failure of vanco rx or vanco allergy, linezolid 600 mg IV/po q12h. If MRSE or MRSA rate in hospital. Nafcillin/oxacillin for vanco. Culture removed catheter. With "roll" method, 15 colonies (NEJM 312:1142, 1985) suggests infection. Lines do not respond to "antibiotic lock" rx & changing when not infected. (When infected, do not insert new catheter over a wire. New antibiotic-coated catheters and other technologies may ↓ infection risk (EID 7:174, 2001; CID 34:1232, 2002). If S. epidermidis & catheter left in, vanco can cure 80% of infections limited to exit site but only 25% cure if infection in subcutaneous tunnel between skin and subclavian vein. If S. aureus & catheter left in, vanco cure rate 10% at exit site & 0% with tunnel infection (AJM 89:137, 1990). Similar statistics for infected "ports" (CID 29:1102, 1999). Infected hemodialysis access catheters should be removed (AnIM 127:275, 1997).
Tunnel type indwelling venous catheters and ports (Broviac, Hickman, Groshong, Quinton), dual lumen hemodialysis catheters (Perma-cath)	Staph. epidermidis, Staph. aureus, (Candida sp.). Rarely: leuconostoc or lactobacillus—both resistant to vanco (see Table 2)			
Impaired host (burn, neutropenic)	As above + Pseudomonas sp., Enterobacteriaceae, Corynebacterium jeikeium, aspergillus, rhizopus	(Vanco + P Ceph 3 AP) or (P Ceph 3 + APAG) (Dosage, see page 42)	(vanco + AP Pen) or IMP	Usually have associated septic thrombophlebitis. Biopsy of vein to rule out fungi. If fungal, surgical excision + amphotericin B. Surgical drainage, ligation or removal often indicated.
Hyperalimentation	As with tunnel + Candida sp. common (see Table 10, resistant Candida species)	If candida, amphotericin B 0.3–0.6 mg/kg qd IV, total dose 5.0 mg/kg or fluconazole 400 mg IV x7 d, then po for 14 d. after last positive blood culture		Remove venous catheter and discontinue antimicrobial agents if possible. Rx all patients with + blood cultures. Amphotericin B (many authorities have recommended 3 mg/kg total dose but less active than C. albicans than others reported) for those with hepatic abscesses. Ophthalmologic consultation recommended. Rx all patients with endophthalmitis; some would prefer to use 7 mg/kg total dose especially if patient is neutropenic. In a multicenter trial, fluconazole = amphoB (NEJM 331:1325, 1994).
Intravenous lipid emulsion	Staph. epidermidis, Malassezia furfur	Vanco 1.0 gm q12h IV. Amphotericin B		Discontinue intralipid (AJM 90:129, 1991
Septic pelvic vein thrombophlebitis with or without septic pulmonary (emboli) Postpartum or postabortion or postpelvic surgery	Streptococci, bacteroides, Enterobacteriaceae	Metro + P Ceph 3, cefoxitin CL, PIP/TZ or AM/SB	IMP or MER or ertapenem or (aztreonam or CIP) + [clinda + APAG]	Use heparin during antibiotic regimen. Continued oral anticoagulation not recommended. Clostridium perfringens less active than clinda vs non-fragilis bacteroides. Cefotetan and cefmetazole have methyltetrazole side-chain which is associated with hypoprothrombinemia (prevent with vitamin K).

(Footnotes and abbreviations on page 45) NOTE: All dosage recommendations are for adults (unless otherwise indicated) and assume normal renal function

TABLE 1 (44): FOOTNOTES AND ABBREVIATIONS

* **Dosages suggested are for adults** (unless otherwise indicated) with clinically severe (often life-threatening) infections. Dosages also assume normal renal function, and not severe hepatic dysfunction. See Table 1B, page 26, for pediatric dosages.

§ **Alternative therapy** includes these considerations: allergy, pharmacology/pharmacokinetics, compliance, costs, local resistance profiles.

AG = aminoglycoside
AHA = American Heart Association
AM/CL = amoxicillin (Augmentin); **AM/CL-ER** (Augmentin XR)
AM/SB = ampicillin/sulbactam (Unasyn)
AMP = ampicillin
APAG = antipseudomonal aminoglycosidic antibiotics
AP Pen = antipseudomonal β-lactamase susceptible penicillins, e.g. piperacillin. See Table 4, page 52 for details.
ARDS = adult respiratory distress syndrome
ARF = acute rheumatic fever
ASA = acetylsalicylic acid (aspirin)
Azithro = azithromycin
AztICP Ceftaz = ceftazidime
CFP = cefepime
Chloro = chloramphenicol
CIP = ciprofloxacin; **CIP-ER** = ciprofloxacin extended release
Clarithro = clarithromycin; **clarithro ER** = clarithromycin extended release
Clinda = clindamycin
C&S = culture and sensitivities
DIC = disseminated intravascular coagulation
Doxy = doxycycline
DRSP = drug-resistant Streptococcus pneumoniae
EBV = Epstein-Barr virus
EDC = expected date of confinement
EES = erythromycin ethyl succinate
ERTA = ertapenem
ETB = ethambutol
FQ = fluoroquinolone

GAS = Group A streptococcus
Gati = gatifloxacin
GC = gonorrhea (N. gonorrhoeae)
GNB = Gram-negative bacilli
HHV-2 = human herpesvirus 2
HIV-1 = human immunodeficiency virus type 1
HLGR = high-level gentamicin resistance
HLR = high-level resistance
I = investigational
IMP = imipenem cilastatin (Primaxin)
INH = isoniazid
IVDU = intravenous drug users
IVIG = intravenous immune globulin
LCM = lymphocytic choriomeningitis virus
LCR = ligase chain reaction
Levo = levofloxacin
LRTI = lower resp/ratory tract infection
Macrolides = erythro, azithro, clarithro, dirithro
MER = meropenem
Metro = metronidazole
Moxi = moxifloxacin
MOTT = mycobacteria other than M. tuberculosis
MQ = mefloquine
MRSA/MRSE = methicillin-resistant/methicillin-resistant Staph. aureus
MSSA/MSSE = methicillin-sensitive/methicillin-resistant Staph. epidermidis
MTb = Mycobacterium tuberculosis
NF = nitrofurantoin
NSAIDs = nonsteroidal anti-inflammatory drugs
NUS = not available in the United States

O Ceph 1, 2, 3 = oral cephalosporins—see Table 9B, page 65
Oflox = ofloxacin
P Ceph 1, 2, 3 = parenteral cephalosporins—see Table 9B.
P Ceph 3 AP = third generation with enhanced antipseudomonal activity
P Ceph 4 = third generation with antistaphylococcal and antipseudomonal activity
PCR = polymerase chain reaction
Pefox = pefloxacin
PIP/TZ = piperacillin/tazobactam
PVE = prosthetic valve endocarditis
Q/D = quinupristin/dalfopristin
Rick = rickettsia (spotted fever, Q fever)
RIF = rifampin
R/O = rule out
SA = Staph. aureus
Skin/SC = skin and related skin structures
SM = streptomycin
Spar = sparfloxacin
STD = sexually transmitted diseases
TBc = tuberculosis
TC/CL = ticarcillin/clavulanate (Timentin)
TEE = transesophageal echocardiography
Telithro = telithromycin
TMP/SMX = trimethoprim/sulfamethoxazole
Tobra = tobramycin
Toxo = toxoplasmosis
Trova = trovafloxacin
UTI = urinary tract infection
Vanco = vancomycin

ABBREVIATIONS OF JOURNAL AND TEXT TITLES

AAC Antimicrobial Agents & Chemotherapy
Adv PID Advances in Pediatric Infectious Diseases
Adv Par. Advances in Parasitology
AHJ American Heart Journal
AIDS AIDS
AJDC American Journal of Diseases of Children
AJG American Journal of Gastroenterology
AJM American Journal of Medicine
AJRCCM American Journal of Respiratory Critical Care Medicine
AJTMH American Journal of Tropical Medicine & Hygiene
AnEM Annals of Emergency Medicine
AnIM Annals of Internal Medicine
AnNY Annals of Internal Medicine
ArIM Archives of Internal Medicine
ARRD American Review of Respiratory Disease
CCM Critical Care Medicine
CID Clinical Infectious Diseases

COID Current Opinion in Infectious Disease
CTID Clinical Topics in Infectious Diseases
DMID Diagnostic Microbiology and Infectious Disease
EID Emerging Infectious Diseases
EJCMID European Journal of Clin. Micro. & Infectious Diseases
Gastro. Gastroenterology
ICHE Infection Control and Hospital Epidemiology
IDCNA Infectious Disease Clinics of North America
IDCP Infectious Diseases in Clinical Practice
J Clin Micro. Journal of Clinical Microbiology
J Ped. Journal of Pediatrics
JAC Journal of Antimicrobial Chemotherapy
JAMA Journal of the American Medical Association
JAVMA Journal of the Veterinary Medical Association
JID Journal of Infectious Diseases
JNS Journal of Neurosurgery

JTMH Journal of Tropical Medicine and Hygiene
JTP Journal of Tropical Pediatrics
Ln Lancet
Ln Inf Dis Lancet Infectious Disease
Med Lett Medical Letter
MMWR Morbidity & Mortality Weekly Report
NEJM New England Journal of Medicine
Peds Pediatrics
PIDJ Pediatric Infectious Disease Journal
QJM Quarterly Journal of Medicine
SGO Surgery, Gynecology and Obstetrics
SMJ Southern Medical Journal
TRSM Transactions of the Royal Society of Medicine
WJM Western Journal of Medicine

TABLE 1B: PROPHYLAXIS AND TREATMENT OF ORGANISMS OF POTENTIAL USE AS BIOLOGICAL WEAPONS

DISEASE	ETIOLOGY	SUGGESTED EMPIRIC TREATMENT REGIMENS		SPECIFIC THERAPY AND COMMENTS
		PRIMARY	**ALTERNATIVE**	
Anthrax **Cutaneous, inhalational, gastrointestinal** Refs: *JAMA* 281:1735, 1999; *MMWR* 50:909, 2001; *NEJM* 345:1621, 2001; *CID* 35:851, 2002 or www.bt.cdc.gov See Table 1, pages 28 & 34 To report bioterrorism event: 770-488-7100	*Bacillus anthracis* **Post-exposure prophylaxis** Ref: *Med Lett* 43:91, 2001 **Treatment—** **Cutaneous** anthrax *NEJM* 345:1611, 2007 **Treatment—** **Inhalational,** gastrointestinal, or oropharyngeal Refs: *JAMA* 286: 2549, 2554 & 2595, 2001; *NEJM* 345: 1607, 2001	**Adults (including pregnancy): Doxy** 100 mg po bid x60 d. **Children: CIP** 20–30 mg/kg/d div q12h x60 d. **Adults (including pregnancy): CIP** 500 mg po bid x60 d. **Children: CIP** 500 mg po bid x60 d. **Adults (including pregnancy): CIP** 400 mg IV q12h) + **RIF** 300 mg IV q8h or **clinda** 900 mg IV q8h. Switch to po when able & ↓ **CIP** to 500 mg po bid. Treat x60 days. See Table 2, page 48 for other alternatives.	**Adults (including pregnancy): Doxy** 100 mg po bid x60 d. **Children (see Comment): Doxy** >8 y/o & >45 kg: 100 mg po bid; >8 y/o & ≤45 kg: 2.2 mg/kg po bid; ≤8 y/o: 2.2 mg/kg po bid x60 d. **Adults (including pregnancy): Doxy** 100 mg po bid x60 d. **Children: Doxy** >8 y/o & >45 kg: 100 mg po bid; >8 y/o & ≤45 kg: 2.2 mg/kg po bid; ≤8 y/o: 2.2 mg/kg po bid. All for 60 days. **Children: (CIP** 10–15 mg/kg IV q12h or (**Doxy** >8 y/o & >45 kg: 100 mg IV q12h; >8 y/o & ≤45 kg: 2.2 mg/kg IV q12h; ≤8 y/o: 2.2 mg/kg IV q12h) **plus clindamycin** 7.5 mg/kg IV q6h **plus RIF** 20 mg/kg (max. 600 mg) IV qd. Treat x60 days. See Table 16, page 126 for oral dosage.	1. Once organism shows susceptibility to penicillin, switch children to amoxicillin 80 mg/kg/d (max. 500 mg q8h); switch pregnant pt to **amoxicillin** 500 mg po tid. 2. Do not use cephalosporins or TMP/SMX. 3. Other **FQs** (gati, levo, moxi) & clarithro should work but no clinical experience. 1. If penicillin-susceptible: **Adults: Amox** 500 mg q8h x60 d. **Children: Amox** 80 mg/kg/d div q8h (max. 500 mg q8h). 2. Usual treatment of cutaneous anthrax is 7–10 d; 60 d in setting of bioterrorism with presumed aerosol exposure. 1. Clinda may block toxin production. 2. Rifampin penetrates CSF & intracellular sites. 3. If statile shown penicillin-susceptible: a. **Adult: Pen G** 4 mU IV q4h b. **Child:** <12 y/o: 50,000 U/kg IV q6h; >12 y/o: 4 mU IV q4h Do not use pen or amp alone. 4. Do not use cephalosporins or TMP/SMX. 5. Erythro, azithro active borderline; clarithro active. 6. No person-to-person spread.
Botulism Refs: *JAMA* 285:1059, 2001 Food-borne See Table 1, page 28	*Clostridium botulinum*	Purge GI tract if no ileus. **Trivalent antitoxin** (types A, B, & E), single 10 ml vial/pt, diluted in saline IV (slowly)	Antibiotics have no effect on toxin	Supportive care for all types. Follow vital capacity. Submit suspect food for toxin testing.
Hemorrhagic fever viruses Ref: *JAMA* 287:2391, 2002	Ebola, Lassa, Hanta, yellow fever, & others	Fluid/electrolyte balance Optimize circulatory volume.	For Lassa & Hanta: **Ribavirin** dose same as Adults. Pregnancy, Children: LD 30 mg/kg (max. 2 gm) IV x1, then 16 mg/kg IV q6h (max. 1 gm/dose) x4 d., then 8 mg/kg IV (max. 500 mg) q8h x6 d	Ribavirin active in vitro, not FDA-approved for this indication. NOTE: Ribavirin contraindicated in pregnancy. However, in this setting, the benefits outweigh the risks.
Plague Ref: *JAMA* 283:2281, 2000 Inhalation pneumonic plague[1] See Table 1, page 39	*Yersinia pestis* **Treatment** **Post-exposure prophylaxis**	**Gentamicin** 5 mg/kg IV qd or **streptomycin** 15 mg/kg IV bid Tobramycin should work **Doxy** 100 mg po bid x7 d	(**Doxy** 200 mg IV x1, then 100 mg IV bid or (**CIP** 500 mg po bid x7 d (po q12h) **CIP** 500 mg po bid x7 d	1. **Chloro** also active: 25 mg/kg IV qid. 2. In mass casualty situation, may have to treat po. Pediatric doses: see Table 16, page 126. 3. Pregnancy: As for non-pregnant adults Isolate first 48 hrs. of treatment For community with pneumonic plague epidemic. Pediatric doses: see Table 16, page 126. Pregnancy: As for non-pregnant adults
Smallpox Ref: *NEJM* 346:1300, 2002 See Comment	*Variola* virus	Smallpox vaccine up to 4 days after exposure; isolation, gloves, gown; & NAS respirator	Cidofovir protected mice against aerosol cowpox (*JID* 181:10, 2000)	**Immunize:** DoD & State notifies CDC 770-488-7100). Vaccinia immune globulin of no benefit. For vaccination complications, see *JAMA* 288:1901, 2002.
Tularemia Inhalational tularemia[1] Ref: *JAMA* 285:2763, 2001 See Table 1, page 40	*Francisella tularensis* **Treatment** **Post-exposure prophylaxis**	(**Streptomycin** 15 mg/kg IV bid) or (**gentamicin** 5 mg/kg IV qd) x10 d. **Doxy** 100 mg po bid x14 d	**Doxy** 100 mg po bid x14–21 d. or **CIP** 400 mg IV (or 750 mg po) bid x14–21 d **CIP** 500 mg po bid x14 d.	For pediatric doses: see Table 16, page 126. Pregnancy: As for non-pregnant adults **Tobramycin** should work. For pediatric doses: see Table 16, page 126. Pregnancy: As for non-pregnant adults

[1] There are other clinical forms of botulism, plague, and tularemia, but the inhalation form seems most probable in bioterrorism.

TABLE 1C
TEMPORAL APPROACH TO DIFFERENTIAL DIAGNOSIS OF INFECTION AFTER ORGAN TRANSPLANTATION*

USUAL HOSPITAL-ACQUIRED INFECTIONS	OPPORTUNISTIC INFECTIONS	COMMUNITY-ACQUIRED OR CHRONIC INFECTIONS

VIRAL:
— HSV
— CMV
— CMV retinitis or colitis ‡
— EBV, VZV, Influenza, RSV, Adenovirus
— Onset of Hepatitis B or C
— Papillomavirus, PTLD[1] ‡

BACTERIAL:
— Pneumonia, IV line, UTI, Wound...
— Nocardia
— Listeria, Tuberculosis

FUNGAL:
— Pneumocystis
— Aspergillus
— Cryptococcus
— Coccidioidomycosis, Histoplasmosis ‡

PARASITIC
— Candida
— Leishmania
— Toxoplasma
— Strongyloides
— Trypanosoma cruzi

MONTHS AFTER TRANSPLANTATION

1 2 3 4 5 6

[1] PTLD = Post-transplant lymphoproliferative disease. * Adapted from Fishman and Rubin, *NEJM* 338:1741, 1998. For hematopoietic stem cell transplant recipients, see *MMWR* 49:RR-10, 2000. ‡ Solid lines indicate usual time period for onset of infection; dotted lines indicate risk at reduced level

BACTERIAL SPECIES	ANTIMICROBIAL AGENT (See footnote[2] for abbreviations)		
	RECOMMENDED	ALTERNATIVE	ALSO EFFECTIVE[1] (COMMENTS)
Alcaligenes xylosoxidans (Achromobacter xylosoxidans)	IMP, MER, AP Pen	TMP/SMX. Some strains susc. to ceftaz (AAC 32: 276, 1988)	Resistant to P Ceph 1, 2, 3, 4; aztreonam; FQ (AAC 40:772, 1996)
Acinetobacter calcoaceticus– baumannii complex	IMP or MER or [FQ + (amikacin or ceftaz)]	AM/SB (CID 24:932, 1997). Sulbactam[NUS] also effective (JAC 42: 793, 1998)	Up to 5% isolates resistant to IMP; resistance to FQ, amikacin increasing. Doxy + amikacin effective in animal model (JAC 45:493, 2000). (See Table 5, page 55)
Actinomyces israelii	AMP or Pen G	Doxy, ceftriaxone	Clindamycin, erythromycin
Aeromonas hydrophila	FQ	TMP/SMX or (P Ceph 3, 4)	APAG; erta; IMP; MER; tetracycline (some resistant to carbapenems)
Arcanobacterium (C.) haemolyticum	Erythromycin	Benzathine Pen G	Sensitive to most drugs, resistant to TMP/SMX (AAC 38:142, 1994)
Bacillus anthracis (anthrax): inhalation See Table 1B, page 46	CIP or doxy. For systemic infections, add 1 or 2 of: (RIF, clinda)	If Pen G susceptible: Pen G or amox	Also active: IMP, MER, vanco, chloramphenicol, clarithro. Resistant to expanded-spectrum cephalosporins (MMWR 50: 909, 2001; NEJM 345:1621, 2001; JAMA 287:2236, 2002).
Bacillus cereus, B. subtilis	Vancomycin, clindamycin	FQ, IMP	
Bacteroides fragilis (ssp. fragilis)	Metronidazole	Clindamycin	Cefoxitin, erta, IMP, MER, TC/CL, PIP/TZ, AM/SB, cefotetan, AM/CL, trovafloxacin
"DOT" group of bacteroides[3]			(not cefotetan)
Bartonella (Rochalimaea) henselae, quintana See Table 1, pages 30, 38	Erythro or doxy (bacillary angiomatosis) or azithro (cat-scratch)	Clarithro or CIP	Other drugs: TMP/SMX (IDC No. Amer 12:137, 1998). Consider doxy + RIF for severe bacillary angiomatosis (PIDJ 17:447, 1998) for severe bacillary angiomatosis (IDC No Amer 12:137, 1998)
Bordetella pertussis	Erythromycin	TMP/SMX	An erythro-resistant strain reported in Arizona (MMWR 43:807, 1994)
Borrelia burgdorferi, B. afzelii, B. garinii	Ceftriaxone, cefuroxime axetil, doxy, amox (See Comments)	Penicillin G (HD), cefotaxime	Clarithro. Choice depends on stage of disease, Table 1, page 39
Borrelia recurrentis	Doxy	Erythromycin	Penicillin G
Brucella sp.	Doxy + either gentamicin or streptomycin	(Doxy + RIF) or (TMP/SMX + gentamicin)	FQ + RIF (AAC 41:80, 1997; Emerg ID 3:213, 1997; CID 21:283, 1995)
Burkholderia (Pseudomonas) cepacia	TMP/SMX or MER or CIP	Minocycline or chloramphenicol	(Usually resistant to APAG, IMP) (AAC 37: 123, 1993 & 43:213, 1999) (Some resistant to carbapenems). Combination rx may be necessary (AJRCCM 161:1206, 2000).
Burkholderia (Pseudomonas) pseudomallei	Ceftaz (continuous IV) (AAC 39: 2356, 1995) or AM/CL	TMP/SMX, IMP (CID 29: 381, 1999), chloramphenicol	(In Thailand, 12–80% strains resistant to TMP/SMX). FQ active in vitro. Combination of chloro, TMP/SMX, doxy more effective than doxy alone for maintenance rx (CID 29:375, 1999). Combinations of ceftazidime or cefoperazone/ sulbactam[NUS] + TMP/SMX have also been reported effective in Thailand, but no comparison with monotherapy (CID 33:29, 2001).
Campylobacter jejuni	Erythromycin	FQ († resistance, NEJM 340:1525,1999)	Clindamycin, doxy, azithro, clarithro (see Table 5, page 55)
Campylobacter fetus	IMP	Gentamicin	AMP, chloramphenicol, erythromycin
Capnocytophaga ochracea (DF-1) and canimorsus (DF-2)	Clindamycin or AM/CL	CIP, Pen G	P Ceph 3, IMP, cefoxitin, FQ, (resistant to APAG, TMP/SMX)
	AM/CL		
Chlamydia pneumoniae	Doxy	Erythromycin, FQ	Azithro, clarithro, telithro
Chlamydia trachomatis	Doxy or azithro	Erythromycin or ofloxa	Levofloxacin
Chryseobacterium (Flavobacterium) meningosepticum	Vancomycin ± RIF (CID 26:1169, 1998)	CIP, levofloxacin	In vitro susceptibilities may not correlate with clinical efficacy (AAC 41: 1301, 1997; CID 26:1169, 1998)
Citrobacter diversus (koseri), C. freundii	CARB	FQ	APAG
Clostridium difficile	Metronidazole (po)	Vancomycin (po)	Bacitracin (po)
Clostridium perfringens	Pen G ± clindamycin	Doxy	Erythromycin, chloramphenicol, cefazolin, cefoxitin, AP Pen, CARB
Clostridium tetani	Metronidazole or Pen G	[Doxy	CARB
Corynebacterium jeikeium	Vancomycin	Pen G + APAG	
C. diphtheriae	Erythromycin	Clindamycin	RIF. Penicillin reported effective (CID 27:845, 1998)
Coxiella burnetii (Q fever) acute disease	Doxy	Erythromycin	In meningitis consider FQ (CID 20:489, 1995)
chronic disease	(CIP or doxy) + RIF	FQ + doxy x3 yrs (CID 20:489,1995)	Chloroquine + doxy (AAC 37:1773, 1993). ? gamma interferon (Ln 20:546, 2001)
Ehrlichia chaffeensis, Ehrlichia ewingii, Anaplasma (Ehrlichia) phagocytophila	Doxy	Tetracycline, RIF (CID 27:213, 1998)	CIP, ofloxa, chloramphenicol also active in vitro. Resistant to clinda, TMP/SMX, IMP, AMP, erytho, & azithro (AAC 41: 76, 1997).

TABLE 2 (2)   49

BACTERIAL SPECIES	ANTIMICROBIAL AGENT (See footnote[2] for abbreviations)		
	RECOMMENDED	ALTERNATIVE	ALSO EFFECTIVE[1] (COMMENTS)
Eikenella corrodens	Penicillin G or AMP or AM/CL	TMP/SMX, FQ	Doxy, cefoxitin, cefotaxime, IMP (Resistant to clindamycin, cephalexin, erythromycin, and metronidazole)
Enterobacter spp. (aerogenes, cloacae)	CARB or (AP Pen + APAG)	TC/CL or PIP/TZ or CIP	P Ceph 4. As many as 40% strains from ICUs may be ceftaz-resistant
Enterococcus faecalis	Penicillin G or AMP	Vancomycin	Linezolid. For UTI, nitrofurantoin, fosfomycin effective. High-level gentamicin, vancomycin resistance increasing (see footnote p. 19). (See Table 5, p. 55)
	Add gentamicin for endocarditis or meningitis		
Enterococcus faecium, β-lactamase +, high-level aminoglycoside resist., vancomycin resist.	No regimen of proven efficacy. Consultation recommended if pt has endocarditis or other life-threatening infection. (See Endocarditis, Table 1, page 19, & Table 5, page 55)		See discussion, page 19, page 67, and Table 5, page 55; quinu/dalfo, linezolid
Erysipelothrix rhusiopathiae	Penicillin G or AMP	P Ceph 3, FQ	IMP, AP Pen (vancomycin, APAG, TMP/SMX resistant)
Escherichia coli	Sensitive to BL/BLI, cephalosporins, FQ, TMP/SMX, APAG, nitrofurantoin, CARB. Selection of drug depends on site of infection, i.e., UTI multiple po agents; meningitis P Ceph 3 or MER. See Table 1 for infections due to E. coli 0157:H7 & related strains.		
Francisella tularensis (tularemia) See Table 1B, page 46	Gentamicin, tobramycin, or streptomycin	Doxy or CIP	Chloramphenicol, RIF. Doxy/chloro bacteriostatic → relapses.
Gardnerella vaginalis (bacterial vaginosis)	Metronidazole	Clindamycin	See Table 1, page 17 for dosage
Hafnia alvei	Same as Enterobacter spp.		
Helicobacter pylori	See Table 1, page 13		Drugs effective in vitro often fail in vivo.
Hemophilus aphrophilus	[(Penicillin or AMP) + gentamicin] or [AM/SB + gentamicin]	P Ceph 2, 3 ± gentamicin	(Resistant to vancomycin, clindamycin, methicillin)
Hemophilus ducreyi (chancroid)	Azithro or ceftriaxone	Erythromycin, CIP	Most strains resistant to tetracycline, amox, TMP/SMX
Hemophilus influenzae Meningitis, epiglottitis & other life-threatening illness	Cefotaxime, ceftriaxone	TMP/SMX, FQs (AMP if β-lactamase negative) (U.S. 25–30% AMP resistance, Japan 35%)	Chloramphenicol (downgraded from 1st choice because of hematotoxicity). 9% of U.S. strains resistant to TMP/SMX (AAC 41:292, 1997)
non-life threatening illness	AM/CL, O Ceph 2/3, TMP/SMX, AM/SB		Azithro, clarithro, telithro
Klebsiella pneumoniae, Klebsiella oxytoca	P Ceph 3, FQ	APAG, TC/CL, AM/SB, PIP/TZ	AP Pen, CARB, aztreonam. Outbreaks of ceftaz-resistance reported (AnIM 119:353, 1993) (See Table 4, page 53)
Klebsiella ozaenae/rhinoscleromatis	FQ	RIF + TMP/SMX	(Lancet 342:122, 1993)
Lactobacillus sp.	(Pen G or AMP) ± gentamicin	Clindamycin, erythromycin	**May be resistant to vancomycin**
Legionella sp. (42 species & 60 serotypes recognized) (Sem Resp Inf 13:90, 1998)	FQ, or azithro, or (erythromycin ± RIF)	Clarithro, telithro	TMP/SMX, doxy. Most active FQs in vitro: gemi, gati, levo, moxi. See AnIM 129:328, 1998
Leptospira interrogans	Penicillin G	Doxy	
Leuconostoc	Pen G or AMP	Clindamycin, erythromycin, minocycline	APAG **NOTE: Resistant to vancomycin**
Listeria monocytogenes	AMP	TMP/SMX	Erythromycin, penicillin G (high dose), APAG may be synergistic with β-lactams. **Cephalosporin-resistant!**
Moraxella (Branhamella) catarrhalis	AM/CL or O Ceph 2/3, TMP/SMX	Azithro, clarithro, dirithromycin, telithro	Erythromycin, doxy, FQs
Morganella sp.	CARB or P Ceph 3 or 4 or FQ	Aztreonam, BL/BLI	APAG
Mycoplasma pneumoniae	Erythro, azithro, clarithro, dirithro, or FQ	Doxy	(Clindamycin and β lactams NOT effective)
Neisseria gonorrhoeae (gonococcus)	Ceftriaxone, cefixime, cefpodoxime	Ofloxacin & other FQs (Table 1, page 15), spectinomycin	Kanamycin (used in Asia). FQ resistance in Asia, rare in U.S. (MMWR 47:405, 1998)
Neisseria meningitidis (meningococcus)	Penicillin G	Ceftriaxone, cefuroxime, cefotaxime	Sulfonamide (some strains), chloramphenicol. Chloro-resistant strains found in SE Asia (NEJM 339:868, 1998) (Prophylaxis: page 5)
Nocardia asteroides	TMP/SMX, sulfonamides (high dose)	Minocycline	Amikacin + (IMP or ceftriaxone or cefuroxime) for brain abscess
Nocardia brasiliensis	TMP/SMX, sulfonamides (high dose)	AM/CL	Amikacin + ceftriaxone
Pasteurella multocida	Pen G, amox	Doxy, AM/CL, P Ceph 2, TMP/SMX	Ceftriaxone, cefpodoxime, FQ (active in vitro), azithro (active in vitro) (DMID 30:99, 1998; AAC 43:1475, 1999)
Plesiomonas shigelloides	CIP	TMP/SMX	AM/CL, P Ceph 1,2,3,4, IMP, MER, tetracycline, aztreonam
Proteus mirabilis (indole–)	AMP	TMP/SMX	Most agents except nafcillin/oxacillin. β-lactamase (including ESBL) production now being described in P. mirabilis (JCM 40:1549, 2002)
vulgaris (indole +)	P Ceph 3 or FQ	APAG	CARB, aztreonam, BL/BLI

BACTERIAL SPECIES	ANTIMICROBIAL AGENT (See footnote[2] for abbreviations)		
	RECOMMENDED	ALTERNATIVE	ALSO EFFECTIVE[1] (COMMENTS)
Providencia sp.	Amikacin or P Ceph 3 or FQ	TMP/SMX	AP Pen + amikacin, IMP
Pseudomonas aeruginosa	AP Pen, AP Ceph 3, IMP, MER, tobramycin, CIP, aztreonam. For serious inf., use AP β-lactam + tobramycin or CIP	For UTI, single drugs usually effective: AP Pen, AP Ceph 3, cefepime, IMP, MER, APAG, CIP, aztreonam	Resistance to ß-lactams (IMP, ceftaz) may emerge during rx. β-lactam inhibitor adds nothing to activity of TC or PIP against P. aeruginosa. Clavulanic acid has been shown to antagonize TC in vitro (AAC 43:882, 1999). (See also Table 5)
Rhodococcus (C. equi)	IMP, APAG, erythromycin, vancomycin, or RIF (consider 2 agents)	CIP (variable) [resistant strains SE Asia (CID 27: 370, 1998)], TMP/SMX, tetracycline, or clindamycin	Vancomycin active in vitro but intracellular location of R. equi may impair efficacy (Sem Resp Inf 12:57, 1997; CID 34:1379, 2002)
Rickettsiae species	Doxy	Chloramphenicol	FQ
Salmonella typhi	FQ, ceftriaxone	Chloramphenicol, amox, TMP/SMX, azithro (for uncomplicated disease: AAC 43: 1441, 1999)	Multi drug resistant strains (chloramphenicol, AMP, TMP/SMX) common in many developing countries, seen in immigrants
Serratia marcescens	P Ceph 3, erta, IMP, MER, FQ	Aztreonam, gentamicin	TC/CL, PIP/TZ
Shigella sp.	FQ or azithro	TMP/SMX and AMP (resistance common in Middle East, Latin America). Azithro ref.: AnIM 126:697, 1997	
Staph. aureus, methicillin-susceptible	Oxacillin/nafcillin	P Ceph 1, vancomycin, clindamycin	Erta, IMP, MER, BL/BLI, FQ, erythromycin, clarithro, dirithromycin, azithro, quinu/dalfo, linezolid
Staph. aureus, methicillin-resistant	Vancomycin	Teicoplanin[NUS], TMP/SMX (some strains resistant), quinu/dalfo, linezolid, daptomycin	Fusidic acid[NUS], >60% CIP-resistant in U.S. (Fosfomycin + RIF), novobiocin. Partially vancomycin-resistant strains isolated (MMWR 27:624, 1997).
Staph. epidermidis	Vancomycin ± RIF	RIF + (TMP/SMX or FQ)	Cephalothin or nafcillin/oxacillin if sensitive to nafcillin/oxacillin but 75% are resistant. FQs. (See Table 5)
Staph. haemolyticus	TMP/SMX, FQ, nitrofurantoin	Oral cephalosporin	Recommendations apply to UTI only.
Stenotrophomonas (Xanthomonas, Pseudomonas) maltophilia	TMP/SMX	TC/CL or (aztreonam + TC/CL) (AAC 41:2612, 1997)	Minocycline, doxy, ceftaz. [In vitro synergy (TC/CL + TMP/SMX) and (TC/CL + CIP), AAC 39:2220, 1995; CMR 11:57, 1998]
Streptobacillus moniliformis	Penicillin G or doxy	Erythro, clindamycin	
Streptococcus, anaerobic (Peptostreptococcus)	Penicillin G	Clindamycin	Erythromycin, doxy, vancomycin
Streptococcus pneumoniae penicillin-susceptible penicillin-resistant (MIC ≥2.0)	Penicillin G (Vancomycin ± RIF) or (gati, levo, or moxi) See footnote page 4 and Table 5, page 55	Multiple agents effective, e.g., amox	See footnote, page 4 For non-meningeal infections: P Ceph 3/4, CARB, quinu/dalfo, linezolid
Streptococcus pyogenes, Groups A, B, C, G, F. Strep. milleri (constellatus, intermedius, anginosus)	Penicillin G or V (some add gentamicin for serious Group B strep infections)	All ß lactams, erythromycin, azithro, dirithromycin, clarithro, telithro	In France, Finland & Japan: resistance to macrolides up to over 50%, but ↓ in Japan to <1% (Arch Ped 148:67, 1994).
Vibrio cholerae	Doxy, FQ	TMP/SMX	Strain 0139 is resistant to TMP/SMX
Vibrio parahemolyticus	Antibiotic rx does not ↓ course		Sensitive in vitro to FQ, doxy
Vibrio vulnificus, alginolyticus, damsela	Doxy + ceftaz	Cefotaxime, FQ (e.g., levo, AAC 46;3580, 2002)	APAG often used in combination with ceftaz
Yersinia enterocolitica	TMP/SMX or FQ	P Ceph 3 or APAG	CID 19:655, 1994
Yersinia pestis (plague) See Table 1B, page 46	Streptomycin, gentamicin, or tobramycin	Chloramphenicol, doxy, or CIP	Susceptible to FQ, cefixime, ceftriaxone, TMP/SMX in vitro (AAC 44: 1995, 2000)

[1] These agents are more variable in effectiveness than the "Recommended" or "Alternative". Selection of "Alternative" or "Also Effective" agents is based on in vitro susceptibility testing, pharmacokinetics, host factors such as auditory, renal, hepatic function, and cost.

[2] **AM/CL:** amoxicillin clavulanate; **Amox:** amoxicillin; **AMP:** ampicillin; **AM/SB:** ampicillin sulbactam; **APAG:** antipseudomonal aminoglycosides; **AP Pen:** antipseudomonal penicillin (see page 53); **Azithro:** azithromycin; **BL/BLI:** ß-lactam/ß-lactamase inhibitor (AM/CL, TC/CL, AM/SB, or PIP/TZ); **CARB:** carbapenems (ertapenem, imipenem, or meropenem); **Ceftaz:** ceftazidime; **CIP:** ciprofloxacin; **Clarithro:** clarithromycin; **DORI group:** B. distastonis, B. ovatus B. thetaiotaomicron; **Doxy:** doxycycline; **Erta:** ertapenem; **FQ:** fluoroquinolones (ciprofloxacin, ofloxacin, lomefloxacin, enoxacin, pefloxacin, levofloxacin); **IMP:** imipenem + cilastatin; **MER:** meropenem; **NUS:** not available in the U.S.; **P Ceph:** parenteral cephalosporins; **PIP/TZ:** piperacillin/tazobactam; **Quinu/dalfo:** quinupristin/dalfopristin; **RIF:** rifampin; **TC/CL:** ticarcillin clavulanate; **Telithro:** telithromycin; **TMP/SMX:** trimethoprim/sulfamethoxazole

CLINICAL SITUATION		DURATION OF THERAPY
SITE	**CLINICAL DIAGNOSIS**	**(Days)**
Bacteremia	Bacteremia with removable focus (no endocarditis)	10–14 (Clin Inf Dis 14:75, 1992) (See Table 1)
Bone	Osteomyelitis, adult; acute	42
	adult; chronic	Until ESR[6] normal (often > 3 months)
	child; acute; staph. and enterobacteriaceae[3]	21
	child; acute; strep., meningococci, hemophilus[3]	14
Ear	Otitis media with effusion	10 (or 1 dose ceftriaxone)
	Recent metanalysis suggests 5 days of "short-acting" antibiotics effective for uncomplicated otitis media (JAMA 279:1736, 1998).	
Endocardium	Infective endocarditis, native valve	
	Viridans strep	14 or 28 (See Table 1, page 19)
	Enterococci	28 or 42 (See Table 1, page 19)
	Staph. aureus	14 (R-sided only) or 28 (See Table 1, page 19)
Gastrointestinal Also see Table 1	Bacillary dysentery (shigellosis)/traveller's diarrhea	3
	Typhoid fever (S. typhi): Ceftriaxone	14[*]
	FQ[6]	5–7
	Chloramphenicol	14
		*[Short courses less effective (AAC 44:450, 2000)]
	Helicobacter pylori	10–14
	Pseudomembranous enterocolitis (C. difficile)	10
Genital	Non-gonococcal urethritis or mucopurulent cervicitis	7 days doxy[6] or single dose azithro[6]
	Pelvic inflammatory disease	14
Heart	Pericarditis (purulent)	28
Joint	Septic arthritis (non-gonococcal) Adult	14–28 (Ln 351:197, 1998)
	Infant/child	Rx as osteomyelitis above
	Gonococcal arthritis/disseminated GC infection	7 (See Table 1, page 15)
Kidney	Cystitis (bladder bacteriuria)	3
	Pyelonephritis	14 (7 days if CIP used)
	Recurrent (failure after 14 days rx)	42
Lung	Pneumonia, pneumococcal	Until afebrile 3–5 days (minimum 5 days)
	Pneumonia, enterobacteriaceae or pseudomonal	21, often up to 42
	Pneumonia, staphylococcal	21–28
	Pneumocystis carinii, in AIDS;	21
	other immunocompromised	14
	Legionella, mycoplasma, chlamydia	14–21
	Lung abscess	Usually 28–42[4]
Meninges[5]	N. meningitidis	5–7 (IDCP 7:370, 1998)
	H. influenzae	7
	S. pneumoniae	10–14
	Listeria meningoencephalitis, gp B strep, coliforms	14–21 (longer in immunocompromised)
Multiple systems	Brucellosis (See Table 1, page 40)	42 (add SM[6] or GM[6] for 1st 7–14 days)
	Tularemia (See Table 1, pages 29, 30, 40)	7–14
Muscle	Gas gangrene (clostridial)	10
Pharynx Also see Pharyngitis, Table 1, page 32	Group A strep pharyngitis	10 (O Ceph 2/3, azithromycin effective at 5 d.) (JAC 45, Topic T1 23, 2000)
	Diphtheria (membranous)	7–14
	Carrier	7
Prostate	Chronic prostatitis (TMP/SMX)[6]	30–90
	(FQ)	28–42
Sinuses	Acute sinusitis	10–14[7]
Skin	Cellulitis	Until 3 d. after acute inflammation disappears
Systemic	Lyme disease	See Table 1, page 39
	Rocky Mountain spotted fever (See Table 1, page 39)	Until afebrile 2 days

[1] It has been shown that early change from parenteral to oral regimens (about 72 hours) is cost-effective with many infections, i.e., intra-abdominal (AJM 91:462, 1991)

[2] The recommended duration is a minimum or average time and should not be construed as absolute

[3] These times are with proviso: sx & signs resolve within 7 days and ESR[6] is normalized (J.D. Nelson, APID 6:59, 1991)

[4] After patient afebrile 4-5 days, change to oral therapy

[5] In children relapses seldom occur until 3 days or more after termination of rx. Practice of observing in hospital for 1 or 2 days after rx is expensive and non-productive. For meningitis in children, see Table 1, page 4.

[6] **Azithro** = azithromycin; **CIP** = ciprofloxacin; **Doxy** = doxycycline; **ESR** = erythrocyte sedimentation rate; **FQ** = fluoroquinolones; **GM** = gentamicin; **rx** = treatment; **SM** = streptomycin; **TMP/SMX** = trimethoprim/sulfamethoxazole

[7] If pt not sx-free at 10 d., sinus puncture and/or rx for 7 more days (NEJM 326:319, 1992). One study reports 3 days of TMP/SMX effective (JAMA 273:1015, 1995).

TABLE 4
COMPARISON OF ANTIMICROBIAL SPECTRA*

(These are generalizations; there are major differences between countries, areas and hospitals depending upon antibiotic usage patterns—verify for individual location. See Table 5 for resistant bacteria)

Column groups: **PENICILLINS, CARBAPENEMS, AZTREONAM, FLUOROQUINOLONES** — Penicillins (Penicillin G, Penicillin V); Anti-staphylococcal Penicillins (Methicillin, Nafcillin/Oxacillin, Cloxacillin/Dicloxacillin); Amino-Penicillins (Amp/Amox, Amox/Clav, Amp/Sulb); Anti-Pseudomonal Penicillins (Ticarcillin, Ticar/Clav, Pip/Tazo, Mezlocillin, Piperacillin); Carbapenems (Ertapenem, Imipenem, Meropenem); Aztreonam; Fluoroquinolones (Ciprofloxacin, Ofloxacin, Lomefloxacin, Pefloxacin, Levofloxacin, Trovafloxacin, Moxifloxacin, Gatifloxacin)

Organisms	Pen G	Pen V	Meth	Naf/Oxa	Clox/Diclox	Amp/Amox	Amox/Clav	Amp/Sulb	Ticar	Ticar/Clav	Pip/Tazo	Mezlo	Piper	Erta	Imi	Mero	Aztreonam	Cipro	Oflox	Lome	Peflox	Levo	Trova	Moxi	Gati
GRAM-POSITIVE:																									
Strep, Group A,B,C,G	+	+	+	+	+	+	+	+	+	+	+	+	+	+	+	+	0	±	±			+	+	+	+
Strep. pneumoniae	+	+	+	+	+	+	+	+	+	+	+	+	+	+	+	+	0	±	±	0	0	+	+	+	+
Viridans strep	±	±	±	±	±	±	±	±	±	±	±	±	±	+	+	+	0	0	0			+	+	+	+
Strep. milleri	+	+	±	+	+	+	+	+	+	+	+	+	+	+	+	+	0	0	0			+	+	+	+
Enterococcus faecalis	+	+	0	0	0	+	+	+	±	±	±	±	±	±	+	0	0	**	**			0	+	+	+
Enterococcus faecium	±	±	0	0	0	+	+	+	±	±	±	±	±	±	0	0	0	0	0			0	0	±	±
Staph. aureus (MSSA)	0	0	+	+	+	0	+	+	0	+	0	0	0	+	+	+	0	+	+			+	+	+	+
Staph. aureus (MRSA)	0	0	0	0	0	0	0	0	0	0	0	0	0	0	0	0	0	0	0	0	0	0	±	±	±
Staph. epidermidis	0	0	±	±	±	0	±	±	±	±	±	±	±	+	+	0	0	±	±			+	+	+	+
C. jeikeium	0	0	0	0	0	0	0	0	0	0	0	0	0	0	0	0	0	0	0			+			
L. monocytogenes	+	0	0	0	0	+	+	+	±	±	±	±	±	+	+	+	0	±	+			+	+		
GRAM-NEGATIVE:																									
N. gonorrhoeae	0	0	0	0	0	±	+	+	±	+	+	+	+	+	+	+	+	+	+	+	+	+	+	+	+
N. meningitidis	+	0	0	0	0	+	+	+	+	+	+	+	+	+	+	+	+	+	+	+	+	+	+	+	+
M. catarrhalis	0	0	0	0	0	±	+	+	0	+	+	±	±	+	+	+	±	+	+	+	+	+	+	+	+
H. influenzae	0	0	0	0	0	±	+	±	±	+	+	±	±	+	+	+	+	+	+	+	+	+	+	+	+
E. coli	0	0	0	0	0	±	+	+	±	+	+	+	+	+	+	+	+	+	+	+	+	+	+	+	+
Klebsiella sp.	0	0	0	0	0	0	+	+	0	+	+	±	±	+	+	+	+	+	+	+	+	+	+	+	+
Enterobacter sp.	0	0	0	0	0	0	0	0	0	0	+	+	+	+	+	+	+	+	+	+	+	+	+	+	+
Serratia sp.	0	0	0	0	0	0	0	0	0	0	+	+	0	+	+	+	+	+	+	+	+	+	+	+	+
Salmonella sp.	0	0	0	0	0	±	+	+	±	+	+	+	+	+	+	+	+	+	+	+	+	+	+	+	+
Shigella sp.	0	0	0	0	0	±	+	+	±	+	+	+	+	+	+	+	+	+	+	+	+	+	+	+	+
Proteus mirabilis	0	0	0	0	0	+	+	+	+	+	+	+	+	+	+	+	+	+	+	+	+	+	+	+	+
Proteus vulgaris	0	0	0	0	0	0	+	+	+	+	+	+	+	+	+	+	+	+	+	+	+	+	+	+	+
Providencia sp.	0	0	0	0	0	0	+	+	+	+	+	+	+	+	+	+	+	+	+	+	+	+	+	+	+
Morganella sp.	0	0	0	0	0	0	±	+	±	+	+	+	+	+	+	+	+	+	+	+	+	+	+	+	+
Citrobacter sp.	0	0	0	0	0	0	0	0	+	+	+	+	+	+	+	+	+	+	+	+	+	+	+	+	+
Aeromonas sp.	0	0	0	0	0	0	±	+	+	+	+	+	+	+	+	+	+	+	+	+	+	+	+	+	+
Acinetobacter sp.	0	0	0	0	0	0	0	0	±	+	+	±	±	+	+	+	0	±	±			±	±	±	±
Ps. aeruginosa	0	0	0	0	0	0	0	0	+	+	+	+	+	0	+	+	+	±	±	±		±	±	±	±
B. (Ps.) cepacia§	0	0	0	0	0	0	0	0	0	±	±			0	0	±	0						0	0	0
S. (X.) maltophilia§	0	0	0	0	0	0	0	0	0	±	±			0	0	0	0	±	+			0	0		
Y. enterocolitica	0	0	0	0	0	0	±	+	±	+	+	+	+	+	+	+	+	+	+	+	+	+	+	+	+
Legionella sp.	0	0	0	0	0	0	0	0	0	0	0	0	0	0	0	0	0	+	+	+	+	+	+	+	+
P. multocida	+	+	0	0	0	+	+	+	+	+				+	+	+		+	+	+	+	+	+	+	+
H. ducreyi	+					0	+	+																	
MISC.:																									
Chlamydia sp.	0	0	0	0	0	0	0	0	0	0	0	0	0	0	0	0	0	+	+			+	+	+	+
M. pneumoniae	0	0	0	0	0	0	0	0	0	0	0	0	0	0	0	0	0	+	+	0		+	+	+	+
ANAEROBES:																									
Actinomyces	+	±				+	+	+						+				0	0			±			
Bacteroides fragilis	0	±	0	0	0	0	+	+	0	+	+	0	+	+	+	+	0	0	0	0	0	0	±	+	±
P. melaninogenica§	+	0	0	0	0	+	+	+	+	+	+	+	+		+	+	+	0							
Clostridium difficile	+¹						+¹							+¹	+¹	+¹	0	0	0						
Clostridium (not difficile)	+	+				+	+	+	+	+	+	+	+	+	+	+	0	±	±	0		+	+	+	+
Peptostreptococcus sp.	+	+	+	+	+	+	+	+	+	+	+	+	+	+	+	+	0	±	±	0		+	+	+	+

+ = usually effective clinically or >60% susceptible; ± = clinical trials lacking or 30–60% susceptible; 0 = not effective clinically or <30% susceptible; blank = data not available

§ B. melaninogenicus → Prevotella melaninogenica, Pseudomonas cepacia → Burkholderia cepacia, Xanthomonas → Stenotrophomonas

** Most strains ±, can be used in UTI, not in systemic infection

Ticar/Clav = ticarcillin clavulanate; Amp/Sulb = ampicillin sulbactam; Amox/Clav = amoxicillin clavulanate; MSSA = methicillin-sensitive Staph. aureus; MRSA = methicillin-resistant Staph. aureus; Pip/Tazo = piperacillin/tazobactam

¹ No clinical evidence that penicillins or fluoroquinolones are effective for C. difficile enterocolitis (but they may cover this organism in mixed intra-abdominal and pelvic infections)

TABLE 4 (2)

Organisms	Cefazolin	Cefotetan	Cefoxitin	Cefuroxime	Cefotaxime	Ceftizoxime	Ceftriaxone	Cefoperazone	Ceftazidime	Cefepime	Cefadroxil	Cephalexin	Cefaclor/Loracarbef*	Cefprozil	Cefuroxime axetil	Cefixime	Ceftibuten	Cefpodox*/Cefdinir/Cefditoren
CEPHALOSPORINS group	1st Gen	2nd Generation			3rd/4th Generation						1st Gen (Oral)		2nd Generation (Oral)			3rd Generation (Oral)		
GRAM-POSITIVE:																		
Strep, Group A,B,C,G	+	+	+	+	+	+	+	+	+[1]	+	+	+	+	+	+	+	+	+
Strep. pneumoniae[1]	+	+	+	+	+	+	+	+	+[1]	+	+	+	+	+	+	+	±	+
Viridans strep	+	+	+	+	+	+	+	+	±[1]	+	+	+	+	0	+	+	+	+
Enterococcus faecalis	0	0	0	0	0	0	0	0	0	0	0	0	0	0	0	0	0	0
Staph. aureus (MSSA)	+	+	+	+	+	+	+	+	±	+	+	+	+	+	+	0	0	+
Staph. aureus (MRSA)	0	0	0	0	0	0	0	0	0	0	0	0	0	0	0	0	0	0
Staph. epidermidis	±	±	±	±	±	±	±	±	0	±	±	±	±	±	±	0	0	±
C. jeikeium	0	0	0	0	0	0	0	0	0	0	0	0	0	0	0	0	0	0
L. monocytogenes	0	0	0	0	0	0	0	0	0	0	0	0	0	0	0	0	0	0
GRAM-NEGATIVE:																		
N. gonorrhoeae	+	±	±	±	±	±	+	±	±	±	0	0	±	±	±	+	±	+
N. meningitidis	0	±	±	+	+	+	±	+	±	+	0	0	±	±	±	±	±	
M. catarrhalis	±	±	+	+	+	+	+	+	+	+	0	0	0	+	+	+	+	+
H. influenzae	+	±	+	+	+	+	+	+	+	+	0	+	+	+	+	+	+	+
E. coli	+	+	+	+	+	+	+	+	+	+	+	+	+	+	+	+	+	+
Klebsiella sp.	+	+	+	+	+	+	+	+	+	+	+	+	+	+	+	+	+	+
Enterobacter sp.	0	±	0	±	+	+	+	+	+	+	0	0	0	0	0	0	±	+
Serratia sp.	0	+	0	0	+	+	+	+	+	+	0	0	0	0	0	±	±	0
Salmonella sp.					+		+	+			0							
Shigella sp.					+						0							
Proteus mirabilis	+	+	+	+	+	+	+	+	+	+	+	+	+	+	+	+	+	+
Proteus vulgaris	0	+	+	+	+	+	+	+	+	+	0	0	0	0	+	+	+	±
Providencia sp.	0	+	+	0	+	+	+	+	+	+	0	0	0	0	+	+	+	
Morganella sp.	0	+	±	±	+	+	+	+	+	+	0	0	0	0	±	0	0	+
C. freundii	0	0	0	0	0	0	0	0	0	0	0	0	0	0	0	0	0	+
C. diversus	0	±	±	±	+	+	+	+	+	+	0	0	0	0	±	0	0	+
Citrobacter sp.	0	±	±	±	+	+	+	+	+	+	0		±	0	±	+	+	
Aeromonas sp.	0	±	±	+	+	+	+	+	+	+						+	+	
Acinetobacter sp.	0	0	0	0	+	+	+	0	+	±	0	0	0	0	0	0	0	0
Ps. aeruginosa	0	0	0	0	±	±	±	+	+	+	0	0	0	0	0	0	0	0
B. (Ps.) cepacia§	0	0	0	0	±	±	±	+	+	±	0	0	0	0	0	0	0	+
S. (X.) maltophilia§	0	0	0	0	0	0	0	±	±	0	0	0	0	0	0	0		
Y. enterocolitica	0	±	±	±	+	+	+	±	±	+						+	+	
Legionella sp.	0	0	0	0	0	0	0	0	0	0	0	0	0	0	0	0	0	0
P. multocida					+	+	+				0				+			+
H. ducreyi				+	+	+	+									+		
ANAEROBES:																		
Actinomyces					+	+												
Bacteroides fragilis	0	+[2]	+	0	0	±	0	0	0	0	0		0	0	0	0	0	
P. melaninogenica§		+	+	+	+	+	±	+	+	0			+	+	+			+
Clostridium difficile			0		0	0								0	0			
Clostridium (not difficile)		+	+	+	+	+	+	+						+	+	0		
Peptostreptococcus sp.	+	+	+	+	+	+	+	+	+	+		+	+	+	+			

+ = usually effective clinically or >60% susceptible; ± = clinical trials lacking or 30–60% susceptible; 0 = not effective clinically or <30% susceptible; blank = data not available.

§ B. melaninogenicus → Prevotella melaninogenica, P. cepacia → Burkholderia cepacia, Xanthomonas → Stenotrophomonas

* A 1-carbacephem best classified as a cephalosporin

1 Ceftaz 8–16x less active than cefotax/ceftriax, effective only vs Pen-sens. strains (AAC 39:2193, 1995). Oral cefuroxime, cefprozil, cefpodoxime most active in vitro vs resistant S. pneumo (PIDJ 14:1037, 1995).

2 Cefotetan is less active against B. ovatus, B. distasonis, B. thetaiotamicron

3 Cefpodox = Cefpodoxime proxetil

MSSA = methicillin-sensitive Staph. aureus; MRSA = methicillin-resistant Staph. aureus

TABLE 4 (3)

Organisms	Gentamicin	Tobramycin	Amikacin	Netilmicin[AUS]	Chloramphenicol	Clindamycin	Erythro/Dirithro	Azithromycin	Clarithromycin	Telithromycin (Ketolide)	Doxycycline	Minocycline	Vancomycin	Teicoplanin	Fusidic Acid	Trimethoprim	TMP/SMX	Nitrofurantoin	Fosfomycin	Enoxacin	Rifampin	Metronidazole	Quinupristin/dalfopristin	Linezolid	Daptomycin
GRAM-POSITIVE:																									
Strep Group A,B,C,G	0	0	0	0	+	±	+	+	+	+	±	±	+	+	±	±	+[2]	+		0	+	0	+	+	+
Strep. pneumoniae	0	0	0	0	+	+	+	+	+	+	±	+	+	+	+	±	±	+		±	+	0	+	+	+
Enterococcus faecalis	S	S	S	S	±	0	0	0	0	±	0	0	+	+	±	+	+[2]	+	+	0	±	0	±	+	+
Enterococcus faecium	S	0	0	0	±	0	0	0	0	±	0	0	±	±	0	0	0	+	+	0	0	0	+	+	
Staph.aureus(MSSA)	+	+	+	+	±	+	±	+	+	+	±	+	+	+	+	±	+	+	+	0	+		+	+	+
Staph.aureus(MRSA)	0	0	0	0	0	0	0	0	0	0	0	0	+	+	+	+	0	0	0	0	+		+	+	+
Staph. epidermidis	±	±	±	±	0	0	±	0	0	±	±	±	+	+	+	±	±	±			+		+	+	+
C. jeikeium	0	0	0	0	0	0	0	0	0	0	+	+	+	+	0	+	0	0			+		+	+	+
L. monocytogenes	S	S	S	S	+		+	+	+	+	+	+	+	+		+	+				+		+	+	+
GRAM-NEGATIVE:																									
N. gonorrhoeae	0	0	0	0	+	0	±	±	±		±	±			+	0	+	+			+	0	+		
N. meningitidis	0	0	0	0	+	0	+	+			+	+	0	0		±	+				+	0	0	0	
M. catarrhalis[§]	+	+	+	+	+	0	+	+	+	+	+	+			±		+				+	0	±	±	
H. influenzae	+	+	+	+	+	0	±	+	+	+	+	+				±	±			+	+	0	±	±	
Aeromonas	0														0		+	+			+		0	0	
E. coli	+	+	+	+	+	0	0	0	0	0	+		0	0	0	+	+	+	+	+	0	0	0	0	0
Klebsiella sp.	+	+	+	+	±	0	0	0	0	0	±	±	0	0	0	0	±	±	±	+	+	0	0	0	0
Enterobacter sp.	+	+	+	+	±	0	0	0	0	0	0	0	0	0	0	0	0	0	±	+	+	0	0	0	0
Salmonella sp.	+	+	+	+	+	0	±	0	0	0	±	±	0	0	0	±	±	±	+	+	+	0	0	0	0
Shigella sp.	+	+	+	+	+	0	±	0	0	0	±	±	0	0	0	±	±	±	+	+	+	0	0	0	0
Serratia marcescens	+	+	+	+	0	0	0	0	0	0	±	0	0	0	0	0	±	0	±	0	+	0	0	0	0
Proteus vulgaris	+	+	+	+	+	0	0	0	0	0	0	0	0	0	0	0	0	0		±	+	0	±	±	+
Acinetobacter sp.	0	+	0		0	0	0	0	0	0	0	0	0	0	0	0	0			±	±		0	0	
Ps. aeruginosa	+	+	+	+	0	0	0	0	0	0	0	±	0	0	0	0	0	0	0	+	+	0	0	0	0
B. (Ps.) cepacia[§]	0	0	0	0	+	0	0	0	0	0	±		0	0	0	+	+	0				0	0	0	0
S. (X.) maltophilia[§]	0	0	0	0	+	0	0	0	0	0	0	0	0	0	0	+	+	0				0	0	0	0
Y. enterocolitica	+	+	+		0	0	0	0	0	0	0	0	0	0	0	0	0				0		0	0	0
F. tularensis	+				+			0							+						+		0	0	
Brucella sp.	+				0	0	0	0	0		+				+	+					+	0	0		
Legionella sp.							+	+	+	+	+	+			±	+					0	+	±		
H. ducreyi	+	+	±				+	+								0					±				
V. vulnificus	±	±	±								+	+				0							0		
MISC.:																									
Chlamydia sp.	0	0	0	0	+	±	+	+	+	+	+	+				0	0				+	0	+	+	
M. pneumoniae	0	0	0	0	+	0	+	+	+	+	+	+				0	0					0	+	+	
Rickettsia sp.	0	J	0		+		±			+	+	+	0	0		0									
Mycobacterium avium		+					+	+	+														0	0	+
ANAEROBES:																									
Actinomyces	0	0	0	0	+	+	+	+	+	+	+	+	+			+					0				
Bacteroides fragilis	0	0	0	0	+	+	0	0	0		±	±	0			0		+	0		0	+	+	±	
P. melaninogenica[§]	0	0	0	0	+	+		+	+		±	+	0		+				0		+	+	+		
Clostridium difficile	0	0	0	0	±								+	+					0		+	±	+		
Clostridium (not difficile)**		+			±	±	+		+	+	+	+			0						+	+	+		
Peptostreptococcus sp.	0	0	0	0	+	+	±	±	+	+	+	+	0			+					+	+	+		

+ = usually effective clinically or >60% susceptible; ± = clinical trials lacking or 30–60% susceptible; 0 = not effective clinically or <30% susceptible; S = synergistic with penicillins (ampicillin); blank = data not available. Antimicrobials such as azithromycin have high tissue penetration and some such as clarithromycin are metabolized to more active compounds, hence in vivo activity may exceed in vitro activity.

[1] In vitro results discrepant, + in one study, 0 in another [JAC 31(Suppl. C):39, 1993]

[2] Although active in vitro, TMP/SMX is not clinically effective for Group A strep pharyngitis or for infections due to E. faecalis.

§ B. melaninogenicus → Prevotella melaninogenica, P. cepacia → Burkholderia cepacia, Xanthomonas → Stenotrophomonas

** Vancomycin, metronidazole given po active vs C. difficile; IV vancomycin not effective

Dirithro = dirithromycin; **Erythro** = erythromycin; **TMP/SMX** = trimethoprim/sulfamethoxazole; **MSSA** = methicillin-sensitive Staph. aureus; **MRSA** = methicillin-resistant Staph. aureus; **S** = potential synergy in combination with penicillin, ampicillin, vancomycin, or teicoplanin

TABLE 5: TREATMENT OPTIONS FOR SELECTED HIGHLY RESISTANT BACTERIA (NEJM 335:1445, 1996)

ORGANISM/RESISTANCE	THERAPEUTIC OPTIONS	COMMENT[1]
E. faecalis. Resistant to:		
Vanco, streptomycin (MIC >500 µg/ml), β-lactamase neg. (JAC 40:161, 1997)	Penicillin G or AMP (systemic infections); Nitrofurantoin, fosfomycin (UTI only). Usually resistant to Synercid	Non BL strains of E. faecalis resistant to penicillin and AMP recently described in Spain, but unknown (except BL+ strains) so far in U.S. and elsewhere (AAC 40:2420, 1996). Linezolid also effective in 60-70% of cases (AHM, in press, 2002).
Penicillin (β-lactamase producers)	Vanco, AM/SB	Appear susceptible to AMP and penicillin by standard in vitro methods. Most use direct test for β-lactamase with chromogenic cephalosporin (nitrocefin) to identify in lab (JCM 31:1905, 1993).
E. faecium. Resistant to:		
Vanco and high levels (MIC >500 µg/ml) of streptomycin and gentamicin.	Penicillin G or AMP (systemic infections); fosfomycin, nitrofurantoin (UTI only)	For strains with pen/AMP MICs of >8 ≤64 µg/ml there is anecdotal evidence that high-dose (300 mg/kg/day) AMP ± may be effective.
Penicillin, AMP, vanco, & high-level resist. to aminoglycosides and gentamicin (NEJM 342:710, 2000)	Linezolid (Zyvox) 600 mg po or IV q12h and quinu/dalfo (Synercid) 7.5 mg/kg q8h are the only FDA-approved drugs; most strains of E. faecium susceptible. Can try combinations of cell wall-active antibiotics with other agents (including FQs, chloramphenicol, RIF or doxy), chloramphenicol alone effective in some cases of bacteremia (CM 7:17, 2001). Nitrofurantoin or fosfomycin may work for UTI.	For strains with Van B phenotype (vanco R, teico S), teicoplanin[NUS] preferably in combination with streptomycin is the drug of choice if only AG resistant may be effective. Synercid roughly 70% effective in clinical trials (CID 30:790, 2000, & 33:1816, 2001). Linezolid shows similar efficacy. Emergence of resistance with therapeutic failure has occurred during monotherapy with either quinu/dalfo or linezolid (CID 36:790, 2000; Ln 357:1179, 2001). Nosocomial spread of linezolid-resistant E. faecium possible (NEJM 346:867, 2002).
		Infectious disease consultation imperative!
S. aureus. Resistant to:		
Methicillin (Ln 349:1901, 1997; Clin Micro Rev 10:781, 1997; CID 32:108, 2001)	Vanco	Other alternatives include teicoplanin[NUS] 2002). TMP/SMX (test susceptibility first), minocycline & doxy (some strains), linezolid, or quinu/dalfo (CID 34:1481, 2002). Fusidic acid[NUS] 780-880 mg/kg/day. P.O may be active but must be used in combination regimens to prevent in vivo emergence of resistance. **Investigational agents with activity against MRSA include oritavancin (LY333328), dalbavancin.**
Vanco-intermediate (VISA) (NEJM 340:493, 1999; MMWR 46:813, 1997)	Unknown - but high-dose vanco may fail. Linezolid, quinu/dalfo active in vitro.	Oritavancin (LY3333288, 781-860-8660), gatifloxacin (781-860-8660), dalbavancin
(NEJM 339:520, 1998; CID 32:108, 2001)		Vanco added to nafcillin at high level doses MMWR 36 (q4)h), or vanco-resistance (MMWR 27:624, 1997; JAC 41:95, 1997). Some call these strains VISA or GISA. Only anecdotal data on therapeutic regimens, most susceptible to TMP/SMX, minocycline, doxycycline, RIF and AGs (CID 32:108, 2001). RIF should always be combined with another active agent. First emergence of RIF resistance during therapy to the 1st clinical isolate truly vancomycin resistant (MIC 128) MRSA described. Organism still susceptible to TMP/SMX, chloro, linezolid, minocycline, tetracycline (MMWR 51:565, 2002)
S. epidermidis. Resistant to:		
Methicillin, glycopeptides	Vanco (+ RIF and gentamicin for prosthetic valve endocarditis). Quinu/dalfo (see comments on E. faecium generally active in vitro as is linezolid	Vanco more active than teicoplanin[NUS] (Clin Microbiol Rev 8:585, 1995). New FQs (levofloxacin, gatifloxacin, moxifloxacin) in vitro, but development of resistance is a potential problem.
S. pneumoniae. Resistant to:		
Penicillin G (MIC >0.1 ≤1.0)	Ceftriaxone or cefotaxime. High-dose penicillin (≥10 million units/day) or AMP (amox) likely effective for non-meningeal sites of infection (e.g. pneumonia)	IMP, erta, cefepime, cefpodoxime, cefuroxime also active (IDCP 3:75, 1994). MER less active than IMP (AAC 38:898, 1994). Gati, levo, moxi also have good activity (AAC 38:698, 1994; DMID 31:45, 1998; Exp Open Invest Drugs 8:123, 1999).
Penicillin G (MIC ≥2.0)	(Vanco ± RIF) or an active FQ: gati, levo, moxi. Alternatives if non-meningeal infection: ceftria/ cefotax. High-dose AMP, IMP, MER	High-dose cefotaxime (300 mg/kg/day, max. 24 gm/day) effective in meningitis due to strains with cefotaxime MICs as high as 2 µg/ml (AAC 40:218, 1996). Review IDCP 6(Suppl 2):S21, 1997.
Penicillin, erythro, tetracycline, chloramphenicol. TMP/SMX	Vanco ± RIF	60-80% of strains resistant to clindamycin (Diag Microbiol Inf Dis 26:201, 1996). Levo, gati, moxi active in vitro (AAC 42:2431, 1996)
Acinetobacter baumannii. Resistant to: IMP, AP Ceph 3, AP Pen, APAG, FQ	AM/SB (sulbactam alone is active against some A. baumannii, JAC 42:793, 1998)	68 patients with A. baumannii, combinations of FQs (7 organisms) cured with AM/SB (CID 24:932, 1997). Various combinations of FQs and AGs, IMP and AGs, or AP Ceph 3s with AGs may be effective. If susceptible against multiresistant strains (AAC 41:881, 1997; AAC 41:1073, 1997). IV colistin also effective (CID 36:1008, 1999).
Campylobacter jejuni. Resistant to: FQs	Erythro, azithro, clarithro, doxy, clindamycin	Strains resistant to **both FQs & macrolides** have been reported from Thailand (CID 22:868, 1996)
Klebsiella pneumoniae (producing ESBL)		
Resistant to: Ceftazidime, P Ceph 3, aztreonam	IMP, MER, FQ	Strains resistant in vitro activity, but have not been proven entirely effective in animal models (IJAA 8:37, 1997) and some strains which hyperproduce ESBLs are primarily resistant to TC/CL and PIP/TZ (JAC 43:358, 1996). Note that these are strains of ESBL-producing Klebsiella only susceptible to P Ceph 2 or 3 (JCM 39:2206, 2001)
	IP Ceph 1, TC/CL, PIP/TZ show in vitro activity, but have not been proven entirely effective in animal models (IJAA 8:37, 1997) and some strains which hyperproduce ESBLs are primarily resistant to TC/CL and PIP/TZ (JAC 43:358, 1996). Note that these are strains of ESBL-producing Klebsiella only susceptible to P Ceph 2 or 3 (JCM 39:2206, 2001). Infections due to such	

TABLE 5 (2)

ORGANISM/RESISTANCE	THERAPEUTIC OPTIONS	COMMENT[1]
Pseudomonas aeruginosa. Resistant to: IMP, MER	CIP (check susceptibility), APAG (check susceptibility)	Many strains remain susceptible to aztreonam & ceftazidime or AP Pens. Combinations of (AP Pen & APAG) or (AP Ceph 3 + APAG) may show in vitro activity (AAC 39:2411, 1995). IV colistin may have some utility (CID 28:1008, 1999).

[1] Guideline on prevention of resistance. CID 25:584, 1997. **Abbreviations: AGs** = aminoglycosides, **AMP** = ampicillin, **Amox** = amoxicillin, **AM/SB** = ampicillin/sulbactam, **AP Ceph 3** = third generation parenteral cephalosporin with enhanced antipseudomonal activity, **AP Pen** = antipseudomonal penicillins, **APAG** = antipseudomonal aminoglycosidic antibiotics, **Azithro** = azithromycin, **BL** = beta-lactamase, β-L = β-lactamase, **Clarithro** = clarithromycin, **Doxy** = doxycycline, **Erta** = ertapenem, **Erythro** = erythromycin, **ESBLs** = extended spectrum β-lactamases, **FQ** = fluoroquinolone, **Gati** = gatifloxacin, **Levo** = levofloxacin, **Moxi** = moxifloxacin, **P Ceph** = parenteral cephalosporin, **PIP/TZ** = piperacillin/tazobactam, **Quinu/dalfo** = quinupristin/dalfopristin, **R** = resistant, **RIF** = rifampin, **S** = sensitive, **TC/CL** = ticarcillin/clavulanate, **Vanco** = vancomycin, **VISA** = vancomycin intermediately-resistant Staph. aureus, **VRMRSA** = vancomycin-resistant, methicillin-resistant Staph aureus

TABLE 6: RISK CATEGORIES OF ANTIMICROBICS IN PREGNANCY

DRUG	FDA PREGNANCY RISK CATEGORIES[*]	DRUG	FDA PREGNANCY RISK CATEGORIES[*]	DRUG	FDA PREGNANCY RISK CATEGORIES[*]
Antibacterial Agents		**Antifungal Agents:** (CID 27:1151, 1998)		**Antimycobacterial Agents** (continued)	
Aminoglycosides:		Amphotericin B preparations	B	Ethionamide	"do not use"[1]
Amikacin, gentamicin, isepamicin[N/I,S]		Caspofungin	C	INH, pyrazinamide, rifampin	B
Amikacin, gentamicin, streptomycin & tobramycin	D	Fluconazole, itraconazole, ketoconazole	C	Rifabutin	B
Beta Lactams (CPh 27:49, 1994)		flucytosine	C	**Antiviral Agents:**	
Penicillins, pens + BLI; cephalosporins, aztreonam	B	Terbinafine	B	Abacavir	C
Imipenem/cilastatin	C	Voriconazole	D	Acyclovir, famciclovir, valacyclovir	B
Meropenem, ertapenem	B	**Antiparasitic Agents:**		Amantadine, rimantadine	C
Chloramphenicol	C	Albendazole/mebendazole	C	Atazanavir, indinavir	C
Ciprofloxacin, oflox, levofloxa, gatiflox, moxiflox	C	Atovaquone/proguanil	C	Cidofovir	C
Clindamycin	B	Chloroquine, eflornithine	C	Delavirdine, efavirenz, nevirapine	C
Fosfomycin	B	Ivermectin	C	Didanosine (ddI)	B
Linezolid	C	Mefloquine	C	Foscarnet	C
Macrolides:		Pentamidine	C	Ganciclovir, valganciclovir	C
Erythromycin/azithromycin	B	Praziquantel	B	Interferons	C
Clarithromycin	C	Pyrimethamine/pyrisulfadoxine	C	Lamivudine/stavudine	C
Metronidazole	B	Quinine	X	Lopinavir/ritonavir	C
Nitrofurantoin	B	**Antimycobacterial Agents:**		Nelfinavir, ritonavir, saquinavir	B
Sulfonamides/trimethoprim	C		C	Oseltamivir	C
Telithromycin	C	Clofazimine/cycloserine	C	Ribavirin	X
Tetracyclines	D	Dapsone	C	Tenofovir	B
Vancomycin	C	Ethambutol	"avoid"[1]	Valacyclovir	B
			C	Zalcitabine/zidovudine	C
		INH	"safe"[1]	Zanamivir	B
		Thalidomide	X		

TABLE 7: ANTIMICROBIALS ASSOCIATED WITH PHOTOSENSITIVITY

The following drugs are known to cause photosensitivity in some individuals. There is no intent to indicate relative frequency or severity of reactions.

Source: 1998 Drug Topics Red Book, Medical Economics, Montvale, NJ. Listed in alphabetical order:

Amantadine, azithromycin, benznidazole, ciprofloxacin, clofazimine, dapsone, doxycycline, erythromycin ethyl succinate, flucytosine, ganciclovir, griseofulvin, interferons, levofloxacin, ofloxacin, pefloxacin, pyrazinamide, saquinavir, sparfloxacin, sulfonamides, tetracyclines, tretinoins, trovafloxacin, trimethoprim.

* **FDA Pregnancy Categories: A**—studies in pregnant women, no risk; **B**—animal studies no risk, but human not adequate or animal toxicity but human studies no risk; **C**—animal studies show toxicity, human studies inadequate but benefit of use may exceed risk; **D**—evidence of human risk, but benefits may outweigh; **X**—fetal abnormalities in humans, risk > benefit.

Abbreviations: BLI = B-lactamase inhibitor; **FQ** = fluoroquinolones.
[1] From CDC: TB Core Curriculum, 3rd Ed., 1994

The approximate phototoxic potential among fluoroquinolones (from CID 28:352, 1999) is: lomefloxacin, fleroxacin > sparfloxacin > enoxacin > pefloxacin[N/I,S] > ciprofloxacin, [levofloxacin, ofloxacin, trovafloxacin]

8A: PHARMACOKINETICS: Route, Half-life, Protein-binding (See Table 8B for serum levels)

DRUG	ROUTES OF ADMIN.	ORAL WC	ORAL % AB	SERUM t/2 hrs[1]	PROTEIN BOUND %
PENICILLINS					
Natural					
Penicillin G	IV,IM,PO	N	15	0.5	65
Pen'ase Resist.					
Clox,Dicloxacil.	PO	N	35	0.5	95-98
Nafcillin	IV,IM			0.5	90
Oxacillin	IV,IM,PO	N	30	0.5	94
Aminopenicillins					
Amoxicillin	PO	Y	75	1.2	17
AM/CL	PO	Y	75	1.4/1.1	20/30
Ampicillin	IV,IM,PO	N	40	1.2	18-22
AM/SB	IV,IM			1.2	28/28
Antipseudomonal					
Indanyl carb.	PO	N	35	1.0	50
Mezlo;Piperacil.	IV			1.1	16-48
PIP/TZ	IV			1.0	16-48
Ticarcillin;TC/CL	IV			1.2	45/30
CEPHALOSPORINS					
1st Generation					
Cefadroxil	PO	Y	90	1.5	20
Cefazolin	IV,IM			1.9	73-87
Cephalexin	PO	Y	90	1.0	5-15
Cephradine	PO	N	90	1.3	6-20
2nd Generation					
Cefaclor	PO	N	93	0.8	22-25
Cefaclor-CD	PO			0.8	22-25
Cefamandole	IV,IM			1.0	56-78
Cefditoren	PO	Y	16	1.6	88
Cefotetan	IV,IM			4.2	78-91
Cefoxitin	IV,IM			0.8	65-79
Cefprozil	PO	Y	95	1.3-1.8	36-37
Cefuroxime	IV,IM			1.5	33-50
Cefurox -axetil	PO	Y	52	1.5	50
Loracarbef[3]	PO	N	~90	1.2	25
3rd Generation					
Cefdinir	PO	N	25	1.7	60-70
Cefixime	PO	Y	50	3.1	65
Cefoperazone	IV,IM			1.9	82-93
Cefotaxime	IV,IM			1.5	30-51
Cefpodoxime proxetil	PO	Y	46	~2.3	40
Ceftazidime	IV,IM			1.8	< 10
Ceftibuten	PO	N	–	2.4	65
Ceftizoxime	IV,IM			1.7	30
Ceftriaxone	IV,IM			8	85-95
4th Generation					
Cefepime	IV			2.0	20
CARBAPENEMS					
Ertapenem	IV,IM			4	95
Imipenem	IV,IM			1.0	15-25
Meropenem	IV			1.0	
MONOBACTAMS					
Aztreonam	IV,IM			2.0	56
AMINOGLYCOSIDES					
Parenteral: amikacin, gentamicin, isepamicin[NUS], kanamycin, netilmicin[NUS], sisomicin[NUS], tobramycin have similar pharmacokinetics:					
Neomycin	IV,IM			2.5	0-10
	PO		<3		0-10

DRUG	ROUTES OF ADMIN.	ORAL WC	ORAL % AB	SERUM t/2 hrs[1]	PROTEIN BOUND %
MACROLIDES					
Azithromycin	PO	Y	37	12/68	12-50
	IV			12/68	7-51
Clarithromycin	PO	Y	50	5-7	65-70
Dirithromycin	PO	Y	10	8	15-30
Erythromycins	PO	N	18-45	2-4	70-74
MISCELLANEOUS					
Chloramphenicol	PO,IV,IM	N	80	4.1	25-50
Clindamycin	PO,IV,IM	Y	90	2.4	85-94
Doxycycline	PO,IV	Y	93	18	93
Fosfomycin	PO	N	30-37	5.7	<10
Linezolid	PO,IV		100	5	31
Metronidazole	PO,IV		90	6-14	20
Minocycline	PO	Y	95	16	76
Rifabutin	PO	Y	≥20	45	85
Rifampin	PO	N	100	2-5	80
Quinu/dalfo (Synercid)	IV			1.5	
Telithromycin	PO	Y	57	10	60-70
TMP/SMX	PO,IV		90-100	11/9	40-70
Vancomycin	IV			4-6	<10-55
FLUOROQUINOLONES					
Ciprofloxacin (ER)[2]	PO,IV	Y	70	4 (6.6)	20-40
Gatifloxacin	PO,IV	N	96	7-8	20
Levo; Ofloxacin	PO,IV	N	98	7	24-38
Lomefloxacin	PO	Y	>95	8	10
Moxifloxacin	PO,IV	N	89	10-14	50
Trovafloxacin	PO,IV	Y	88	11	76
ANTIVIRALS					
Abacavir	PO	Y	>95	1.5	50
Acyclovir	PO,IV	Y	15-30	2.5	9-33
Adefovir	PO	Y		7.5	
Amantadine	PO	Y	90	15	67
Amprenavir	PO	Y	63	7-10	90
Cidofovir	IV			3-4	<6
Delavirdine	PO		85	5.8	98
Didanosine (ddI)	PO	N	37	1.6	<5
Efavirenz	PO	N	42	40-55	99
Famciclovir	PO	Y	77	2.3-3.0	20
Foscarnet	IV			3	17
Ganciclovir	PO/IV	Y	6-9	2.9	1-2
Valganciclovir	PO	Y	60	4	1-2
Indinavir	PO		80	2	60
Lamivudine (3TC)	PO	Y	86	5-7	36
Lopinavir	PO	Y	?	5-6	98-99
Nelfinavir	PO	Y	20-80	3.5-5.0	>98
Nevirapine	PO	Y	>90	25-30	60
Oseltamivir	PO	Y	75	1-3/ 6-105	60
Ribavirin	PO	Y	52	30-60	0
Rimantadine	PO	Y	>90	27-36	
Ritonavir	PO		Good	3-5	98-99
Saquinavir—softgel	PO		>4	--	98
Stavudine (d4T)	PO	Y	86-99	1.0	<1
Tenofovir	PO	Y	35		<7
Valacyclovir	PO	Y	54	2.5	13-18
Zalcitabine (ddC)	PO	Y	>80	1.2	<4
Zidovudine (ZDV)	PO,IV	N	65	1.1	10-30

Abbreviations: WC = with meals, Y = yes, N = no, % AB = absorption (oral) (bioavailability), AM/CL = amoxicillin clavulanate, AM/SB = ampicillin sulbactam, NUS = not licensed in the U.S., I = investigational, TC/CL = ticarcillin clavulanate, TMP/SMX = trimethoprim/sulfamethoxazole, PIP/TZ = piperacillin tazobactam, Quinu/dalfo = quinupristin/dalfopristin

1. Assumes creatinine clearance >80 ml/min.
2. Extended release ciprofloxacin
3. A 1-carbacephem but classified as a cephalosporin
4. A 1-carbacephem but classified as a cephalosporin
5. Oseltamivir/oselt. carboxylate

TABLE 8B: PHARMACOKINETICS: Peak Serum Levels[1] and Biliary Excretion

DRUG	DOSE/ROUTE	PEAK SERUM LEVEL (μg/ml)	BILIARY EXCRETION[2] %	DRUG	DOSE/ROUTE	PEAK SERUM LEVEL (μg/ml)	BILIARY EXCRETION[2] %
PENICILLINS				**CARBAPENEMS**			
Natural				Ertapenem	1 gm IV	154	10
Benzathine Pen G	1.2 million U IM	0.15		Imipenem	500 mg IV	40	Minimal
Penicillin G	12 million U qd IV	20	500	Meropenem	500 mg IV	26	3–300
Penicillin V	500 mg PO	5–6		**MONOBACTAMS**			
Pen'ase Resistant				Aztreonam	1 gm IV	125	115–450
Clox;Dicloxacillin	500 mg PO	7–18		**AMINOGLYCOSIDES**			
Nafcillin/Oxacillin	500 mg IV	40–576	>100/20–30	Amikacin	7.5 mg/kg IV	38	30
Aminopenicillins				Genta;Tobramy-cin	1.25 mg/kg IV	4–8	10–60
Amoxicillin	250 mg PO	4–5	100–3000				
AM/CL (875/125)	875 mg PO	11.6/2.2	100–3000	Kanamycin	500 mg IM	14–29	1
AM/CL-ES;AM/CL-ER[3]	45 mg/kg PO	17/2		**FLUOROQUINOLONES**			
Ampicillin	500 mg PO	3–6	100–3000	Ciprofloxacin	750 mg PO	1.8–2.8	2800–4500
	2 gm IV	47			400 mg IV	4.6	
AM/SB (2 gm/1gm)	3 gm IV	109–150		Gatifloxacin	400 mg PO/IV	4.2–4.6	
Antipseudomonal				Levofloxacin	500 mg PO/IV	5.7	
Indanyl carb (382 mg)	1 tab (382mg) PO	6.5			750 mg PO/IV	8.6	
Mezlocillin	3 gm IV	263	1000–6000	Moxifloxacin	400 mg PO/IV	4.5	
Piperacillin	4 gm IV	400	100–6000	Ofloxacin	400 mg PO/IV	4.6/5.2–7.2	
PIP/TZ (3/0.375 gm)	3.375 gm IV	209	>100				
4/0.5 gm	4.5 gm IV	209	>100	Trovafloxacin	200 mg PO/IV	3.1/3.1	1500
Ticarcillin	3 gm IV	260		**MACROLIDES**			
TC/CL (3/0.1 gm)	3.1 gm IV	324		Azithromycin	500 mg PO	0.4	High
CEPHALOSPORINS					500 mg IV	3.6	
1st Generation				Clarithromycin	500 mg PO	2–3	7000
Cefadroxil	500 mg PO	16	22	Dirithromycin	500 mg PO	0.4	
Cefazolin	1 gm IV	188	29–300	Erythromycin oral[4]			
Cephalexin	500 mg PO	18–38	216	base	500 mg PO	0.1–2	
Cephradine	1 gm IV	86	10–400	estolate	500 mg PO	2	
	500 mg PO	16		lacto/glucep	500 mg IV	3–4	
2nd Generation				**MISCELLANEOUS**			
Cefaclor	500 mg PO	9.3	≥60	*Antibacterial*			
Cefaclor-CD	500 mg PO	8.4		Chloramphenicol	1.0 gm PO	11–18	
Cefamandole	2 gm IV	165	300–400	Clindamycin	150 mg PO	2.5	250–300
Cefditoren	400 mg PO	4			600 mg IV	10	250–300
Cefprozil	500 mg PO	10.5		Doxycycline	100 mg PO	1.5–2.1	200–3200
Cefuroxime	1.5 gm IV	100	35–80	Fosfomycin	3.0 gm PO	26	
Cefuroxime axetil	250 mg PO	4.1			20 mg/kg IV	130	
Loracarbef[5]	200 mg PO	8		Linezolid	600 mg PO/IV	15–20	
Cephamycins				Metronidazole	500 mg PO	20–25	100
Cefotetan	1 gm IV	124	2–21		500 mg IV	20–25	100
Cefoxitin	1 gm IV	110	280	Minocycline	200 mg PO	2.0–3.5	200–3200
3rd Generation				Polymyxin B	30,000 u/kg IV	1–8	
Cefdinir	300 mg PO	1.6		Quinu/dalfo (Synercid)	7.5 mg/kg IV	Approx. 3	
Cefixime	400 mg PO	3–5	800	Rifampin	600 mg po	7.0	10,000
Cefoperazone	1 gm IV	153	800–1200	Sulfisoxazole	2–4 gm PO	11–25	40–70
Cefotaxime	1 gm IV	100	15–75		2–4 gm IV	11–25	40–70
Cefpodoxime proxetil	200 mg PO	2.9	115	Tetracycline	250 mg PO	1.5–2.2	200–3200
Ceftazidime	1 gm IV	60	13–54	Telithromycin	800 mg PO	2.3	7
Ceftibuten	400 mg PO	15		TMP/SMX–DS (160 mg TMP/800 mg SMX)	1 tab po	TMP 1–2 SMX 40–60	100–200
Ceftizoxime	1 gm IV	132	34–82				
Ceftriaxone	1 gm IV	150	200–500	(160 mg TMP/800 mg SMX)	2 ampuls IV	TMP: 9 SMX: 105	40–70
4th Generation							
Cefepime	2 gm IV	193	≈5	Vancomycin	1 gm IV	20–50[6]	50

---

[1] Traditionally, peak serum levels are determined on serum obtained 1 hr after the start of the infusion of the 3rd dose. However, if dosing is qd and the pt is critically ill, it is reasonable to measure the peak level after the 1st or 2nd dose.

[2] Peak concentration in bile divided by peak concentration in serum x 100. If blank = no data

[3] AM/CL-ES = Amox/Clav extra-strength peds suspension. 600 mg AM & 43 mg CL per 5 ml; 2 adult ER tabs: 2000 mg AM/125 mg CL

[4] Erythromycin oral includes base, stearate, ethyl succinate, lactobionate, and glucaptate

[5] A 1-carbacephem but classified as a cephalosporin

[6] In renal failure pts, assay method (fluorescent polarization immunoassay) may overestimate serum level; use enzyme mult. immunoassay (*JAC 36:411, 1995*).

DRUG	DOSE/ROUTE	PEAK SERUM LEVEL (µg/ml)	DRUG	DOSE/ROUTE	PEAK SERUM LEVEL (µg/ml)
ANTIFUNGAL			**ANTIVIRAL**		
Ampho B—standard	0.4–0.7 kg/kg IV	0.5–3.5	Abacavir	300 mg po	2.9
ABLC[1]	5 mg/kg IV	1.7 ± 0.8	Acyclovir	5 mg/kg IV	9.8
AB chole. complex[1]	4 mg/kg IV	2–9	Adefovir	10 mg po	0.02
Liposom. AB[1]	2.5 mg/kg IV	31 ± 18	Aman/Rimantadine	100 mg po	0.1–0.4
Fluconazole	400 mg po	20–30	Amprenavir	1200 mg po	5.4
	800 mg po	40–60	Delavirdine	400 mg po	19 ± 11
Flucytosine	2.5 gm po	30–45	Didanosine (ddI)	300 mg po	1.6
Itraconazole,oral soln	200 mg po	2 (fasting)	Efavirenz	600 mg po	4.1
ANTIMYCOBACTERIAL			Famciclovir	500 mg po	3–4
Ethambutol	25 mg/kg po	2–6	Foscarnet	57 mg/kg IV	155 (517 µM)
Ethionamide	1 gm po	20	Ganciclovir	5 mg/kg IV	8.3
Isoniazid	300 mg po	3–5	Valganciclovir	900 mg po	5.6
Pyrazinamide	20–25 mg/kg po	30–50	Indinavir	800 mg po	12.6 µM
Rifampin	600 mg po	8–24	Lamivudine (3TC)	2 mg/kg po	1.5
Streptomycin	1 gm IV	25–50	Lopinavir	400 mg po	9 µg/ml
ANTIPARASITIC			Nelfinavir	750 mg po	3–4
Albendazole	400 mg po	1.3	Nevirapine	200 mg po	2
Dapsone	100 mg po	1.8	Oseltamivir	75 mg po	0.65/3.5[2]
Ivermectin	12 mg po	46	Ribavirin	400 mg po	0.6
Mefloquine	1.0 gm po	0.5–1.2	Ritonavir	300 mg po	7.8
Pentamidine	4.0 mg/kg IV	0.5–3.4	Saquinavir (gel)	1200 mg po	Not clear
Pyrimethamine	25 mg po	0.1–0.3	Stavudine (d4T)	70 mg po	1.4
Praziquantel	20 mg/kg po	0.2–2.0	Tenofovir	300 mg po	0.12
Quinine	650 mg po	3–10	Valacyclovir	1000 mg po	5.6
			Zalcitabine (ddC)	0.5 mg po	7.6 ng/ml
			Zidovudine (ZDV)	200 mg po	1.2

[1] **Abbreviations: ABLC** = ampho B lipid complex; **AB chole** = ampho B cholesterol complex; **Liposom. AB** = liposomal ampho B   [2] Oseltamivir/oselt. carboxylate

TABLE 8C: CEREBROSPINAL FLUID CONCENTRATIONS OF ANTIMICROBIALS (see footnotes)[1]

DRUG	CSF/BLOOD (%)	CSF LEVEL POTENTIALLY THERAPEUTIC[1]	DRUG	CSF/BLOOD (%)	CSF LEVEL POTENTIALLY THERAPEUTIC[1]
Antibacterial Drugs			Erythro/Clarithro/Azithromycin	2–13 for erythro	0
			Metronidazole	30–100	+
Penicillins			Sulfisoxazole	∞80	+[6]
Ampicillin	13–14	+	TMP/SMX	<41	+[6]
Nafcillin	9–20	+	Vancomycin, HD[7]	7–14	+[7]
Penicillin G, high dose	5–10	+[2]			
Piperacillin	30	±[3]	**Antifungal Drugs**		
Ticarcillin	40	±[3]	Ampho B, Itraconazole	0	0
Cephalosporins (no activity vs listeria)			Fluconazole	50–94	+
Cefazolin	1–4	0	Flucytosine	60–100	+
Cefepime	10	+	**Antimycobacterial Drugs**		
Cefotaxime	10	+	Cycloserine	80–100	+
Cefoxitin	3	±[3]	Ethambutol	25–50	0
Ceftazidime	20–40	+	Isoniazid	20–90	+
Ceftriaxone	8–16	+	Pyrazinamide	85–100	+
Cefuroxime	17–88	+	Rifampin	7–56	+
Other beta-lactams			**Antiviral Drugs[8]**		
Aztreonam	3–52	±	Abacavir	18	No data
Imipenem	8.5	+	Acyclovir	50	+
Meropenem	21	+	Didanosine	12–85	+
Aminoglycosides	0–30	0[3]	Foscarnet	13–103	+
Chloramphenicol, IV	45–89	+	Ganciclovir	41	+
Clindamycin	<1	0	Lamivudine	6–11	No data
Fluoroquinolones			Saquinavir	Negligible	0
Ciprofloxacin	26	+[5]	Stavudine	16–97	+
Gatifloxacin	36	Under study	Zalcitabine	9–37	+
Levofloxacin	30–50	+	Zidovudine	60	+
Trovafloxacin	23	Under study	No data for delavirdine, indinavir, nelfinavir, nevirapine, or ritonavir		

[1] CSF concentrations are those reported with inflammation. "Therapeutic CSF level" is a judgment based on drug dose and organism susceptibility. As a rule, CSF concentration should be ≥10x above MBC for bactericidal effect. [2] Does not apply to penicillin-resistant S. pneumoniae. [3] Does not apply to P. aeruginosa meningitis; levels borderline for coliforms; may need to add intrathecal gentamicin 5–10 mg. [4] Avoid for meningitis rx due to seizure potential. [5] Concentration inadequate for streptococci, can get to 1 µg/ml in CSF with 400 mg IV q8h (*CID* 31:1131, 2000). [6] Most neisseria resistant. Not cidal vs coliforms. [7] Need high doses for resistant pneumococci (*PJID* 16:895, 1997). [8] Data do not imply inflamed meninges. Ref.: *CID* 27:1117, 1998.

TABLE 9A
SELECTED ANTIBACTERIAL AGENTS—ADVERSE REACTIONS—OVERVIEW

Adverse reactions in individual patients represent all-or-none occurrences, even if rare. After selection of an agent, the physician should read the manufacturer's package insert [statements in the product labeling (package insert) must be approved by the FDA].

Numbers = frequency of occurrence (%); + = occurs, incidence not available; ++ = significant adverse reaction; 0 = not reported; R = rare, defined as <1%. NOTE: Important reactions in bold print

ADVERSE REACTIONS	Penicillin G,V	Cloxacillin	Dicloxacillin	Nafcillin	Oxacillin	Amoxicillin	Amox/Clav	Ampicillin	Amp/Sulb	Piperacillin	Pip/Taz	Ticarcillin	Ticar/Clav	Ertapenem	Imipenem	Meropenem	Aztreonam	Aminoglycosides (Amikacin, Gentamicin, Kanamycin, Netilmicin[NUS], Tobramycin)	Linezolid	Telithromycin
Local, phlebitis	+			++	+				3	4	1		3	4	3	1	4			
Hypersensitivity	+														3	3				
Fever	+	+	+	+	+	+	+	+	+	+	2		+	++	++		2		+	
Rash	**3**	4	4	4	4	5	3	5	2	1	4	3	2	+	+	+	**2**			
Photosensitivity	0	0	0	0	0	0	0	0	0	0	0	0	0		0		0			
Anaphylaxis	R	0	0	R	R	0	R	R	+	0	0	+	+		+		+			
Serum sickness	4									+	+	+	+		+		+			
Hematologic																				
+ Coombs	3	0	0	R	R	+	0	+	0	+	+	0	+		2	+	R			
Neutropenia	R	0	0	+	R	+	+	+	+	6	+	0	+		+		+			1.1
Eosinophilia	+	+	+	22	22	2	+	22	22	+	+	+	5	1	+		8			
Thrombocytopenia	R	0	0	R	R	R	R	R	R	+	+	R	R		+	+	+			3–10
↑ PT/PTT	R	0	0	+	0	+	0	+	0	+	+	+	+		R		R			
GI																				
Nausea/vomiting		+	+	0	0	2	3	2	+	+	7	+	1	3	2	4	R			3/1 6/2
Diarrhea		+	+	0	0	**5**	**9**	**10**	**2**	2	11	3	1	6	2	5	R		4	8
C. difficile colitis		R	R	R	R	R	+	R	+	+	+	+	+		+		+		+	+
Hepatic, LFTs	R	R	R	R	0	+	R	+	R	6	+	+	0	+	6	4	4	2		1.3
Hepatic failure	0	0	0	0	0	0	0	0	0	0	0	0	0		0		1			
Renal: ↑ BUN, Cr	R	0	0	0	0	R	0	R	R	+	+	0	0		+	0		**5–25[1]**		
CNS																				
Headache	R	0	0	R	R	0	0	R	R	R	8	R	R	2	+	3	+		2	1.5
Confusion	R	0	0	R	R	0	0	R	R	R	R	R	R		+		+			
Seizures	R	0	0	0	+	0	R	R	0	0	R	R	+	See footnote[2]			+			
Special Senses																				
Ototoxicity	0	0	0	0	0	0	0	0	0	0	0	0	0		R		0	**3–14[1]**		
Vestibular	0	0	0	0	0	0	0	0	0	0	0	0	0		0		0	**4–6[1]**		
Cardiac																				
Dysrhythmias	R	0	0			0	0	0	0	0	0	0	0		0		+			
Miscellaneous, Unique (Table 9B)	+		+	+	+	+	+	+	+	+				+	+		+			+
Drug/drug interactions, common (Table 21)	0	0	0	0	0	0	0	0	0	0	0	0	0		0		0	**+**	+	+

[1] Varies with criteria used

[2] **All β-lactams in high concentration can cause seizures** (JAC 45:5, 2000). In rabbit, IMP 10x more neurotoxic than benzylpenicillin (JAC 22:687, 1988). In clinical trial of IMP for pediatric meningitis, trial stopped due to seizures in 7/25 IMP recipients; hard to interpret as purulent meningitis causes seizures (PIDJ 10:122, 1991). Risk with IMP less with careful attention to dosage (Epilepsia 42:1590, 2001).
Postulated mechanism: Drug binding to $GABA_A$ receptor. IMP binds with greater affinity than MER.
Package insert, percent seizures: ertapenem 0.5, IMP 0.4, MER 0.7. However, in 3 clinical gtrials of MER for bacterial meningitis, no drug-related seizures (Scand J Inf Dis 31:3, 1999; Drug Safety 22:191, 2000). In febrile neutropenic cancer pts, IMP-related seizures reported at 2% (CID 32:381, 2001; Peds Hem Onc 17:585, 2000).

ADVERSE REACTIONS	Cefazolin	Cephapirin	Cefotetan	Cefoxitin	Cefuroxime	Cefoperazone	Cefotaxime	Ceftazidime	Ceftriaxone	Cefepime	Cefpirome[NUS]	Cefaclor/Cef.ER[1]/Loracarb	Cefadroxil	Cefdinir	Cefixime	Cefpodoxime	Cefprozil	Ceftibuten	Cefditoren	Cefuroxime-axetil	Cephalexin
Local, phlebitis	+	+	R	R	2	1	5	1	4	2	1	2									
Hypersensitivity	5		1				2			+		+									
Fever	+	+	+	+		R		R	+		+		+		R	+				R	R
Rash	+	+		2	R	2	2	2	2	2	1	1	+	R	1	1	1		R	R	1
Photosensitivity	0	0	0	0	0	0	0	R	0	0											
Anaphylaxis	R	R	+					R					R			R					R
Serum sickness												≤0.5[2]	+								+
Hematologic																					
Anemia			10		5			R				+								2	R
+ Coombs	3	+	+	2	R	2	6	8		14	3		R							R	+
Neutropenia	+	+		2	R	2	+	1	+	2	1		+	+	R	R	R	R			3
Eosinophilia		+	+	3	7	10	1	8	4	6	1			R	R	3	2	5	R	1	9
Thrombocytopenia	+	+						+	+	+		2			R	R	+	R			
↑ PT/PTT		+	++	+		++	+	+	+	+	+										
GI																					
Nausea/vomiting			2	1			R		R	1	+	3		13	7	4	4	2	6	3	
Diarrhea			4		R	3	1	1	3	1	+	1-4		15	16	7	3	3		14	4
AAC	+	+	+	+	+	+	+	+	+	+	+	+	+	+	+	+	+	+	+	+	+
Hepatic, ↑ LFTs	+	+	1	3	4	8	1	6	4	+	+	3	+	1	R	4	2	R	2		+
Hepatic failure	0	0	0	0	0	0	0	0	0	0	0										
Renal, ↑ BUN, Cr	+	R		3		6		R	1	+		+		R	+	4	R	R	R		+
CNS																					
Headache	0					R		2		2		3		2		1	R			R	+
Confusion	0											+				R					+
Seizures	0		+																		
Special Senses																					
Ototoxicity	0	0	0	0		0	0	0	0			0	0	0	0	0	0	0	0	0	0
Vestibular	0	0	0	0		0	0	0	0			0	0	0	0	0	0	0	0	0	0
Cardiac																					
Dysrhythmias	0	0	0	0		0	0	0	0			0	0	0	0	0	0	0	0	0	0
Miscellaneous, Unique (Table 9B)							+		+			+[2]									
Drug/drug interactions, common (Table 21)	0	0	0	0	0	0	0	0	0			0	0		0	0	0	0		0	0

[1] Cefaclor extended release tablets

[2] Serum sickness requires biotransformation of parent drug plus inherited defect in metabolism of reactive intermediates (*Ped Pharm & Therap 125.805, 1994*)

* See note at head of table, page 60

TABLE 9A (3)

ADVERSE REACTIONS (AE)	MACROLIDES				QUINOLONES[1]							OTHER AGENTS								
	Azithromycin	Clarithromycin, Reg. & ER*	Dirithromycin	Erythromycin	Ciprofloxacin	Gatifloxacin	Levofloxacin	Lomefloxacin	Moxifloxacin	Ofloxacin	Trovafloxacin	Chloramphenicol	Clindamycin	Metronidazole	Minocycline	Quinupristin/dalfopristin[2]	Rifampin	Tetracycline/Doxycycline	TMP/SMX	Vancomycin
Rx stopped due to AE	1	3	3		3.5	2.9	4	3	3.8	4	5									
Local, phlebitis			+			5									+	++		+		13
Hypersensitivity																	1	++	++	8
Fever																	+	+	+	1
Rash	R		R	+	3	R	1.7	R	R	2	1	+	+	+	+	R		+	+	3
Photosensitivity	R				R				2	R	R				4	R		+	+	0
Anaphylaxis				+			R	R		R	R									R
Serum sickness														+						
Hematologic																				
Anemia					R						R	++								+
Neutropenia	R	1			R	R				1		+	+	+			+	+	+	2
Eosinophilia			1		R					1			+	+				+	+	+
Thrombocytopenia	R	R	R		R							+	+			R	+	+	+	+
↑ PT/PTT																				0
GI			6	++																
Nausea/vomiting	3	3[5] (25)	8	20–	5	8/2	1.2	4	7/2	7	7	+		12	+	+		3	+	+
Diarrhea	5	3–6	8	8	2	4	1.2	1	6	4	2	+	7	+	+		+		+	3
AAC		+		+	R	R	R	R		R	R		++				R	+	+	
Hepatic, LFTs	R	R	R	+	2	R	+		R	2	≥1			+			2	+	+	0
Hepatic failure	0	0	0								R						+	+	+	0
Renal																				
↑ BUN, Cr	+	4	1		1					R				0			+	+	+	5
CNS																				
Dizziness, lightheadedness					R	3	2.5	2.3	3	3	4				++					
Headache	R	2	4		1	4	5.4	6	2		5	+	+	+					+	+
Confusion				+			+		R	R	2	+		+	+		+		+	
Seizures				+	+		+	+		R	R			+						
Special senses																				
Ototoxicity	+			+	0					R					+					R
Vestibular															21					
Cardiac																				
Dysrhythmias				+	R	+[3]	+[3]		+[3]	+[3]	+[3]		R							0
Miscellaneous, Unique (Table 9B)	+			+	R	+	+	+	+	+	+	+	+	+	+	+	+	+	+	+
Drug/drug interactions, common (Table 21)	+	+	+	+	+	+	+	+	+	+	+						++	+	+	

[1] Concern expressed that quinolones may be associated with episodes of tendonitis.

[2] Quinupristin/dalfopristin = Synercid

[3] Fluoroquinolones as class assoc. with QT, prolongation: ↑ QT, can cause torsades de pointes which can lead to ventricular fibrillation. ↑ risk with concomitant ↓ K+, ↓ Mg++. or concomitant class Ia or IIIa antiarrhythmic agents. Ref.: CID 34:861. 2002.

[4] Regular and extended-release formulations

[5] Less GI upset/abnormal taste with ER formulation

* See note at head of table, page 60

TABLE 9B: SUMMARY OF CURRENT ANTIBIOTIC DOSAGE[*] AND SIDE-EFFECTS

CLASS, AGENT, GENERIC NAME (TRADE NAME)	USUAL ADULT DOSAGE (Cost)	ADVERSE REACTIONS, COMMENTS (See Table 9A for Summary)
NATURAL PENICILLINS		**Most common adverse reactions are hypersensitivity.** Anaphylaxis in up to 0.05%, 5-10% fatal. Commercially available skin test antigen (penicillyl polylysine) does not predict anaphylactic reactions. Hematologic: renal. CNS (seizures) reactions usually seen with high dose (>20 million units/day) and renal failure. With procaine pen G and benzathine pen G, an immediate but transient (5-30 min. after injection) toxic reaction with bizarre behavior and neurologic reactions can occur (Hoignes syndrome). Coombs test positive hemolytic anemias are rare but typically severe; in contrast, the Coombs test is often positive with cephalosporin therapy, but clinically significant hemolysis is rare. Penicillin allergy ref. *JAMA 278:1895, 1997*
Benzathine penicillin G (Bicillin)	600,000-1.2 million u IM q2-4 wks Cost: 1.2 mU $26.34	
Penicillin G	Low: 600,000-1.2 million u/d IM High: ≥20 million u q d IV (= 12 gm)	
Penicillin V	0.25-0.5 gm po tid, qid before meals & hs Cost: 500 mg G $0.14, NB $0.18	
	Cost: 5 mU $3.14	
PENICILLINASE-RESISTANT PENICILLINS		
Cloxacillin (Cloxapen)	0.25-0.5 gm q6h ac, po. Cost: 500 mg, G $0.65	Blood levels ~2x greater than cloxacillin. Acute hemorrhagic cystitis reported. Acute abdominal pain with GI bleeding without antibiotic-associated colitis also reported.
Dicloxacillin (Dynapen)	0.125-0.5 gm q6h ac. po. Cost: 500 mg G $0.73	
Flucloxacillin[x,8] (Floxapen, Lutropin, Staphcil)	0.25-0.5 gm q6h po	In Australia, cholestatic hepatitis (women predominate, age >65, rx mean 2 weeks, onset 3 weeks from starting rx) (Ln 339:679, 1992). 16 deaths since 1980; recommendation: use only in severe infection (Ln 344:676, 1994).
Nafcillin (Unipen, Nafcil)	1.0-2.0 gm q4-6h IV, IM. Cost: 1.0 gm $2.79	Extravasation can result in tissue necrosis. With dosages (over 10% with ≥21-day rx, occasionally WBC <1000/mm³). **Reversible neutropenia (over 10% with ≥21-day rx, occasionally WBC <1000/mm³).**
Oxacillin (Prostaphlin)	1.0-2.0 gm q4-6h IV, IM. Cost: 2.0 gm IV $5.44	**Hepatic dysfunction with ≥12 gm/d.** LFTs usually ↑ 2-24 days after start of rx, reversible. ↑ SGOT in 9/11 HIV+ pts (An M 120:1048, 1994). In children, more rash and lower toxicity with oxacillin as compared to nafcillin (CID 34:50, 2002).
AMINOPENICILLINS		
Amoxicillin (Amoxil, Polymox)	0.5 gm q8h po or 0.875 gm q12h. Cost: 500 mg G $0.16, NB $0.40	IV available in UK, Europe. IV amoxicillin rapidly converted to ampicillin. Rash with infectious mono—see *Ampicillin.*
Amoxicillin/clavulanate (Augmentin)	875/125 mg bid po. Cost: 875/125 mg NB $5.40. Extended release: 1000/125 mg tabs. Dose: 2 tabs po bid	With bid regimen, less clavulanate & less diarrhea (PIDJ 16:463, 1997). Clavulanate assoc. with rare reversible cholestatic hepatitis, esp. men >60 yrs. on rx >2 weeks (AIM 156:1327, 1996). 2 cases anaphylactic reaction to clavulanic acid (J All Clin Immun 96:748, 1995). Comparison **adult** Augmentin products:
AM/CL extra-strength peds suspension	600/42.9 per 5 ml. Dose: 90/6.4 mg/kg/d po. Cost: 75 ml $38.00	Augmentin 500/125 1 tab po tid Augmentin 875/125 1 tab po bid
AM/CL-ER—extended release adult tabs	1000/62.5	Augmentin-XR 1000/62.5 2 tabs po bid
Ampicillin (Principen)	0.25-0.5 gm q6h po. Cost: 500 mg G $0.13, NB $0.17	A maculopapular rash occurs (not urticarial), **not true penicillin allergy**, in 65-100% pts with infectious mono. 90% with chronic lymphocytic leukemia, and 15-20% with allopurinol therapy.
Ampicillin/sulbactam (Unasyn)	1.5-3.0 gm q6h IV. Cost: 3.0 gm NB $16.72 (see Comment)	Supplied in vials: ampicillin 1.0 gm, sulbactam 0.5 gm or amp 2.0 gm, sulbactam 1.0 gm. Antibiotic is not active vs pseudomonas. Total daily dose sulbactam ≤4 gm.
ANTIPSEUDOMONAL PENICILLINS NOTE: Ureidopenicillins (piperacillin, mezlocillin) (congeners of aminopenicillins) have better activity vs enterococci & klebsiella than carboxypenicillins (ticarcillin)		
Mezlocillin (Mezlin)	3.0 gm q4h IV. Cost: 2.0 gm $8.94 1.85 mEq Na⁺/gm	For urinary tract infection: 2.0 gm q6h IV. Cost: 3.0 gm/21 1.85 mEq Na⁺/gm
Piperacillin (Pipracil)	3.0-4.0 gm q4-6h IV (200-300 mg/kg/d up to 500 mg/kg/d). 1.85 mEq Na⁺/gm	
Piperacillin/tazobactam (Zosyn)	3.375 gm q6h IV Cost: 3.375 gm NB $16.52 4.5 gm/8h NB $22.12	Supplied in vials: piperacillin 3.0 gm, tazobactam (TZ) 0.375 gm. In Europe, studied mostly as 4.0 gm pip/0.5 gm tazo. TZ is similar to clavulanate and more active than sulbactam vs β-lactamase inhibitor. Has ↑ activity over pip alone vs gram-negatives and anaerobes. PIP/TZ 3.375 gm q6h is monotherapy **not adequate for serious pseudomonas infections.** Ok when combined with an aminoglycoside (tobramycin).

---

* NOTE: all dosage recommendations are for adults (unless otherwise indicated) and assume normal renal function.

TABLE 9B (2)

CLASS, AGENT, GENERIC NAME (TRADE NAME)	USUAL ADULT DOSAGE (Cost)	ADVERSE REACTIONS, COMMENTS (See Table 9A for Summary)
ANTIPSEUDOMONAL PENICILLINS (continued)		
Ticarcillin disodium (Ticar)	3.0 gm q4-6h IV. Cost: 3.0 gm NB $13.43	Coagulation abnormalities common with large doses, interferes with platelet function, ↑ bleeding times; may be clinically significant in pts with renal failure. (4.75–5.0 mEq Na⁺/gm)
Ticarcillin/clavulanate (Timentin)	3.1 gm q4-6h IV. Cost: 3.1 gm NB $15.40	Supplied in vials: ticarcillin 3.0 gm, clavulanate 0.1 gm/vial. 4.75–5.0 mEq Na⁺/gm. Diarrhea due to clavulanate secondary to clavulanate. Rare reversible cholestatic hepatitis secondary to clavulanate.
CARBAPENEMS		
Ertapenem (Invanz)	1.0 gm qd IV/IM. Cost: 1.0 gm NB $47.69	Lidocaine diluent for IM use; ask about lidocaine allergy.
Imipenem + cilastatin (Primaxin)	0.5 gm q6h IV. Cost: 500 mg NB $33.10	For seizure comment, see footnote 2, Table 9A, page 60. Cross-reactivity in ½ pts with anaphylaxis to penicillin (J All Clin Imm 82:213, 1988). Resistance of P. aeruginosa reported (see Table 5).
Meropenem (Merrem)	0.5–1.0 gm q8h IV Cost: 0.5 gm NB $27.41	For seizure incidence comment, see Table 9A, page 60. Comments: Does not require a dehydropeptidase inhibitor (cilastatin). Activity vs aerobic gm-neg. slightly ↑ over IMP, activity vs staph & strep slightly ↓; anaerobes = to IMP. B. ovatus, B. distasonis more resistant to meropenem.
MONOBACTAMS		
Aztreonam (Azactam)	1.0 gm q8h–2.0 gm q6h IV Cost: 1.0 gm NB $18.89	Can be used in pts with allergy to penicillins/cephalosporins. Animal data and a letter raise concern about cross-reactivity with ceftazidime (Rev Inf Dis 7:613, 1985), side-chains of aztreonam and ceftazidime are identical.
CEPHALOSPORINS (1st parenteral, then oral drugs).		**NOTE:** Prospective data demonstrate correlation between use of cephalosporins (esp. 3rd generation) and ↑ risk of C. difficile toxin-induced diarrhea. May also ↑ risk of colonization with vancomycin-resistant enterococci.
1st Generation, Parenteral		
Cefazolin (Ancef, Kefzol)	0.25 gm q8h–1.5 gm q6h IV. IM. Cost: 1.0 gm G $1.90, NB $5.59	Do not give into lateral ventricles—seizures!
2nd Generation, Parenteral		
Cefamandole (Mandol)	0.5 gm q8h–2.0 gm q4h IV. IM. Cost: 1.0 gm NB $9.06	Mild ↑ in BUN, creatinine esp. in pts >50 yrs. Concurrent furosemide may ↑ reaction rates (34%). Rare disulfiram-like reactions after alcohol. Contains Al⁺⁺⁺: toxic levels can occur, esp. with renal insufficiency.
Cefotetan (Cefotan)	1–3 gm q12h IV. IM. (Max. dose not >6 gm qd). Cost: 1.0 gm NB $11.16	3 cases anaphylaxis after 2.0 gm IV over 15 min. (Am J Ob Gyn 59:125, 1988). Active vs B. fragilis, Prevotella bivius. Prevotella disiens (most common in pelvic infections).
Cefoxitin (Mefoxin)	1.0 gm q6h–2.0 gm q4h IV. IM. Cost: 1.0 gm IV, 1.0 gm G $10.44, NB $11.38	In vitro may induce ↑ β-lactamase, esp. in Enterobacter sp.; clinical significance ?
Cefuroxime (Kefurox, Zinacef)	0.75–1.5 gm q8h IV/IM. Cost: 1.5 gm IV NB $13.13–$13.80	More stable vs staphylococcal β-lactamase than ceftazidime.
3rd Generation, Parenteral—One study correlated use of P Ceph 3 drugs with incidence of C. difficile toxin diarrhea (Am J Gastro 89:519, 1994)		
Cefoperazone (Cefobid)	2.0 gm q12h–4 gm q6h IV. Pyelonephritis: 1.0 gm q12h IV. Cost: 2.0 gm NB $34.94	Maximum dose 8.0 gm qd. Q8h dosage required for Pseudomonas sp. Disulfiram-like reactions after alcohol, up to 48 hrs after completion of antibiotic rx.
Cefotaxime (Claforan)	1.0 gm q8-12h to 2.0 gm q4h IV. Cost: 2.0 gm NB $22.00	Maximum daily dose: 12 gm.
Ceftazidime (Ceptaz, Fortaz, Tazicef, Tazidime)	1.0 gm q8-12h to 2.0 gm q6h IV. Cost: 2.0 gm NB $28.45–43.30	Excessive use may result in ↑ incidence of C. difficile-assoc. diarrhea and/or selection of vancomycin-resistant E. faecium. Ceftaz is susceptible to extended-spectrum cephalosporinases (CID 27:76 & 81, 1998).
Ceftizoxime (Cefizox)	1.0 gm q8–12h to 4.0 gm q6h IV. Cost: 2.0 gm NB $24.64	Maximum daily dose 12 gm in vitro active vs B. fragilis, dependent on testing method.

* NOTE: all dosage recommendations are for adults (unless otherwise indicated) and assume normal renal function.

(See page 68 for footnotes and abbreviations)

TABLE 9B (3)

CLASS, AGENT, GENERIC NAME (TRADE NAME)	USUAL ADULT DOSAGE (Cost)	ADVERSE REACTIONS, COMMENTS (See Table 9A for Summary)
CEPHALOSPORINS, 3rd Generation, Parenteral (continued)		
Ceftriaxone (Rocephin)	Commonly used IV dosage in adults: < Age 65: 2.0 gm once daily > Age 65: 1.0 gm once daily Purulent meningitis: 2.0 gm q12h. Can give **IM** in 1% lidocaine. Cost: 1.0 gm NB $40.18	Dosage: 2.0 gm IV qd gives better tissue levels than 1.0 gm q12h (overcomes protein binding) (see footnote[1]). "Pseudocholethiasis" "2" to sludge in gallbladder by ultrasound (50%), symptomatic (9%) (NEJM 322:1821, 1990). More likely with ≥2 gm/d with pt on total parenteral nutrition and not eating (AnIM 115:712, 1991). Clinical significance still unclear but has led to cholecystectomy (JID 17:356, 1995) and gallstone pancreatitis (Ln 17:662, 1998).
4th Generation, Parenteral		
Cefepime (Maxipime)	1.0–2.0 gm q12h IV Cost: 2.0 gm NB $32.25	Active vs P. aeruginosa and many strains of Enterobacter, serratia, C. freundii resistant to ceftazidime, cefotaxime, aztreonam (CID 20:56, 1995). More active vs S. aureus than 3rd generation cephalosporins.
Cefpirome[AUS] (HR 810)	1.0–2.0 gm q12h IV	Similar to cefepime: ↑ activity vs enterobacteriaceae, P. aeruginosa, Gm + organisms. Anaerobes less active than cefoxitin, more active than cefotax or ceftaz.
Oral Cephalosporins		
1st Generation, Oral		
Cefadroxil (Duricef)	0.5–1.0 gm q12h po. Cost: 0.5 gm G $3.32. NB $4.73	The oral cephalosporins are generally safe. **Patients with a history of IgE-mediated allergic reactions to a penicillin (e.g. anaphylaxis, angioneurotic edema, immediate urticaria) should not receive a cephalosporin.** If the history is a "measles-like" rash to a penicillin, available data suggest a 5–10% risk of rash in such patients; there is no enhanced risk of anaphylaxis.
Cephalexin (Keflex, Keftab, generic)	0.25–0.5 gm q6h po. Cost: 0.5 gm NB $3.40, G $0.21	Any of the cephalosporins can result in C. difficile toxin-mediated diarrhea/enterocolitis. The reported frequency of nausea/vomiting and non-C. difficile toxin diarrhea is summarized in Table 9A.
Cephradine (Velosef, generic)	0.25–0.5 gm q6h po. Cost: 0.5 gm NB $1.86, G $1.00	There are few drug-specific adverse effects, e.g. **Cefaclor**: Serum sickness-like reaction 0.1 –0.5%—arthralgia, rash, erythema multiforme but no adenopathy, proteinuria or demonstrable immune complexes. Anecdotal reports of similar reaction to loracarbef. Appear due to mixture of drug
2nd Generation, Oral		
Cefaclor (Ceclor)	0.25–0.5 gm q8h po. Cost: 0.25 gm NB $3.30.	biotransformation and genetic susceptibility (Ped Pharm & Therap 125:805, 1994).
Cefaclor-ER (Ceclor CD)	0.375–0.5 gm q12h po. Cost: 0.5 gm $4.40	**Cefdinir**: Drug-iron complex causes red stools in roughly 1% of pts.
Cefprozil (Cefzil)	0.25–0.5 gm q12h po. Cost: 0.5 gm NB $7.65	**Cefditoren**: Use increases renal excretion of carnitine. **potential carnitine deficiency**. Contains caseinate (milk protein): **avoid if milk allergy**. Need gastric acid for optimal absorption.
Cefuroxime axetil po (Ceftin)	0.125–0.5 gm q12h po. Cost: 0.5 gm NB $8.00	**Cefpodoxime**: There are rare reports of acute liver injury, bloody diarrhea, pulmonary infiltrates with eosinophilia.
Loracarbef (Lorabid)	0.4 gm q12h po. Cost: 0.4 gm NB $5.90	
Cefdinir (Omnicef)	300 mg q12h or 600 mg qd. Cost: 300 mg $4.12	
3rd Generation, Oral		
Cefditoren (Spectracef)	200–400 mg bid po. Cost: 200 mg $[? $?]	
Cefixime (Suprax)	0.2–0.4 gm q12–24h po. Cost: 0.4 gm NB $8.53	
Cefpodoxime proxetil (Vantin)	0.1–0.2 gm q12h po. Cost: 0.2 gm NB $4.25	
Ceftibuten (Cedax)	0.4 gm qd po. Cost: 0.4 gm NB $8.25	

AMINOGLYCOSIDES AND RELATED ANTIBIOTICS—See Table 9C, page 70, and Table 17, page 127

[1] The age-related dosing of ceftriaxone is based on unpublished pharmacokinetic data that show an age-related reduction in hepatic clearance of ceftriaxone; hence, there is possible underdosing in younger pts, therefore the suggested 2 gm/day dose.
(See page 68 for footnotes and abbreviations) * NOTE: all dosage recommendations are for adults (unless otherwise indicated) and assume normal renal function.

TABLE 9B (4)

CLASS, AGENT, GENERIC NAME (TRADE NAME)	USUAL ADULT DOSAGE (Cost)	ADVERSE REACTIONS, COMMENTS (See Table 9A for Summary)
GLYCOPEPTIDES		
Teicoplanin[NUS] (Targocid)	For septic arthritis—maintenance dose 12 mg/kg/d; for endocarditis—trough serum levels >20 µg/ml required (12 mg/kg q12h x3 loading dose, then 12 mg/kg/d)	Hypersensitivity: fever (at 3 mg/kg 2.2%, at 24 mg/kg 8.2%), Marked ↓ platelets (high dose ≥15 mg/kg/d). Red neck syndrome less common than with vancomycin (JAC 32:792, 1993)
Vancomycin (Vancocin)	15 mg/kg q12h IV; 125 mg q6h po; intrathecal 5–10 mg q48–72h; Cost: 500 mg IV G $7.31, NB $17.53. Oral 125 mg (capsule) Cost $8.35. For intrathecal use, see Comment. One report on safety & efficacy of once-daily vanco, 30 mg/kg (JAC 49:155, 2002).	Measure serum levels if: planned dose ≥20 gm/d, rapidly changing renal function, chronic renal failure. Target levels: peak 20–50 µg/ml, trough 5–10 µg/ml. Rapid infusion (over <1 hr) can cause non-specific histamine release manifest as angioedema, flushed skin ("red neck syndrome"), or hypotension. Can continue vanco but infuse over 1–2 hrs. Ototoxicity and nephrotoxicity now rare unless vanco given with an aminoglycoside; aminoglycoside amplifies the risk of nephrotoxicity. Neutropenia, rash occur. Rarely, association with linear IgA bullous dermatosis (AnIM 129:507, 1998). **Intrathecal vanco** occ. used for meningitis and/or ventriculitis/shunt infections. **Initial** dosing ranges from 5–10 mg/d (infants) to 10–20 mg/d (children/adults) adjusted to achieve trough CSF conc. of 10–20 µg/ml (AnPharmacotherapy 27:912, 1993).
CHLORAMPHENICOL, CLINDAMYCIN(S), ERYTHROMYCIN GROUP, KETOLIDES, OXAZOLIDINONES, QUINUPRISTIN/DALFOPRISTIN (SYNERCID)		
Chloramphenicol (Chloromycetin)	0.25–1 gm po/IV q6h to max. of 4 gm/day. Cost: 1.0 gm IV $7.95; po $0.86	No oral drug distributed in U.S. Hematologic: (↓ RBC – 1/3 pts, aplastic anemia 1:21,600 courses). Gray baby syndrome in premature infants, anaphylactoid reactions, optic atrophy or neuropathy (very rare), digital paresthesias, minor disulfiram-like reactions.
Clindamycin (Cleocin)	0.15–0.45 gm q6h po; 600–900 mg q8h IV, IM. Cost: 150 mg po NB $1.19, 600 mg IV NB $3.94	Lincomycin (Lincocin)	0.5 gm q6–8h po, 0.6 gm q8h IV, IM. Based on number of exposed pts, these drugs are the most frequent cause of C. difficile toxin-mediated diarrhea. In most severe form can cause pseudomembranous colitis/toxic megacolon
Erythromycin Group (Review drug interactions before use) Ref. Mayo Clin Proc 74:613, 1999		Motilin is gastric hormone that activates duodenal/jejunal receptors to initiate peristalsis. Erythro (E) esters, both po and IV (esp. estolate), stimulate motilin receptors and cause uncoordinated peristalsis with resultant 20–25% incidence of anorexia, nausea and vomiting (Gut 33:397, 1992). Less binding and GI distress with azithromycin/clarithromycin.
Azithromycin (Zithromax)	po: 0.5 gm on day 1, then 0.25 gm po qd on days 2–5 po. Cost: 250 mg $6.96. IV: 0.5 gm/d. Cost: $25.23	Systemic erythro in 1st 2 wks of life associated with infantile hypertrophic pyloric stenosis (J Peds 139:380, 2001). Frequent drug-drug interactions: see Table 21, page 138. Ex: Cisapride + erythro or clarithro can prolong QT interval, ↑ Q-t intervals, torsades de pointes, or ventricular tachycardia. Erythro alone can prolong QT interval (Chest 115:983, 1999), esp. in women (JAMA 280:1774, 1998).
Base and esters (Erythro, Ilosone) IV name: E. lactobionate	0.25 gm q6h–0.5 gm q6h po. IV 15–20 mg/kg up to 4.0 gm od. Infuse over 30 or more minutes. Cost: po 250 mg base G $0.18, stearate $0.18, estolate $0.31; ESS 400 $0.23 IV 1.0 gm NB $17.58	Cholestatic hepatitis in approx. 1:1000 adults (not children) given E. estolate. Transient reversible tinnitus or deafness with ≥4 gm/d of erythro IV in pts with renal or hepatic impairment. Reported with ≥600 mg/d of azithro (CID 24:76, 1997).
Clarithromycin (Biaxin) or clarithro extended release (Biaxin XL)	0.5 gm q12h po. Cost: 500 mg $4.15 Extended release: Two 0.5 gm tabs po/d Cost: 500 mg ER $4.42	Dosages of oral erythro preparations expressed as base equivalents. With differences in absorption/biotransformation, variable amounts of erythro required to achieve same free erythro serum level, e.g. 400 mg E ethyl succinate = 250 mg E base.
Dirithromycin (Dynabac)	0.5 gm po qd. Cost: 250 mg $3.87	Macrolide-induced Churg-Strauss syndrome reported in an atopic pt (Ln 350:563, 1997). Dirithromycin available as once-daily macrolide. **Very low serum levels; do not use if potential for bacteremic disease.**
Ketolide		
Telithromycin (Ketek)	Two 400 mg tabs po qd—anticipated dose. 400 mg tabs.	First available antimicrobial. Diarrhea, nausea/vomiting, & dizziness most common side-effects. Drug-drug interactions with cisapride, digoxin, itraconazole, and ketoconazole—see Table 21, page 140. No dosage adjustment necessary for age or hepatic insufficiency; dose reduction for severe renal insufficiency (see Table 17).

(See page 68 for footnotes and abbreviations)   *NOTE: all dosage recommendations are for adults (unless otherwise indicated) and assume normal renal function.*

TABLE 9B (5)

CLASS, AGENT, GENERIC NAME (TRADE NAME)	USUAL ADULT DOSAGE (Cost)	ADVERSE REACTIONS, COMMENTS (See Table 9A for Summary)
CHLORAMPHENICOL, CLINDAMYCIN(S), ERYTHROMYCIN GROUP, KETOLIDES, OXAZOLIDINONES, QUINUPRISTIN/DALFOPRISTIN (SYNERCID) (continued)		
Linezolid (Zyvox)	PO or IV dose: 600 mg q12h all indications except 400 mg q12h for uncomplicated skin infections. Available as IV solution, oral suspension (100 mg/ml), & IV solution. 600 mg po $56, 600 mg IV $76	First oxazolidinone. Nausea/vomiting & diarrhea most common adverse effects. **Rx duration dependent reversible thrombocytopenia, neutropenia, & anemia: monitor blood counts if rx beyond 2 weeks** (CID 34:695, 2002). Tongue discoloration (CID 35:1321, 2002). Inhibitor of monoamine oxidase; risk of severe hypertension if taken with foods rich in tyramine. Be careful with drugs containing pseudoephedrine, phenylpropanolamine. SSRIs.* Serotonin syndrome (fever, agitation, mental status changes, tremors) reported (CID 34:1651, 2002)
Quinupristin + dalfopristin (Synercid)	Dosage: 7.5 mg/kg q8h IV q21–72 d. Cost: 350 mg–150 mg $107.43	Venous irritation (5%), none with central venous line. Asymptomatic * in unconjugated bilirubin. Arthralgia 2%. Drug-drug interactions: Cyclosporine, nifedipine, midazolam
TETRACYCLINES (Mayo Clin Proc 74:727, 1999)		
Doxycycline (Vibramycin, Doryx, Monodox)	0.1 gm po or IV q12h. Cost IV q12h po $0.08–0.11, NB $2.34; 100 mg IV NB $4.16	Similar to other tetracyclines. ↑ nausea on empty stomach. Erosive esophagitis, esp. if taken hs. Phototoxicity + but less than with tetracycline. Deposition in teeth less. Can be used in patients with renal failure.
Minocycline (Minocin)	0.1 gm q12h po. Cost: 100 mg 53 $0.80; NB $3.60	Comments: Effective in treatment and prophylaxis of malaria, syphilis, and typhus fevers. Similar to other tetracyclines. Vestibular symptoms (30–90%) in some groups; none in others). (Vertigo 33%, ataxia 43%; nausea 50%, vomiting 3%), women more frequently than men. Hypersensitivity pneumonitis, reversible. –34 cases reported (BMJ 310:1520, 1995).
Tetracycline, Oxytetracycline (Terramycin)	0.25–0.5 gm q6h po. 0.5–1.0 gm q12h IV. 250 mg po $0.06	Comments: More effective than other tetracyclines vs staph and in prophylaxis of meningococcal disease. P. acnes: many resistant to other tetracyclines., not to mino.; Active vs Nocardia asteroides. Mycobacterium marinum. **Toxicity:** GI (oxy 19%, tetra 4%), anaphylactoid reaction (rare), deposition in teeth, negative N balance, hepatotoxicity, enamel ageneris, pseudotumor cerebri/encephalopathy. Outdated drug, Fanconi syndrome. See drug-drug interactions, Table 21. **Contraindicated in pregnancy, hepatotoxicity in mother, transplacental to fetus.** Comments: IV dosage over 2.0 gm/d may be associated with fatal hepatotoxicity
FLUOROQUINOLONES (FQs)		
Ciprofloxacin (Cipro) and Ciprofloxacin-extended release (Cipro XL)	400 mg IV q12h. **Urinary tract infection:** 250 mg bid po or Cipro 500 mg bid po. Parenteral rx 200–400 mg q12h IV. Cost: 500 mg po $4.95; 400 mg IV/$39.00. 400 mg IV or po qd. Cost: 400 mg po $8.00; 400 mg IV $38.20	**Children:** No FQ approved for use under age 16 based on cartilage injury in immature animals. No use,,uvocal arthropathy in humans (CID 25:1196, 1997). For use of FQs in children: PIDJ 18:467, 1999. **Tendinitis:** Suggested association of FQs with tendinitis and tendon rupture (NEJM 332:193, 1995; Arth Care & Res 45:235, 2001). Lung transplant recipients may be at ↑ risk (Eur Respir J 19:469, 2002). Achilles tendon most frequent. **QTc (corrected QT) interval prolongation:** QT >500 msec or >60 msec from baseline is considered possible with any FQ. ↑ QTc can lead to torsades de pointes and ventricular fibrillation. Risk varies with specific FQ (data limited); greatest with sparfloxacin, least with ciprofloxacin (Pharmacother 21:1468, 2001; JAC 49:593, 2002; CID 34:861, 2002). Risk ↑ in women, ↓ K+, ↓ Mg++, bradycardia.
Gatifloxacin (Tequin)	250–750 mg po qd	
Levofloxacin (Levaquin)	260–750 mg qd po or IV. Cost: 500 mg po $8.00; 500 mg IV $41.39	Updates online: www.qtdrugs.org, www.torsades.org. **CNS toxicity:** Poorly understood. Varies from mild (lightheadedness) to moderate (confusion) to severe (seizures). May be aggravated by NSAIDs.
Lomefloxacin (Maxaquin)	400 mg qd po. Cost: 400 mg $7.38	
Moxifloxacin (Avelox)	400 mg IV or po qd. Cost: 400 mg po $9.00; IV $44.00	
Ofloxacin (Floxin)	200–400 mg bid po. Cost: 400 mg po $5.44	FQs can cause false-positive urine assay for opiates (JAMA 286:3115, 2001).

Avoid concomitant drugs with potential to prolong QTc:

Antiarrhythmics:	Anti-infectives:	Anti-Hypertensives:	CNS Drugs	Misc.
Amiodarone	Clarithro	Bepridil	Fluoxetine	Naratriptan
Disopyramide	Erythro	Isradipine	Sertraline	Sumatriptan
Dofetilide	Foscarnet	Nicardipine	Tricyclics	Zolmitriptan
Flecainide	Mefloquine	Moexipril	Venlafaxine	Dolasetron
Ibutilide	Pentamidine		Haloperidol	Droperidol
Procainamide			Phenothiazines	Fosphenytoin
Quinidine			Pimozide	Indapamide
Sotalol			Risperidone	Tacrolimus
			Quetiapine	Tizanidine
			Ziprasidone	

[1] SSRI = selective serotonin reuptake inhibitors, e.g., fluoxetine (Prozac).   * NOTE: not all dosage recommendations are for adults (unless otherwise indicated) and assume normal renal function.

(See page 68 for footnotes and abbreviations)

TABLE 9B (6)

CLASS, AGENT, GENERIC NAME (TRADE NAME)	USUAL ADULT DOSAGE (Cost)	ADVERSE REACTIONS, COMMENTS (See Table 9A for Summary)
FLUOROQUINOLONES *(continued)*		
Trovafloxacin (Trovan) Trovafloxacin mesylate tabs po (Trovan) & alatrofloxacin mesylate IV (Trovan IV) **See Comment**	Adult IV dosage is 200–300 mg/d. NOTE: Reduce dose in pts with chronic liver disease *(see package insert)*. Cost: 200 mg IV $40.08, 200 mg po $7.81	In a small number of pts, trova associated with serious liver injury leading to liver transplant and/or death. Reported after both short- & long-term treatment. Rx over 2 wks assoc. with ↑ risk liver injury. Recommended that trova use be reserved for serious life- or limb-threatening infection in pts in hospital or nursing care facility.
MISCELLANEOUS AGENTS		
Daptomycin	4–6 mg/kg given once daily under study	Not FDA-approved. For compassionate use, call 781-860-8660.
Fosfomycin (Monurol)	3.0 gm mixed with water po x1 dose Cost $32.48	Generally well-tolerated. Diarrhea in 9% of study population compared to 6% of pts given nitrofurantoin and 2.3% given TMP/SMX. If given with metoclopramide (Reglan), ↓ serum level.
Fusidic acid[NUS] (Fucidin)	500 mg tid po, IV (Leo Laboratories, Denmark)	Mild GI: occ. skin rash, jaundice (17% with IV, 6% with po). (None in CSF, <1% in urine).
Immune globulin IV therapy	Dosage, frequency vary with the indication. At least 7 manufacturers. Cost by trade name: Sandoglobulin 12 gm-$697, Gammar IV-$800, Gamimune-N 10 gm $900, Gammagard S/D 10 gm $854, Panglobulin 12 gm $990, Venoglobulin 10 gm $900, Iveegam 10 gm $816	At present, 6 FDA-approved indications: primary immune-def., recent bone marrow transplant, B-cell lymphocytic leukemia, Kawasaki syndrome, pediatric HIV. Many other enclosed uses (*MMWR 48:159, 1999*). Reported adverse effects range from 1–15%. Fever, headache, myalgia. N/V relate to rate of infusion, mild, & self-limited. More serious: anaphylactoid reactions, thromboemboli, aseptic meningitis, & renal injury (in 6.7%, *CJM 93:751, 2000*).
Methenamine hippurate (Hiprex, Urex)	1.0 gm q6h po. Cost: 1.0 gm $1.39 (= 480 mg methenamine)	Nausea and vomiting, skin rash or dysuria. Overall ~3%. Methenamine requires (pH ≤5) urine to liberate formaldehyde.
Methenamine mandelate (Mandelamine)	1.0 gm q6h po (480 mg methenamine). Cost: 1.0 gm NB $0.69	Limited place in therapy, useful in suppressive therapy when original infecting organisms have been cleared. Do not use for pyelonephritis. *Comment:* Fluids should not be forced, as concentration of formaldehyde may fall below inhibitory concentrations. Of no value in pts with continuously draining urethral catheter. If urine pH >5.0, co-administer ascorbic acid (1–2 gm q4h) to acidify the urine. Cranberry juice (1200–4000 ml/day) has been used, results ↑.
Metronidazole (Flagyl) *Int'l Mayo Clin Proc 74:825, 1999*	Anaerobic infections, usually IV, 7.5 mg/kg (~500 mg) q6h (not to exceed 4.0 gm/day). With long T½, can use IV at 15 mg/kg q12h. If life-threatening, use loading dose of 15 mg/kg IV. Oral dose: 500 mg tid. Cost: 250 mg tab G $0.33, NB $2.00; 500 mg IV G $2.76, NB $12.38; 70 gm vaginal gel $44.82 Ext. release 750 mg $9.98	Can be given rectally (enema or suppository). In pts with decompensated liver disease (manifest by ↓ alb., ↑ ascites, encephalopathy, ↑ prothrombin time, ↓ serum albumin) ↑½ prolonged, unless dose ↓ by approx. ½, side-effects ↑. Absorbed into serum from vaginal gel. **Neurol:** headache, rare paresthesias or peripheral neuropathy, ataxia, seizures, aseptic meningitis; report of reversible metro-induced cerebellar lesions (*NEJM 346:68, 2002*). **Avoid alcohol during & 48 hrs after (disulfiram-like reaction).** Very dark urine (common but harmless). Skin: urticaria. Mutagenic in Ames test. Tumorigenic in animals (high doses over lifetime). No evidence of risk in man. No teratogenicity.
Mupirocin (Bactroban)	Skin ointment 2%: Apply tid. Cost: Apply bid. Nasal ointment 2%: apply bid. 100 mg q6h po: Cost: 100 mg G $1.28, NB $1.86.	Skin ointment 2%, apply bid. Nasal ointment 2%, apply tid, itching 1%, rash, contact dermatitis <1%.
Nitrofurantoin	for long-term UTI suppression: 50–100 mg at bedtime	Absorption ↑ with meals. Increased activity in acid urine, much reduced activity at pH 8 or over. Not effective in endstage renal disease (*JAC 33/Suppl. A:121, 1994*). Nausea and vomiting, hypersensitivity, peripheral neuropathy. Pulmonary reactions with chronic (30 acute ARDS type; chronic **desquamative interstitial pneumonia**, **pulmonary fibrosis**), elevated cholestasis & possible chronic active hepatitis. Hemolytic anemia in G6PD deficiency.
macrocrystals (Macrodantin)	100 mg qid po. Cost: 100 mg $1.45	Contraindicated in renal failure. Should not be used in infants <1 month of age.
monohydrate/macrocrystals (Macrobid)		Efficacy of Macrobid 100 mg bid = Macrodantin 50 mg qid. Adverse effects 5.6%, less nausea than with Macrodantin.

(See page 68 for footnotes and abbreviations)   *NOTE: all dosage recommendations are for adults (unless otherwise indicated) and assume normal renal function.*

TABLE 9B (7)

CLASS, AGENT, GENERIC NAME (TRADE NAME)	USUAL ADULT DOSAGE (Cost)	ADVERSE REACTIONS, COMMENTS (See Table 9A for Summary)
MISCELLANEOUS AGENTS (continued)		
Sulfonamides [e.g. sulfisoxazole (Gantrisin), sulfamethoxazole (Gantanol)]	Sulfisoxazole (Gantrisin) peds suspension: Cost 500 mg/5 ml: 480 ml $42.22	**Short-acting are best:** high urine concentration and good solubility at acid pH. More active in alkaline urine. **Allergic reactions:** skin rash, drug fever, pruritus, photosensitization. Periarteritis nodosa & SLE, Stevens-Johnson syndrome, serum sickness syndrome, myocarditis. Neurotoxicity (psychosis, neuritis), hepatic toxicity. Blood dyscrasias; usually agranulocytosis. Crystalluria. Nausea & vomiting, headache, dizziness, lassitude, mental depression, acidosis, sulfhemoglobin. Hemolytic anemia in G6PD deficient & unstable hemoglobins (Hb Zurich). Do not use in newborn infants or in women near term, ↑ frequency of kernicterus (binds to albumin, blocking binding of bilirubin to albumin).
Trimethoprim (Trimpex and others)	100 mg tab tab q12h or 200 mg (2 tabs) po q24h. Cost: 100 mg NB $0.90, G $0.15	Frequent side-effects are rash and pruritus. Rash in 3% pts at 100 mg bid; 6.7% at 200 mg qd. Rare reports of photosensitivity, exfoliative dermatitis, Stevens-Johnson syndrome, toxic epidermal necrosis, and aseptic meningitis (CID 19:431, 1994). Check drug interaction with phenytoin. Increases serum K⁺ (see TMP/SMX Comments). TMP can ↑ homocysteine blood levels (LjI 352:1827, 1998).
Trimethoprim (TMP)/ Sulfamethoxazole (SMX) (Bactrim, Septra). Single-strength (SS) is 80 TMP/400 SMX, double-strength (DS) 160 TMP/800 SMX	Standard po rx (UTI, otitis media): 1 DS tablet bid. P. carinii: see Table 12, page 93. IV rx (base on TMP component): standard 8–10 mg/kg/d divided q6h, q8h, or q12h. For shigellosis: 2.5 mg/kg IV q6h. Cost: 160/800 po G $0.09, NB $3.51 SI.61–1.72; 160/800 IV $11.21	Adverse reactions in 10% or more of pts: GI and skin. GI: nausea, vomiting, anorexia. Skin: Rash, urticaria, photosensitivity. Less often but more serious (1–10%): Stevens-Johnson syndrome and toxic epidermal necrolysis. Skin adverse reactions may represent toxic metabolites of SMX and ↓ glutathione rather than allergy (An Pharm 32:381, 1998). See other sulfonamide adverse reactions above. TMP competes with creatinine for tubular secretion and serum creatinine can ↑; TMP also blocks distal renal tubule reabsorption of Na⁺ and secretion of K⁺; ↑ serum K⁺ in 21% of pts (AnIM 124:316, 1996). TMP/SMX suspected etiology of aseptic meningitis, esp. TMP component (CID 19:431, 1994). TMP/SMX contains sulfites and may trigger asthma in sulfite-sensitive pts. One of most frequent drugs to cause thrombocytopenia (AnIM 129:886, 1998).

* Cost to pharmacist according to manufacturer's listing in 2002 DRUG TOPICS RED BOOK, Medical Economics (average wholesale price).

Abbreviations: G = generic, **NB** = name brand, **MRSA** = methicillin-resistant Staph. aureus, **APAG** = antipseudomonal aminoglycoside, **NUS** = not available in the U.S.

* NOTE: all dosage recommendations are for adults (unless otherwise indicated) and assume normal renal function.

TABLE 9C
AMINOGLYCOSIDE ONCE-DAILY AND MULTIPLE DAILY DOSING REGIMENS
(See Table 17, page 127, if estimated creatinine clearance <90 ml/min.)

General: Dosage given as both once-daily (OD) and multiple daily dose (MDD) regimens.
Pertinent formulae:
(1) Estimated creatinine clearance (CrCl): $\frac{140-age)(ideal\ body\ weight\ in\ kg)}{(72)(serum\ creatinine)}$ = CrCl for men in ml/min; multiply answer × 0.85 for CrCl of women

(2) Ideal body weight (IBW)—Females: 45.5 kg + 2.3 kg per inch over 5' = weight in kg
Males: 50.0 kg + 2.3 kg per inch over 5' = weight in kg
(3) Obesity adjustment: use if actual body weight (ABW) is >30% above IBW. To calculate adjusted dosing weight in kg: IBW = 0.4(ABW–IBW) = adjusted weight (CID 25:112, 1997)

DRUG	MDD AND OD REGIMENS/ TARGETED PEAK (P) AND TROUGH (T) SERUM LEVELS	COST Name Brand (NB), Generic (G)	COMMENTS For more data on once-daily dosing, see AJM 105:182, 1998, and Table 17, page 127
Gentamicin (Garamycin), Tobramycin (Nebcin)	MDD: 2 mg/kg load, then 1.7 mg/kg q8h P 4–10 µg/ml, T 1–2 µg/ml ⋯ OD: 5.1 (if critically ill) mg/kg q24h P 16–24 µg/ml, T <1 µg/ml	Gentamicin: 80 mg NB $5.76, G $1.60 Tobramycin: 80 mg NB $7.28, G $11.96	All aminoglycosides have potential to cause tubular necrosis and renal failure, deafness due to cochlear toxicity, vertigo due to damage to vestibular organs, and rarely neuromuscular blockade. Risk minimal with oral or topical application due to small % absorption unless tissues altered by disease.
Kanamycin (Kantrex), Amikacin (Amikin), Streptomycin	MDD: 7.5 mg/kg q12h P 15–30 µg/ml, T 5–10 µg/ml ⋯ OD: 15 mg/kg q24h P 56–64 µg/ml, T <1 µg/ml	Kanamycin: 500 mg NB $0.25 Amikacin: 500 mg NB $32.89, G $8.75 Streptomycin: 1.0 gm $6.90	Risk of nephrotoxicity ↑ with concomitant administration of cyclosporine, vancomycin, ampho B, radiocontrast. Risk of nephrotoxicity ↓ by concurrent AP Pen and perhaps by once-daily dosing method (especially if baseline renal function normal).
Netilmicin[NUS]	MDD: 2.0 mg/kg q8h P 4–10 µg/ml, T 1–2 µg/ml ⋯ OD: 6.5 mg/kg q24h P 22–30 µg/ml, T <1 µg/ml	2 gm NB $28.21	In general, same factors influence risk of ototoxicity. NOTE: There is no known method to eliminate risk of aminoglycoside nephro/ototoxicity. Proper rx attempts to ↓ the % risk. The clinical trial data of OD aminoglycosides have been reviewed extensively by meta-analysis (CID 24:816, 1997).
Isepamicin[NUS]	Only OD: Severe infections 15 mg/kg q24h, less severe 8 mg/kg q24h		Serum levels: Collect serum for a peak serum level (PSL) exactly 1 hr after the start of the infusion of the 3rd dose. In critically ill pts, it is reasonable to measure the PSL after the 1st dose as well as later doses as volume of distribution and renal function may change rapidly.
Spectinomycin (Trobicin)	2.0 gm IM x1–gonococcal infections	500 mg G $0.96	Other dosing methods and references: For once-daily 7 mg/kg of gentamicin—Hartford Hospital method, see AAC 39:650, 1995.
Neomycin—oral	Prophylaxis GI surgery: 1.0 gm po x3 with erythro, see Table 15B, page 123 For hepatic coma: 4–12 gm/d. po		

Tobramycin—inhaled (Tobi): See Cystic fibrosis, Table 1, page 28. Adverse effects few: transient voice alteration (13%) and transient tinnitus (3%). Cost: 300 mg $44.78
Paromomycin—oral: See Entamoeba and Cryptosporidia, Table 12, page 90. Cost: 250 mg $2.81

[1] Estimated CrCl invalid if serum creatinine <0.6 mg/dl. Consultation suggested.

TABLE 10A: TREATMENT OF FUNGAL, ACTINOMYCOTIC, AND NOCARDIAL INFECTIONS—ANTIMICROBIAL AGENTS OF CHOICE[*]

(See Table 10B for Amphotericin B Preparations and Adverse Effects)

TYPE OF INFECTION/ORGANISM/ SITE OF INFECTION	ANTIMICROBIAL AGENTS OF CHOICE		COMMENTS
	PRIMARY	ALTERNATIVE	
Actinomycosis (CID 26:1255, 1998) (A. israelii most common, also A. naeslundii, A. viscosus, A. odontolyticus, A. meyeri, A. gerencseriae)	**Ampicillin** 50 mg/kg/d IV x 4-6 wks, then 0.5 gm **amoxicillin** tid po x 6 mos. **Penicillin G** 10-20 million u/d IV x 4-6 wks, then **penicillin V** 2-4 gm/d po for 6-12 mos	**Doxycycline** or **ceftriaxone** or **clinda-mycin** or **erythromycin** **Chloramphenicol** 50-60 mg/kg/d div q6h IV (or po) has been recommended for CNS infection in pen-allergic pts.	Tuboovarian abscesses may complicate IUDs. Removal of IUD is primary rx. With abscesses or fistulae, surgery often required. While penicillin G and ampicillin IV have been effective, with home IV therapy agents given po, e.g. ceftriaxone, are more practical (CID 19:161, 1994). **Surgery may be necessary for hemoptysis** (An Thor Surg 74:185, 2002)
Aspergillosis (A. fumigatus most common, also A. flavus and others) (CID 30:696, 2000) Allergic bronchopulmonary	**Corticosteroids**	**Itraconazole** 200 mg po qd or bid x8 mos.	Corticosteroids primary rx. Itraconazole, (CID 100:813, 1991) & in 55 pts Itra + steroid requirements, ↑ pulmonary function & exercise tolerance and improved chest x-ray (NEJM 342:756, 2000)
Allergic fungal sinusitis (Laryngoscope 111:1006, 2001): relapsing chronic sinusitis, nasal polyps without bony inva-sion. >50% have hx allergic condition (asthma, eczema or allergic rhinitis), ↑ IgE levels and isolation of Aspergillus sp. or other dematiaceous sp. (Alternaria, Cladosporium, etc.)	Rx controversial: systemic cortico-steroids + surgical debridement (80% respond but 2/3 relapse)	For failures might tv **itra** 200 mg po bid x12 mos. (CID 31:303, 2000)	
Aspergilloma (fungus ball)	Efficacy of antimicrobial agents not proven (po) of benefit in any study. Itraconazole (CID 23:697, 1996). Another case responded to itra 200 mg/d x3		Surgery if hemoptysis becomes massive (post-op complications 25%)
Invasive, pulmonary (IPA) or extrapulmonary Occurs post-transplantation and post-chemotherapy in neutropenic pts (BMT, leukemia, lymphoma, etc.) or late (20-180 days) complication in allogeneic bone marrow transplantation: median survival 36 days, but overall mortality rates vary from 78-94% (CID 28:322, 1998). Typical x-ray/CT lung lesions (halo sign, cavitation, or mycotic lung sequestration) have ~90% positive predictive value for inva-sive pulmonary aspergillosis (CID 31:859, 2000). See CID 26:781, 1998, for excellent review. Test that detects aspergillus galacto-mannan in plasma looks hopeful (Blood 97:1604, 2001)	**Voriconazole** 6 mg/kg IV q12h on day 1, then either (4 mg/kg IV q12h) or (200 mg po q12h for body weight ≥40 kg, cut 100 mg po q12h for body weight <40 kg) or **Ampho B**: Rapid increase to 1 mg/kg (1–1.25 mg/kg if neutropenic) qd IV. Total dose of 2–2.5 gm rec. by some but data to support this lacking. If response good may switch to itra after 2-3 wks. For renal impairment, use lipid-based Ampho B (see footnote) or **Caspofungin** 70 mg IV on day 1, then 50 mg IV qd (reduce to 35 mg for moderate hepatic insufficiency)	**Itraconazole[3]** 200 mg IV q12h x4 doses, then 200 mg IV qd x12 days followed by 200 mg po bid.	**Voriconazole** appears to be better than Ampho B in one large randomized trial of 277 immunosuppressed pts with IPA. 53% responded vs 32% rx with Ampho B. Overall survival better (71 vs 58%) (NEJM 347:408, 2002). In addition, 31% pts with UB refractory or intolerant to ampho B who received voriconazole responded with itra (Chest 106:810, 1994) and clinical responses (ICAAC 2002, Abst. M868). Other studies report response rates of 38 & 43% (CID 34:563, 2002; NEJM 347:2021, 2002). **Ampho B overall success rate 34%** (CID 26:781, 1998) in pulmonary aspergillosis in those pts rx ≥14 days. Dependent on underlying disease: 83% heart/kidney transplant, 54% neutropenic leukemia pts, 33% bone marrow transplant, 20% liver transplant (CID 23:608, 1996). Overall case fatality rate 58% (CID 32:358, 2001). Lipid-based Ampho B generally equally effective with less nephrotoxicity (CID (Supp2):S133, 1996). **Caspofungin.** FDA approval based on 50% response in 40 pts who received ≥7 days of rx. All had significant impairment in host defense (ICAAC 2000, Abst. 1103). Minimal toxicity reported to date (Transpl Inf Dis 25, 2002). **Itraconazole** effective in 1 small series. 15/31 pts (48%) responded to IV x2 wks then po.[3] (CID 34:1160, 2002). Comment: While new drugs may ↑ response and survival, it remains one of the most refractory fungal infections. Some experts have resorted to rx with combinations of antifungal drugs (Am Soc Hematol Abst 1381, 2001; CID 34:1160, 2002).

71

---

[1] Hydration before and after infusion with 500 cc saline shown to reduce renal toxicity.
[2] **Lipid-based Ampho B** May be as effective and less nephrotoxic than standard Ampho B **but much more expensive. Dosages: ABLC** 5 mg/kg IV over 2 hrs. **Ampho B cholesteryl complex** 3–4
[3] **Oral solution preferred to tablets because of ↑ absorption** (see Table 10B, page 80)
  * All dosage recommendations are for adults (unless otherwise indicated) and assume normal renal function

See page 78 for abbreviations.

TABLE 10A (2)

TYPE OF INFECTION/ORGANISM/SITE OF INFECTION	ANTIMICROBIAL AGENTS OF CHOICE		COMMENTS
	PRIMARY	ALTERNATIVE	
Blastomycosis (CID 30:679, 2000) (Blastomyces dermatitidis) Cutaneous, pulmonary or extrapulmonary	**Itraconazole** oral solution 200-400 mg/d po for 6 mos. or **Ampho B**[2] 0.7-1 mg/kg/d to a total dose of ≥1.5 gm for very sick pts	**Fluconazole** 400-600 mg/d for at least 6 mos. 85% + effective for non-life-threatening disease (CID 25:200, 1997)	Itra in patients treated for ≥2 months, 95% cure (AJM 93: 489, 1992). Ampho B successful in >90% when ≥1.5 gm total dose used (CID 2:S102, 1996).

Candidiasis: Candida is a major cause of nosocomial bloodstream infection, has increased dramatically since 1996 to 7.6/10,000 discharges (Mycoses 45:141, 2002), and has demonstrated a decrease in C. albicans and an increase in non-albicans species which show ↓ susceptibility to antifungal agents. These changes have predominantly affected immunocompromised pts (hematological malignancies, transplant and intensive care environments where azoles are used). The pathophysiology of candidemia is only partially understood. For antifungal drugs to date has not undergone testing in in vivo validation studies, and clinical outcomes are often more dependent on host factors (Am J Med 112:380, 2002). Yet it seems prudent to use susceptibility profiles to help select empiric antifungal therapy. The following table attempts to summarize the current, published reports of frequency of candida isolates, and interpretation as to whether a drug is clinically effective (**S = sensitive**) may require dose escalation (**S-DD = sensitive with dose escalation**), or is likely to be ineffective (**R = resistant**) (Ln 359:1135, 2002).

Candida Isolates	% of Candida Isolates	Risk Factors	% Sensitive In Vitro			
			Fluconazole	Itraconazole	Voriconazole	Ampho B
C. albicans	55-65	HIV/AIDS, surgery	97% (S)	93% (S)	99% (S)	>95% (S)
C. glabrata	10-15	Heme malignancies, azole prophylaxis	60% (S-DD)	4% (R)	92% (S)	>95% (S)
C. parapsilosis	15-20	Azole prophylaxis, neonates, foreign bodies	99% (S)	4% (S-DD)	99% (S)	>95% (S)
C. tropicalis	5-10	Neutropenia	98% (S)	58% (S)	99% (S)	>95% (S)
C. krusei	2-10	Heme malignancies, azole prophylaxis	5% (R)	2% (R)	>95% (S)	>95% (S)
C. guilliermondi	1	Azole prophylaxis, previous ampho rx	>95% (S)	? (S)	>95% (S)	? (R)
C. lusitaniae	1	Previous ampho rx	>95% (S)	? (S)	>95% (S)	(R)

TYPE OF INFECTION	PRIMARY	ALTERNATIVE	COMMENTS
Bloodstream: clinically stable with or without venous catheter (no metastatic lesions), non-neutropenic. **All positive blood cultures require therapy!**	**Fluconazole** 400 mg IV or po x 1 d, then po for 14 d after last + blood culture or **Ampho B**[2] 0.5-0.6 mg/kg qd IV, total dose 5-7 mg/kg. (In renal impairment, use lipid-based Ampho B)	In pts who fail to respond or deteriorate, higher doses of either drug (may be used (**ampho B** 1.0 mg/kg/d IV) or **fluconazole** 800 mg/d IV or po) (CID 25:43, 1997). **Be sure catheter is removed.**	**Remove & replace venous catheters** (not "over a wire") if possible (CID 34:591 & 600, 2002). Mortality 21% vs 41% if catheter not removed (AJM 155:2429, 1995). Observe for metastatic lesions (endophthalmitis). In a multicenter trial fluconazole = ampho B but less toxicity with flu (NEJM 331:1325, 1994 AJM 155:2429, 1995); microbiologic failure 10-14% in both. Similar results found in cancer pts (AJM 11:170, 1996).
Bloodstream: neutropenic but clinically stable See Results of 1997 Consensus Conference (CID 25:43, 1997)	**Fluconazole** 400 mg IV or po x 1 d, then neutropenia resolved or **Ampho B**[2] 0.5-0.6 mg/kg qd IV to total dose 6-7 mg/kg (when switch to **fluconazole** 400 mg qd po. Continue flu until neutropenia resolved) (In renal impairment, use lipid-based Ampho B)	**Voriconazole**[NEDA2] loading dose 6 mg/kg q12h x 1 d, IV, then maintenance dose 4 mg/kg IV bid for invasive aspergillosis & serious mold infections, **3 mg/kg bid IV** for serious candida infections **Caspofungin**[NEDA2] 70 mg IV on day 1 followed by 50 mg IV qd (reduce to 35 mg IV qd with moderate hepatic insufficiency)	ABLC successful in some who had failed ampho B (CID 21:1184, 1995; CID 22:S95, 1996). Non-albicans candidemia (therefore more likely to be fluconazole-resistant) more likely in pts with leukemia, neutropenia, and those receiving antifungal prophylaxis (CID 28:1071, 1999). Both voriconazole & caspofungin may have a role in this clinical setting (Euro Con Clin Micro & Inf Dis 2002, Abst. 237; IDSA 2002, Abst. 352).

---

1 **Oral solution preferred to tablets because of ↑ absorption** (see Table 10B, page 80).
2 Hydration before and after infusion with 500 cc saline has been shown to reduce renal toxicity.
See page 78 for abbreviations.   * All dosage recommendations are for adults (unless otherwise indicated) and assume normal renal function

TABLE 10A (3)

TYPE OF INFECTION/ORGANISM/ SITE OF INFECTION	ANTIMICROBIAL AGENTS OF CHOICE		COMMENTS
	PRIMARY	ALTERNATIVE	
Candidiasis (continued)			
Bloodstream: unstable, deteriorating, or with metastatic lesions (pulmonary, eye, hepatosplenic) ± neutropenia For endophthalmitis, see Table 1, pages 9, 10	**Ampho B** 0.8-1 mg/kg/d IV + 5FC 37.5[1] mg/kg/d qdh (in renal impairment, use lipid-based Ampho B) **(b)** OR **Fluconazole** 400-800 mg IV/d If start Ampho B, switch to fluconazole 400 mg po qd for 14 d. after last positive blood culture, resolution of neutropenia & disappearance of signs/symptoms of candidal infection.	**Lipid-based Ampho B** (ABLC) 5 mg/kg/d OR **Voriconazole. Loading dose 6 mg/kg q12h x1 d, then maintenance dose 4 mg/kg bid IV** for invasive aspergillus & serious mold infections. **3 mg/kg bid IV** for serious candida infections OR **Caspofungin** 70 mg IV on day 1 followed by 50 mg IV qd (reduce to 35 mg IV qd with moderate hepatic insufficiency)	ABLC successful in some who had failed ampho B (CID 21:1184, 1995; CID 22:595, 1996). Non-albicans candidemia (therefore more likely to be fluconazole-resistant) more likely in pts with leukemia, neutropenia, and those receiving antifungal prophylaxis (CID 33:1071, 1999). Both voriconazole & caspofungin may have a role in this clinical setting (Euro Con Clin Micro & Inf Dis 2002, Abst. 237; IDSA 2002, Abst. 352)
Chronic mucocutaneous	**Ketoconazole** 400 mg/d po (as single daily dose with food) for 3-9 months	**Fluconazole** 400 mg/d po 1st day then **fluconazole** 3-6 mg/kg/d po as single daily dose	Respond to ampho B but relapse is usual. Fluconazole used and may be less toxic, but expensive limited.
Cutaneous (including paronychia, Table 1, page 18)	Apply topical **ampho B, clotrimazole, econazole, miconazole,** or **nystatin** 3-4x daily for 7-14 days or **Ketoconazole** 400 mg po once daily x14 d. **Ciclopirox olamine** 1% cream/lotion. Apply topically bid x7-14 d.		Cost (30 gm tube cream): AB $29. Clo $13. Eco $19. MIC $21. My $3.56. Clc $18.20
Endocarditis Causes of fungal endocarditis: C. albicans 24%, non-albicans Candida sp. 24%, Aspergillus sp. 24%, others 27% (CID 32:50, 2001)	**Ampho B** 0.6 mg/kg/d IV for 7 days, then 0.8 mg/kg qod IV. Continue 6-10 weeks after surgery + **Flucytosine** 25-37.5 mg/kg po qid.	**Fluconazole** 200-400 mg/d IV or po for chronic suppression may be of value when valve not replaced	**Adjust flucyt dose and interval to produce serum levels; peak 70-80 mg/L, trough 30-40 mg/L.** With nephrotoxicity, dosage of flucyt needs to be ↓. Surgery may not always be required (CID 22:262, 1996) (GGD 242:895, 2001). Caspofungin cidal vs candida & may be of value; no data.
Oral (thrush)—not AIDS patient	**Fluconazole** 200 mg single dose or 100 mg po x5-14 days or **Itraconazole** oral solution 200 mg (20 ml) qd without food >3 days	**Nystatin** pastilles (200,000 u) lozenge qid, 500,000 u (swish & swallow) qid or (500,000 u) tabs tid for 14 d. or **Clotrimazole** troche (10 mg) 5x/d x14d.	**Fluconazole: Single dose 100 mg po; 16/16 clinical cure** 75% mycologic at 2 weeks (AAC 34:2267, 1990). Maintenance not required in non-AIDS pts. Usually improves in 3-4 days, longer rx ↓ relapse. C. krusei fungemia reported in chronic-rx pts (NEJM 325: 1315, 1991).
AIDS patient **Stomatitis, esophagitis, vaginitis** Oral colonization with candida correlates with HIV RNA levels in plasma, less so with CD4 counts (JID 180:534, 1999). Protease inhibitors appear to ↓ recurrent oral candidiasis themselves vs. with antiretroviral agents (p< 0.0001) (J AIDS 21:20, 1999). May be due to direct effect on candida aspartic protease (J AIDS 22:106, 1999).	**Fluconazole** 200 mg po 1st day then 100 mg po x7-14 d. or **Itraconazole** oral solution 200 mg po qd or bid or 100 mg po bid x14 d. or **Caspofungin** 50 mg IV qd. for flu-refractory disease. Some recommend oral topical agents[2] for oral without esophageal involvement if CD4 >50 & receiving (or will receive) HAART	**For fluconazole-refractory disease:** Options include: 1. **Fluconazole** 400-800 mg po qd or bid or 2. **Itraconazole** solution 100 mg po bid or 3. **Parenteral Ampho B** 0.3-0.5 mg/kg/d IV or or 4. **Voriconazole** (see Table 10B, page 81 for dose)	Fluconazole resistance in vitro[1] associated with prolonged use of flu but clinical relevance difficult to establish & >50% of infections caused by resistant isolates respond to flu. **Fluconazole-refractory disease response low** (4%, if CD4 counts in pts with low CD4 counts (<50/mm³). Most will have prior exposure to flu (within previous 6 mos.) daily or qod (p = 0.004), and exhibit in vitro resistance to flu. Some may have acquired new candida species resistant to flu: C. krusei, C. glabrata, but most have C. albicans (CID 30:749, 2000; CID 33:1069, 2001). Flu superior to oral suspension of nystatin (CID 24:1204, 1997). Itra 100 mg po bid x14 d. achieved clinical response in 41/74 (65%) flu unresponsive to flu (AIDS Res Hum Retrovir 15:1413, 1999). Ampho B oral suspension gave 42-55% response to flu, but 0/6 refractory to flu relapsed (AIDS 14:845, 2000). For esophagitis, caspofungin as effective as ampho B IV but less toxic: 74% vs 24% adverse events respectively (CID 33: 1529, 2001). Voriconazole as effective as fluconazole for esophagitis (AAC 46:451, 2002). (CID 33:1447, 2001).

[1] Some experts reduce dose of 5FC to 25 mg/kg q6h.
[2] Oral agents: Nystatin, clotrimazole troche 10 mg 5x/d

See page 78 for abbreviations.   * All dosage recommendations are for adults (unless otherwise indicated) and assume normal renal function

TABLE 10A (4)

TYPE OF INFECTION/ORGANISM/ SITE OF INFECTION	ANTIMICROBIAL AGENTS OF CHOICE		COMMENTS
	PRIMARY	ALTERNATIVE	
Candidiasis/AIDS patient/Stomatitis, esophagitis, vaginitis *(continued)* **chronic suppressive rx** for disabling recurrent oral, esophageal infection). Authors would rx: if sustained CD4 count ^{-see footnote} (>200/ mm³) following HAART.		If fluconazole-refractory esophagitis, failed flu suppression, may be forced to rx with **ampho B** (0.3 mg/kg IV q d) or **1 mg/kg IV q week**	Fluconazole 200 mg qd does reduce risk of candida esophagitis & cryptococcosis *(NEJM 332:700, 1995)*. Disadvantages: Concern of emergence of fluconazole (azole)-resistant Candida species.
Peritonitis (Chronic Ambulatory Peritoneal Dialysis) Based on Peritoneal Dialysis International 20:396, 2000. See Table 19, page 132	[Flucytosine 2 gm po (loading dose) then 1.0 gm qd po + **fluconazole** 200 mg po IP daily] x4-6 weeks.	[Fluconazole 200 mg IP q d at 1.5 mg/L of dialysis fluid x4–6 weeks.	If no clinical improvement in 4–7 d, remove catheter. Oral fluconazole not available in Canada. Fluconazole alone may be preferred to combination of flucon & flucytosine *(Am J Kid Dis 36:1183, 2000).*
Cystitis Refs.: *CID 32:1602, 2001; 20:1152, 1995; 20:1510, 1995; 21:960, 1995; J Urol 154:2032, 1995*	Fluconazole 200 mg 1st day, then 100 mg po qd x4 days *(Ann Pharm 35:369, 2001)*	**Ampho B** (bladder irrigation) with 5 mg/ 100 ml H₂O at 42 ml/hr x1–2 d, or **ampho B** 0.3 mg/kg IV single dose *(J Urol 154: 2032, 1995)*	If poor response, consider fungus "ball" in renal pelvis. If possible, remove urethral catheter.
Vaginitis—Non-AIDS patients Review article: *MMWR 51(RR-6), 2002* (Candida vaginitis in AIDS patients: see above). *(See Table 1, page 17)*	Oral: **Fluconazole** 150 mg po x1 or Itraconazole 200 mg po bid x d.	Intravaginal: Multiple imidazoles with 85–95% cure rates. See doses in footnote¹ ** = over-the-counter preparations	**In general, oral and vaginal rx are similarly effective.** Rx aided by avoiding tight clothing, e.g., pantyhose. Oral drugs → rectal candida and may ↑ relapses. Fluconazole resistance reported in both HIV(−) and HIV(+) pts *(CID 22:726, 1996)* but incidence of flu-refractory disease remains low *(CID 26:557, 1998)*. Boric acid solution intravaginally has also been used *(CID 24: 649, 1997).*
"Candida syndrome"	In a double-blind study, nystatin did not reduce systemic or psychological symptoms vs placebo *(NEJM 323:1717, 1990).*		
Chromomycosis *(J Am Acad Derm 44:585, 2001)* Dematiaceous fungi. Verrucous, crusted lesions usually seen on the feet, legs.	In lesions small and few, surgical excision or cryosurgery. For larger, more chronic, extensive, burrowing: **itraconazole**.	**Itraconazole** 100 mg/kg po x18 months OR **flucytosine** 37.5 mg/kg po q6h. Cures disappointing.	2 relapses (18, 24 mos). 2 responded. In subgroup terbinafine impressive in a small number of pts *(AJTMH 55:45, 1996; Cutis 66:45, 2000).*
Coccidioidomycosis (Coccidioides immitis) *(see AnIM 130:293, 1999; IDCP 8:21, 1999; CID 30:658, 2000)*			**Cure rate (ampho B) 50–70%. Responses to azoles are similar.** Itra may have slight advantage esp. in soft tissue infection. Relapse rates after rx 40%. Relapse rate (RR=4.7) flu ↑ CF titer ≥1:256 (RR = 4.7) or neg. coccidioidin skin test (RR=4.7) *(CID 28:1205, 1997)*. Following CF titers warrants readministration of rx important and rising titers should warrant re-rx *(Am J Med 86:115, 1989)*. In a randomized double-blind study of 198 pts with progressive non-meningeal cocci, 57% responded to flu vs 72% to itra (p=0.05) by 12 mos. Those with skeletal infections responded twice as frequently to itra than flu. Relapse after rx: 28% after flu, 18% after itra *(AnIM 133:676, 2000)*. For maintenance in HIV+ patients: flu 200 mg po qd or itra 200 mg po bid.
Fever, uncomplicated in normal host. Influenza-like illness of 1–2 wks duration	**Antifungal rx not generally recommended** and rx if fever, wt loss and/or fatigue do not resolve within several wks to 2 months *(see below)*		
Primary pulmonary (San Joaquin or Valley Fever), complicated in normal host. Influenza-like illness of 1–2 wks duration			
Primary pulmonary in pts with ↑ risk for complications or dissemination. Rx indicated: • Immunosuppressive disease (AIDS) or therapies (steroids) • Pregnancy in 3rd trimester • Diabetes • complement fixation antibody titer (titer >1:16) • pulmonary infiltrates • hilar adenopathy	Mild to moderate severity: Itraconazole 200 mg po or IV bid OR Fluconazole 400 mg po for 3–12 months Locally severe or extensive disease: **Ampho B** 0.6–1 mg/kg/d x7 d, then 0.8 mg/kg/qod. Total dose 2.5 gm or more, followed by **itra** or **flu**		
Primary pulmonary/non-pulmonary—dissemination (identification of spherules or culture of organism from ulcer, joint effusion, pus from abscess or bone bx, etc.)	Consultation with specialist recommended; surgery may be required		

---

¹ **Butoconazole** 2% cream (5 gm) qd hs x3 d** or 2% cream SR 5 gm x1; or **clotrimazole** 100 mg vaginal tabs (2 qd hs x3 d) or 1% cream (5 gm) qd hs x7 d (14 d max) ↑ cure rate) or 100 mg vaginal tab x7 d or 500 mg vaginal tab x1; or **miconazole** 200 mg vaginal suppos. (qd x7 d) or 2% cream (5 gm) qd hs x7 d or **terconazole** 80 mg vaginal tab (1 qd hs x3 d) or 0.4% cream (5 gm) qd hs x7 d or 0.8% cream 5 gm intravaginal qd x3 d or **tioconazole** 6.5% vag. ointment x1 dose**. ** = over-the-counter product

See page 78 for abbreviations.

All dosage recommendations are for adults (unless otherwise indicated) and assume normal renal function

TABLE 10A (5)

TYPE OF INFECTION/ORGANISM/ SITE OF INFECTION	ANTIMICROBIAL AGENTS OF CHOICE		COMMENTS
	PRIMARY	ALTERNATIVE	
Coccidioidomycosis (continued)			
Meningitis: occurs in 1/3 to 1/2 of pts with disseminated coccidioidomycosis			
Adult	**Fluconazole** 400–800 mg qd po indefinitely	**Ampho B** IV as for pulmonary (above) + 0.1–0.3 mg daily intrathecal (intraventricular) via reservoir device.	**37/47 patients responded to flucon (median rx 3 yrs)** (*AnIM* 119:28, 1993). 14/18 pts rx with azoles relapsed when drug discontinued, therefore recommended that **fluconazole be continued indefinitely** (*AnIM* 124:305, 1996). One study also found flu 400–600 mg qd to be effective (*AnIM* 112:108,1990).
Child	**Fluconazole** (po) (Pediatric dose not established, 6 mg/kg qd used)	**Itraconazole** 200–400 mg solution qd for 6–12 mos OR **Ampho B** 0.3 mg/kg/d qd + **flucytosine** 37.5 mg/kg qid po x6 wks.	
Cryptococcosis (Cryptococcus neoformans) (*CID* 30:710, 2000)			
Non-meningeal (non-AIDS)	**Itraconazole** 400 mg/d IV or po for 8 wks to 6 mos **For more severe disease: Ampho B** 0.5–0.8 mg/kg/d IV till response then change to **fluconazole** 400 mg qd po for 8–10 week course.	**Itraconazole** 37.5 mg/kg/d[3] 37.5 mg/kg/qd IV + **flucytosine** 37.5 mg/kg qid po until pt afebrile and cultures neg (~6 weeks), then stop ampho B/flucyt, start **fluconazole** 200 mg po qd po (*AnIM* 113:183, 1990).	Adjust flucon dose and interval to produce serum levels of peak 70–80 mg/L, trough 30–40 mg/L. **Flucon alone 90% effective for meningeal and non-meningeal forms** (74% on steroid rx). French study suggests fluconazole equally as effective as ampho B (*CID* 22:S154, 1996) and 92% effective in 31 cancer pts (*CID* 32:S145, 2001).
Meningitis (non-AIDS)	Mycoses Study Group recommends: **ampho B** 0.7–1 mg/kg/d IV + **flucytosine[3] 25 mg/kg po q6h x2** wks or until clinically stable followed by flu **400 mg/d. for minimum of 10 wks.** then switch to 200 mg qd (suppression) (see below).	**Fluconazole** 400 mg po qd x6–10 wks, then suppressive rx (see Comments) or **Fluconazole** 400 mg po qd + **flucytosine** 37.5 mg/kg po q6h x10 wks (↑ toxicity) or Liposomal amphotericin 5 mg/kg/d x2 wks followed by fluconazole as above	**Flucytosine levels must be measured:** adjust dose and interval to keep serum: peak 70–80 mg/L, trough 30–40 mg/L. **Flucytosine alone has been used successfully,** comparative clinical trials lacking (*NEJM* 301:126, 1979). Hydrocephalus may be successfully rx with VA[3] or V-P shunting (*CID* 28:629, 1999).
	Ampho B alone 0.7–1.0 mg/kg/d IV x2 wks or until afebrile, headache, nausea and vomiting gone. Then dc ampho B, start **flucon** 400 mg qd for 8–10 weeks. Then maintain on flucon 200 mg qd.	**Ampho B** alone 0.7–1.0 mg/kg/d IV x2 wks or until afebrile, headache, nausea and vomiting gone. Then dc ampho B, start **flucon** 400 mg qd for 8–10 weeks. Then maintain on flucon 200 mg qd. or **Ampho B** lipid complex (V:5 mg/kg/d x2 wks, then 3x/wk x4 wks)[3][V-P][4] (*CID* 22:315, 1996)	If normal mental status, >20 cells/mm³ CSF and CSF crypto antigen <1:1024, flucon alone is reasonable (*CID* 22:322, 1996). Serum cryptococcal antigen useful in dx (95% sens.), no help in monitoring rx. ↑ CSF pressure: lower with CSF removal. Lumbar drains or V-P shunts have been used to control persistent ↑ CSF pressure. (*CID* 28:629, 1999).
HIV+/AIDS Treatment (see *CID* 30:710, 2000). Cryptococcal meningitis Cryln era of HAART (*Neuro* 56:257, 2001)			Must monitor 5-FC levels, peak 70–80 mg/L, trough 30–40 mg/L. Higher levels assoc. with bone marrow toxicity (*CID* 28:329, 1999).
* Cryptococcus in blood culture or positive blood culture or positive test of serum for cryptococcal antigen		**Itraconazole** 200 mg po bid may be used in place of flu in cases of flu intolerance for continuation rx after ampho B. (Not as effective as flu (*AIDS* 6:185, 1992).)	Even with rx (ampho B + 5FC regimen) 29/236 pts died within 1st 2 wks & 62 (26%) by 10 wks; only 129 (55%) were alive & culture-neg at 10 wks (*CID* 30:47, 1997). In Zambia, 230 pts received fluconazole mono rx, all but died by 6 months. None had received HAART (*Postgrad Med J* 77:769, 2001).
With HAART, symptoms of acute meningitis may return, immune reconstitution (*AIDS* 12:1491, 1999). If failure to respond to initial rx, think of infection with tbc, neurosyphilis, toxo, etc. (*Neuro* 51:1213, 1998).		**Ampho B** 1.0 mg/kg IV 1x/week	Itraconazole not as effective as fluconazole. Not recommended as suppressive rx 23% (4%) receiving fluconazole (p = 0.006) (*CID* 28:291, 1999).
Suppression	**Fluconazole** 200 mg/d po; flucon relapsed vs. none (*AIDS* 6:185, 1992)	**Itraconazole** 200 mg po bid if flu intolerant or failure	

---

¹ Some experts would reduce to 25 mg/kg q6h
² **VA** = ventriculoatrial **VP** = ventriculoperitoneal **VA** = ventriculoatrial
³ Flucytosine = 5-FC

See page 78 for abbreviations.

* If blood culture for acute meningitis may be manifest by positive blood culture or positive test of serum for cryptococcal antigen

* *All dosage recommendations are for adults (unless otherwise indicated) and assume normal renal function*

76

TABLE 10A (6)

TYPE OF INFECTION/ORGANISM/ SITE OF INFECTION	ANTIMICROBIAL AGENTS OF CHOICE		COMMENTS
	PRIMARY	ALTERNATIVE	
Dermatophytosis			
Erythrasma (Corynebacterium minutissimum)	Erythromycin 250 mg po qid for 14 days	2% aqueous clindamycin topically	Diff. dx with Tinea versicolor, Tinea cruris. Erythrasma gives coral red fluorescence with Wood's light.
Onychomycosis (Tinea unguium) (see CID 23:305, 1996; Ln 351:541, 1998; J Am Ped Med Assn 91:127, 2001) A "no lacquer" (ciclopirox) has been approved but resulted in cure in only 5-9% after 48 wks (Med Lett 42:51, 2000) but 1 to 50% cure in another study (J Am Acad Derm 44:479, 2001).	**Fingernail Rx Options:** **Terbinafine** 250 mg po qd (children <20 kg: 67.5 mg/d, 20–40 kg 125 mg/d, >40 kg 125 mg/d) x6 wks (79% effective) or **Itraconazole** 200 mg po qd x3 mos or 200 mg po bid x1 wk/mo x2 mos. or **Fluconazole** 150–300 mg po q wk x3–6 mos	**Toenail Rx Options:** **Terbinafine** 250 mg po qd (children <20 kg: 67.5 mg/d, 20–40 kg 125 mg/d) x12 wks (70–81% effective) or **Itraconazole** 200 mg po qd x3 mos (58–66% effective)^NFDAI or 200 mg po bid x1 wk/mo x3–4 mos or **Fluconazole** 150–300 mg po q wk x6–12 mos. (30–40% effective)^NFDAI	All agents with similar cure rates (60–100%) in clinical studies (Red Derm 17:304, 2000). Griseofulvin considered drug of choice by some although concerns for resistance and toxicities. Addition of topical ketoconazole or selenium sulfate shampoo reduces transmissibility (J Derm 39:261, 2000)
	NOTE: For side-effects, see footnotes **1 & 2**		
Tinea capitis ("ringworm") (Trichophyton tonsurans, Microsporum canis, N. America; other sp. elsewhere) (PIDJ 18:191, 1999)	**Terbinafine** 250 mg po qd x4 wks for T. tonsurans, 8 wks for Microsporum canis^NFDAI. Children 125 mg po qd	**Itraconazole**^3 3–5 mg/kg/d po x4–6 wks^NFDAI or **Fluconazole** 8 mg/kg q wk x8–12 wks.^NFDAI **Griseofulvin** adults 500 mg po x4–6 wks, children 10–20 mg/kg/d until hair regrows, usually 6–8 wks.	Keto po often effective in severe recalcitrant infection. Follow for hepatotoxicity. Terbinafine 87% & 5 mos of mycologic cure in double-blind study (32 pts). (J Med Assn Thai 76:388, 1993; Brit J Derm 130(S43):22, 1994) and fluconazole 78% (J Am Acad Derm 40:531, 1999).
Tinea corporis, cruris, or pedis (Trichophyton rubrum, T. mentagrophytes, Epidermophyton floccosum) "Athlete's foot, jock itch," and ringworm	**Topical rx:** Generally applied 2x/d. Available as creams, ointments, sprays, by prescription & "over the counter." Apply 2x/d for 2–3 wks. See footnote^4 for names and prices. Recommend: Lotrimin Ultra or Lamisil AT; contain butenafine & terbinafine—both are fungicidal	**Itraconazole** 200 mg po qd x2 x2 wks^NFDAI OR **fluconazole** 150 mg po 1 x/wk for 2–4 wks^NFDAI **Griseofulvin** adults 500 mg po qd x4–6 wks, children 10–20 mg/kg/d. Duration: 2–4 wks for corporis, 4–8 wks for pedis	Keto 1 x 97% effective in 1 study. Another alternative: Selenium sulfide (Selsun), 2.5% lotion, apply as lather, leave on 10 min then wash off. 1x/d x7 d or 3–5x/week x2–4 weeks 9/21 tx successful; 4 wk 2 bloodstream, 2 sinus & 1 skin.
Tinea versicolor (Malassezia furfur or Pityrosporum orbiculare)	**Ketoconazole** (400 mg po single dose) or (200 mg po qd x7 days) or (2% cream applied 1x qd x2 wks)	**Fluconazole** 400 mg po single dose or **Itraconazole** 400 mg po qd x3–7 days	
Fusariosis Causes infection in eye, skin, sinus and disseminated diseases—increased in transplant patients (CID 34:909, 2002)	**Ampho B** 1–1.2 mg/kg	**Ampho B** 1–1.2 mg/kg	
Histoplasmosis (Histoplasma capsulatum): See CID 30:688, 2000. Best diagnostic test is urinary antigen (ELISA) (CID 22:S102, 1996). MiraVista Diagnostics (1-866-647-2847).	**Mild disease:** My.b., diol. None useful. **Moderate disease:** **Itraconazole** 200 mg/d solution po for 9 months. If life-threatening 200 mg (all) are applied to affected area bid. Dose 200 mg IV bid x4 doses followed by 200 mg IV qd (see Table 10B) **Severe, including meningitis: Ampho B** 0.5–1 mg/kg/d IV x7 d, followed by 0.8 mg/kg IV q other day (See Comments)		With ≥2 months Itra rx, 86% success in chronic pulmonary & cavitary pulmonary (AnIM 93:635, 1980). Antifungal rx not useful for histo fibrosis mediastinitis. Clinical: Severe: Temp >39.5°C, Karnofsky <60; albumin <3 gm/dl; hepatic enzymes >5x normal, WBC <500, platelets <50,000, creatinine >6 mg/dl (CID 23(Suppl 1):S19, 1994). Itra more effective than Itra (CID 23: 996, 1996)
	Prescription drugs: butenafine (Lotrimin) $12, ciclopirox (Loprox) $12, clotrimazole (Lotrimin) $13, Mycelex) $10, econazole (Spectrazole) $13, ketoconazole (Nizoral) NB $5–13, G,$4, naftifine (Naftin) NB 17, oxiconazole (Oxistat) $14, sulconazole (Exelderm) $10, terconazole (Terazol) $9 Non-prescription (over-the-counter): Tolnaftate (Tinactin $5, Ting or Tolnate $2), undecylenic acid (Cruex $5, Desenex $5). Lotrimin AT 1%, 12 gm $6.17, Lamisil AT 1%, 12 gm $6.79		

---

1 **Serious but rare cases of hepatic failure** have been reported in pts receiving terbinafine & should not be used in those with chronic or active liver disease. (See Table 10A) Suggest checking ALT & AST before prescribing (Am J Health Sys Pharm 58:1076, 2001)

2 Itraconazole absorption requires low gastric pH and is enhanced with food & acidic drinks & impaired with onset and progression of renal failure (see Ln 357:1766, 2001)

3 Drug name (trade name) and wholesale price for 15 gm (all are applied to affected area bid. Prescription drugs: butenafine...

4 Oral solution preferred to tablets because of^1 absorption (See Table 10B, page 80).

*All dosage recommendations are for adults (unless otherwise indicated) and assume normal renal/renal function

See page 78 for abbreviations.

TABLE 10A (7)

TYPE OF INFECTION/ORGANISM/ SITE OF INFECTION	ANTIMICROBIAL AGENTS OF CHOICE		COMMENTS
	PRIMARY	ALTERNATIVE	
Histoplasmosis (continued) Immunocompromised patient (AIDS) (CID 24:1195, 1997, & 32:1215, 2001)	For moderate to severe disease: Lipid-based Ampho B or Liposomal Ampho B 3 mg/kg/d IV x14 d, then suppressive therapy with itraconazole 200 mg po qd (AnIM 137:435, 2002) Ampho B 0.5–1 mg/kg/d IV x1 d, followed by 0.8 mg/kg qod (3x/week) to total dose of 10–15 mg/kg, then suppressive therapy as above	For less severe disease: Itraconazole (300 mg bid po x3 d, then 200 mg bid po x12 wks) or (400 mg po x12 wks (85–90% response) then 200 mg qd (see Table on page 76). Not recommended for meningitis. IV if unable to take po	Liposomal Ampho B superior at 2 weeks vs Ampho B (88% vs 64%; clinical success) in 81 patients with a decrease in nephrotoxicity (97% vs 37%). No difference in mortality after 10 additional weeks of itra in both arms (AnIM 137:105, 2002) Itra (ACTG 120) 50/59 (85%) cleared fungemia with only 5% toxicity: 1 pt with meningitis failed, 2 failed because of low serum levels. Avoid rifampin, reduces itra serum concentration (AJM 98:336, 1995). Itra best drug for suppression at 200 mg qd but 3/46 had probable hepatic toxicity (J AIDS & Human Retro 16:100, 1997). Flu less effective than Itra & induces flu resistance (CID 33:1910, 2001).
Madura foot (See Comments)/(See Nocardia, Pseudallescheria boydii, below)	None, unless Nocardia (see below)		In U.S., usually Pseudallescheria boydii or usually Nocardia brasiliensis, in Japan, N. asteroides. [NUB] In Mexico, (Petriellidium spp.). Miconazole IV agent of choice.
Mucormycosis (Zygomycosis—Rhizopus, Rhizomucor, Absidia) Rhinocerebral, pulmonary (AnIM 159:1301, 1999)	Ampho B. Increase rapidly to 0.8–1.5 mg/kg IV, then qod. Total dose usually 2.5–3 gm. Azoles and caspofungin usually inactive (In renal impairment, use lipid-based Ampho B.)		Treatment requires control of underlying condition, esp. diabetic ketoacidosis. Surgical debridement usually required and discontinue deferoxamine if applicable. Deferoxamine ↑ risk of mucormycosis, use hydroxypyridinone chelators, e.g., deferiprone (Phase 3 study, Apotex 847-573-9999). High-dose (10–15 mg/kg/d) liposomal amphotericin successful in 2 cases (J Inf 41:265, 2000).
Nocardiosis (N. asteroides & N. brasiliensis). Culture & sensitivities may be valuable in refractory cases: Reference Labs, R.J. Wallace (903) 877-7680 or CDC (404) 639-3158 (IDCP 8:27, 1999)			
Cutaneous and lymphocutaneous (sporotrichoid)	TMP/SMX 5–10 mg/kg/d of TMP & 25–50 mg/kg/d of SMX in 2–4 div. doses x3, po or IV. After 3–4 wks, ↓ dose to 1/2 dose po (see Comment)	Sulfisoxazole 2 gm po qid or minocycline 100–200 mg po bid	Survival may be excellent with sulfa-containing regimen used (Medicine 68:38, 1999). Measure sulfonamide blood levels early to ensure absorption
Pulmonary, disseminated brain abscess		IMP 500 mg IV q6h) + (amikacin 7.5 mg/kg IV q12h) x3–4 wks & then po regimen	of po rx. Desired peak level 2 hrs 100–150 μg/ml 2 hrs post-dose for most. Some recommend 3 mos. for immunocompetent host (38%) and 6 mos. for immunocompromised (62% organ transplant, malignancy, chronic lung disease, diabetes, ETOH use, steroid rx, and AIDS).
Paracoccidioidomycosis (South American blastomycosis)/P. brasiliensis	Itraconazole 200 mg/d po x 6 months or Ketoconazole 400 mg/d po for 6–18 months	Ampho B 0.4–0.5 mg/kg/d IV to total dose of 1.5–2.5 gm or sulfonamides (doses: see Comment)	Improvement in >90% pts on itra or keto.[NFM] Sulfa: 4–6 gm/d for several weeks, then 500 mg/d for 3–5 yrs also used (CID 14[Suppl.]:S-68, 1992). HIV+ TMP/SMX suppressive rx indefinitely (CID 21:1275, 1995).
Lobomycosis (keloidal blastomycosis)/P. loboi	Surgical excision, clofazimine or ampho B		
Penicilliosis (Penicillium marneffei) Common disseminated fungal infection in AIDS pts in SE Asia (esp. Thailand & Vietnam) (CID 24:1080, 1997; Int J Inf Dis 3:48, 1998)	Ampho B 0.5–1 mg/kg/d IV daily x3 d, then 200 mg po x2 wks, then 400 mg po x 10 wks followed by itraconazole 400 mg/d po indefinitely for HIV-infected pts (CID 26:1107, 1998) See Comment	Itra 200 mg po bid x3 d, then 200 mg po x2 wks, then 200 mg po qd (IV if unable to take po)	3rd most common OI in AIDS pts in SE Asia following TBc and cryptococcal meningitis. May resemble histoplasmosis or TBc (CID 23:125, 1996). Skin nodules are umbilicated (mimic cryptococcal infection or molluscum contagiosum) (JAIDS). In AIDS pts, long-term suppression with itra was effective in pre- venting relapses in 36/36 pts, whereas 20/35 pts receiving placebo relapsed within 6 mos. (NEJM 339:1739, 1998).

¹ Oral solution preferred to tablets because of ↑ absorption (see Table 10B, page 80).

¹ All dosage recommendations are for adults (unless otherwise indicated) and assume normal renal function

See page 78 for abbreviations.

TABLE 10A (8)

TYPE OF INFECTION/ORGANISM/ SITE OF INFECTION	ANTIMICROBIAL AGENTS OF CHOICE		COMMENTS
	PRIMARY	ALTERNATIVE[NFDAi]	
Phaeohyphomycosis (black molds/ dematiaceous fungi) (See CID 34:467, 2002) Sinuses, skin, brain abscess. **Species: Scedosporium prolificans,** Bipolaris, Wangiella, Curvularia, Exophiala, Phialemonium, Scytalidium, Alternaria, & others) Cause of disseminated disease in immuno-suppressed patients (3/4), esp. neutropenia & fungal endocarditis, esp. porcine valve. Blood cultures pos. in ~50%, eosinophilia in 11%	Surgery + **itraconazole** 400 mg/d po. duration not defined. probably 6 months[NFDAi]		Notoriously resistant to antifungal rx including amphotericin and azoles (CID 34:909, 2002). Mortality >80%. **Voriconazole** has some in vitro activity, but clinical experience limited to date vs S. prolificans (AAC 45:2151, 2001). **Itraconazole + terbinafine** synergistic against S. prolificans (AAC 44:470, 2000). No clinical data
Pseudallescheria boydii (Scedosporium apiospermum) (not considered a true dematiaceous mold) Skin, subcutaneous (Madura foot), brain abscess, recurrent meningitis	**Voriconazole** 6 mg/kg IV q12h on day 1, then either (4 mg/kg IV q12h) or (200 mg po q12h for body weight ≥40 kg) but 100 mg po q12h for body weight <40 kg) (PLU 21:240, 2002)	Surgery + **itraconazole** 200 mg po bid until clinically well[NFDAi]. (Many species now resistant or refractory to itra) **or** **Miconazole**[NUS] 600 mg IV q8h	These saprophytic fungi are notoriously resistant to antifungal drugs including amphotericin. In vitro voriconazole was more active than itra (J Clin Micro 39:954, 2001). MIC 2.52 vs 5, 75 for ampho & 7.5 µg/ml for itra. Several case reports of successful rx of disseminated and CNS disease with voriconazole have been reported (CID 31:1499 & 673, 2000). Effective in 5/8 patients (2 pulmonary & 5 CNS, 1 disseminated). 2 that failed had S. prolificans
Sporotrichosis (CID 29:231, 1999; CID 30:684, 2000) Cutaneous/Lymphonodular	**Itraconazole** 100–200 mg/d solution po x3-6 mos. (then 200 mg po bid long-term? for HIV-infected pts[DCbA])	**Fluconazole** 400 mg po qd x6 mos or Sat. soln. potassium iodide (SSKI) (1 gm of KI in 1 ml of H₂O). Start with 5–10 drops tid, gradually ↑ to 40–50 drops tid for 3-6 mos. Take after meals.	Itra ref.: CID 17:210, 1993 Some authorities use ampho B as primary therapy. Ampho B resistant strains reported (AJM 95:279, 1993). Itra rx for up to 24 months effective in multifocal osteoarticular infection (CID 23: 394, 1996) SSKI side-effects: nausea, rash, fever, metallic taste, salivary gland swelling
Extracutaneous: Osteoarticular, pulmonary, disseminated, meningeal	**Osteoarticular, pulmonary: Itraconazole** 300 mg po bid x6-12 mos. then 200 mg po bid (long-term for HIV-infected pts) (IV if unable to take po)	**Disseminated, meningeal: Ampho B** 0.5 mg/kg to total of 1–2 gm, followed by **itra** 200 mg bid or **flu** 800 mg qd	

Abbreviations: AM/CL = amoxicillin clavulanate; **Ampho B** = amphotericin B; **Clot** = clotrimazole; **dc** = discontinue; **Flu** = fluconazole; **Flucy** = flucytosine; **G** = generic; **Griseo** = griseofulvin; **I** = investigational; **IMP** = imipenem; **IT** = intrathecal or intraventricular; **Itra** = itraconazole; **Keto** = ketoconazole; **NB** = name brand; **NFDAi** = not FDA-approved indication; **NUS** = not available in the U.S.; **PSL** = peak serum level; **R/O** = rule out; **TMP/SMX** = trimethoprim/sulfamethoxazole; **vag. oint.** = vaginal ointment

† **Oral solution preferred to tablets because of ↑ absorption** (see Table 10B, page 80).

* All dosage recommendations are for adults (unless otherwise indicated) and assume normal renal function

See page 78 for abbreviations.

TABLE 10B: ANTIFUNGAL DRUGS: ADVERSE EFFECTS, COMMENTS, COST

DRUG NAME, GENERIC (TRADE)/ USUAL DOSAGE/COST	ADVERSE EFFECTS/COMMENTS
Non-lipid amphotericin B (Fungizone) 0.3–1 mg/kg/d as single infusion 50 mg $10 to 25	**Non-lipid amphotericin B (Fungizone)** **Admin.:** Commercial ampho B is a colloidal suspension that must be prepared in electrolyte-free D5W at 0.1 mg/ml to avoid precipitation. No need to protect drug suspension from light. Ampho B infusions often cause chills/fever, myalgia, anorexia, nausea, rarely hemodynamic collapse/hypotension. Postulated due to release of proinflammatory cytokines, hypersensitivity reaction cannot be excluded. Manufacturer recommends a test dose of 1 mg. Can cut the dose in 1/2 & run at low ml/ min for 4 hrs if such reactions occur. Gradually increasing amount of ampho B whether with or without hydrocortisone (25–50 mg) (Am J Hlth Pharm 52:1463, 1995) except chills/fever occurred sooner with 1-hr infusion. Frequency and severity of febrile reactions decrease with repeated doses. Rare pulmonary reactions (severe dyspnea and focal infiltrates suggesting pulmonary edema) appear to be associated with rapid infusion (CID 33:75, 2001). Severe rigors may respond to meperidine (25–50 mg) IV. Premedication with acetaminophen, diphenhydramine, hydrocortisone (25–50 mg) and heparin (1000 units) had not clearly been efficacious; if used, give a half-hour before ampho B. Hydrocortisone postulate correct, NSAIDs or high-dose steroids may prove efficacious but their use may risk worsening infection under rx or increased risk of nephrotoxicity (i.e., NSAIDs). Clinical side effects ↓ with ↑ age (CID 26:334, 1998). **Toxicity:** Major concern is nephrotoxicity (15% of 102 pts surveyed, CID 26:334, 1998). Manifest initially by kaluresis and hypokalemia, then fall in serum bicarbonate (may proceed to renal tubular acidosis), a rise in serum creatinine. Hypomagnesemia may occur. Can reduce risk of renal injury by **(a) pre- and post-infusion hydration with 500 ml saline (if clinical status will allow salt load)**, (b) avoidance of other nephrotoxins, e.g., radiocontrast, cis-platinum, aminoglycosides. Use of low-dose dopamine did not significantly reduce renal toxicity (AAC 42:1303, 1998). In a single randomized controlled trial of 80 neutropenic pts with refractory fever & suspected or proven invasive fungal infection, 0.97 mg/kg/d amphotericin **continuously infused over a 24-hr period** was compared to the classical **rapid infusion of 0.95 mg/kg/d infused over 4 hrs.** Continuous infusion produced less nephrotoxicity (28% vs in max. serum Cr (p=0.0005)), a reduction in fever, chills & vomiting (p <0.02–0.0003) & appeared as effective as rapid infusion but in very few proven fungal infections (BMJ 322:1, 2001). Await trials of efficacy in larger number of proven fungal infections!
Lipid-based ampho B products:[1]	
Amphotericin B lipid complex (ABLC) (Abelcet) (Abelcet): 5 mg/kg/d as single infusion 100 mg IV $230	**Amphotericin B lipid complex (ABLC) (Abelcet):** **Admin.:** Indicated for rx of invasive fungal infections in pts refractory or intolerant to non-lipid ampho B. Consists of ampho B complexed with 2 lipid bilayer ribbons. Compared to standard ampho B, larger volume of distribution, rapid blood clearance and high tissue concentrations (liver, spleen, lung). Dosage: **5 mg/kg once daily**, infuse at 2.5 mg/kg/hr; adult and ped. dose the same. Do NOT use an in-line filter. Do not dilute with saline solution or mix with other drugs or electrolytes (AAC 41:2201, 1997). **Toxicity:** Fever and chills in 14–18%; nausea 9%, vomiting 8%, serum creatinine ↑ in 11%; renal failure 5%; anemia 4%; ↓ K 5%; rash 4%.
Liposomal amphotericin B (L-AmB, AmBisome) (AmBisome): 1–5 mg/kg/d as single infusion 50 mg $188 ($130/350 mg)	**Liposomal amphotericin B (AmBisome):** **Admin.:** Approved for empiric rx for presumed fungal infections in febrile neutropenic pts; rx of pts with aspergillus, candida and/or cryptococcus infections refractory to conventional ampho B, or in pts where renal impairment or unacceptable toxicity precludes the use of conventional ampho B; and rx of visceral leishmaniasis. Consists of a true vesicular bilayer liposome with ampho B intercalated within the membrane. Dosage: **3–5 mg/kg IV** as single dose infused over a period of approx. 120 min. If infusion is well tolerated, infusion time can be reduced to 60 min.[1] 1 mg/kg/d was as effective as 4 mg/kg/d in pts from malignancy (CID 27:1406, 1998). Survival rates 1.5% vs 1.7%, respectively, in pts with invasive aspergillosis complicating bone marrow transplant (J Inf #9, 1999; Bone Marrow Tx 20:39, 1997). **Major toxicity:** Generally less than ampho B deoxycholate. Nephrotoxicity 18.8% vs 33.7% for ampho B, chills 47% vs 75%, nausea 39.7% vs 38.7%, vomiting 31.8% vs 43.9%, rash 24% for both. ↓ Ca 18.4% vs 20.9%, ↓ K 20.4% vs 25.6%, ↓ K 20.4% vs 25.6%.
Amphotericin B cholesteryl complex (amphotericin B colloidal dispersion, ABCD, Amphotec) (Amphotec): 3–4 mg/kg/d as single infusion 100 mg $160	**Amphotericin B cholesteryl complex (Amphotec):** **Admin.:** Approved for rx of aspergillosis in pts who either failed or are intolerant to standard ampho B. Consists of ampho B deoxycholate stabilized with cholesteryl sulfate (forms ampho B in a disc structure). Compared to standard ampho B, larger volume of distribution, rapid blood clearance, high tissue concentrations. Dosage: Initial dose for adults & children: **3–4 mg/kg/day**. If necessary, can ↑ to 6 mg/kg/day. Dilute in D5W & infuse at 1 mg/kg/hr. Do NOT use in-line filter. **Toxicity:** Chills 50%, fever 33%,[1] serum creatinine 12–20%, ↓ Ca 6%, ↓ K 17%.

---

[1] Published data from patients intolerant of or refractory to conventional ampho B deoxycholate (Amp B d). **None of the lipid ampho B preps has shown superior efficacy compared to ampho B in prospective trials. Dosage equivalency has not been established.** Nephrotoxicity ↓ with all lipid ampho B preps (IDCP 7:516, 1998; CID 27:603, 1998; NEJM 340:764, 1999).

[2] Comparisons between Abelcet and AmBisome suggest a higher infusion associated toxicity (rigors) and febrile episodes with Abelcet (70% vs 36%) but ↓ hepatic toxicity with AmBisome (AAC 46:828, 2002). Note: product inserts use the price AWP (average wholesale price) — can differ significantly from actual prices (CID 26:1383, 1998).

* From CURRENT DRUGS (DRUG RED BOOK, Medical Economics Data and Hospital Formulary Pricing Guide. **Price is average wholesale price (AWP).**

All dosage recommendations are for adults (unless otherwise indicated) and assume normal renal function

TABLE 10B (2)

DRUG NAME, GENERIC (TRADE)/ USUAL DOSAGE/COST	ADVERSE EFFECTS/COMMENTS
Caspofungin (Cancidas) 70 mg IV (day 1) followed by 50 mg IV qd (reduce to 35 mg IV qd with moderate hepatic insufficiency) 70 mg $464, 50 mg $360	An echinocandin which inhibits synthesis of β-(1,3)-D-glucan, a critical component of fungal cell walls. Fungicidal against candida (MIC <2 μg/ml) including those resistant to other antifungals & active against aspergillus (MIC 0.4–2 μg/ml). Serum levels on rec. dosages = peak 12, trough 1.3 (24 hrs) μg/ml. Approved for refractory aspergillosis and invasive candida & other mycoses in pts with neutropenia. Indicated for treatment of esophageal candida. Additional uses under study. **Toxicity**: remarkably non-toxic with no nephrotoxicity reported. Only 2% of 263 pts in double-blind trial do to drug-related adverse event (*Transpl Inf Dis 1:25, 2002*). 14% had ↑ transaminases (similar to triazoles). Most common adverse effect: pruritus at infusion site & headache associated with infusion. Drug metabolized in liver & dosage ≈ 35 mg in moderate to severe hepatic failure. Class C for pregnancy (embryotoxic in rats & rabbits), so only use if potential benefits outweigh risks. See *Table 21, page 136 for drug-drug interactions*
Fluconazole (Diflucan) 100 mg tabs $9.25 150 mg tabs $13.17 200 mg tabs $13.50 400 mg IV $142 Oral suspension- 40 mg/ml, $123/35 ml bottle	IV and oral doses of equal efficacy; excellent absorption po, wide tissue distribution; 80% excreted unchanged in urine; good CSF penetration even with non-inflamed meninges. Peak serum levels (see *Table 8B, page 59*) 1/2 22 hrs. 12% protein bound. **CSF levels 50–90% of serum in normals**, 60–80% in meningitis. No effect on mammalian steroid metabolism. **Drug-drug interactions common, see Table 21**. Side-effects overall 16% [more common in HIV+ pts (21%)]. Nausea 3.7% headache 1.9%, skin rash 1.8%, abdominal pain 1.7%, vomiting 1.7%, diarrhea 1.5%. ↑ SGOT 20%. Alopecia (scalp, pubic crest) in 12–20% pts on ≥400 mg/d qd after median of 3 months (reversible in approx. 6 mos.) (*AnIM 123:354, 1995*). Rare: severe hepatotoxicity, exfoliative dermatitis. Anaphylaxis (*CID 13:81, 1993*): thrombocytopenia, leucopenia. Good reference: *NEJM 330:263, 1994*
Flucytosine (Ancobon) 500 mg cap $8.03	AEs: Overall 30%. GI 6% (diarrhea, anorexia, nausea, vomiting); hematologic 22% [leucopenia, thrombocytopenia, when serum level > 100 μg/ml (esp. in azotemic pts)]; hepatotoxicity (asymptomatic ↑ SGOT, reversible); skin rash 7%; aplastic anemia (rare–2 or 3 cases). False ↑ in serum creatinine on EkTACHEM analyzer (*JAC 26:171, 2000*)
Griseofulvin (Fulvicin, Grifulvin, Grisactin) 500 mg G $1.56, susp 125 mg/ml 120 ml $38	Photosensitivity, urticaria, skin rash. Leucopenia (rare). Interferes with warfarin drugs. Increases blood and urine porphyrins, should not be used in patients with porphyria Disulfiram-like reactions. Exacerbation of systemic Lupus erythematosus.
Imidazoles: topical For vaginal and/or skin use	Not recommended in 1st trimester of pregnancy. Local reactions: 0.5–1.5%: dyspareunia, mild vulvar erythema, burning, pruritus, urticaria, rash. Rarely similar symptoms in sexual partner.
Itraconazole (Sporanox), 100 mg cap $7.78 10 mg/ml oral solution (fasting state) (150 ml) $122) (AAC 42: 1862, 1998) IV usual dose 200 mg bid x 4 doses followed by 200 mg qd for a maximum of 14 days ($185,$060 mg)	Cost of treating vaginitis topically. Butoconazole x3 d$33, clotrimazole x7 d$12, miconazole x3 d$30, terconazole x3 d$34, tioconazole x1 dose $24. Oral agents preferred because of convenience, compliance, and cost. Fluconazole 150 mg po x1 dose $12 **Itraconazole tablet and solution forms are not interchangeable, solution preferred.** Many authorities recommend measuring drug serum concentration after 2 weeks of prolonged rx to ensure satisfactory absorption. To obtain the highest plasma concentration, the tablet is given with food and acidic drinks (e.g., cola) while the solution is taken in the fasting state; under these conditions, the peak conc. of the capsule is approx. 3 μg/ml and the solution 5.4 μg/ml. Peak levels are reached faster (2.2 vs 5 hrs) with the solution. **Peak plasma concentrations after IV injection (200 mg) compared to oral capsule (200 mg): 2.8 μg/ml (on day 7 of rx) vs 2 μg/ml (on day 36 of rx)**. Protein-binding for both preparations is over 99%, which explains the virtual absence of penetration into the CSF (**do not use to treat meningitis**). Most common adverse effects are dose-related nausea 10%, diarrhea 8%, vomiting 6%, and abdominal discomfort 5.7%. Allergic rash 1.6%, pruritus 1.5%, edema 3.5% and hypokalemia 2% reported. Rarely, high doses may produce hypokalemia 8% and ↑ blood pressure 3.2%. Thrombocytopenia and leucopenia have been reported (*AnIM 125:157, 1996*). **Reported to produce impairment in cardiac function (see** *footnote 2, page 76*). Other concern, as with fluconazole and ketoconazole, is **drug-drug interactions; see Table 21**. Some interactions can be life-threatening.
Ketoconazole (Nizoral) 200 mg tab $3.86	Gastric acid required for dissolution—cimetidine, omeprazole, antacids block absorption; in achlorhydria, dissolve tablet in 4 ml 0.2N HCl, drink with a straw. Coca-Cola ↑ absorption by 65% (*AAC 39:1671, 1995*). CSF levels "none". **Drug-drug interactions important, see Table 21**. **Some interactions can be life-threatening. Dose-dependent nausea and vomiting.** Liver toxicity of hepatocellular type reported in about 1:10,000 exposed pts—usually after several days to weeks of exposure. Inhibition of testosterone and cortisol synthesis is dose-dependent. With high doses (≥800 mg/d) gynecomastia, decreased libido, and (rarely) adrenal (Addisonian) crisis reported.
Miconazole (Monistat IV) 200 mg—not available in U.S.	IV miconazole indicated in patient critically ill with Pseudallescheria boydii. Used in some centers as prophylaxis in initial rx regimens in febrile neutropenic pts (*AJM 83:1103, 1987; J Clin Onc 8:280, 1990*). Very toxic due to vehicle needed to get drug into solution.
Nystatin (Mycostatin) 30 gm cream $28.52 500,000 u oral tab $0.78	Topical: virtually no adverse effects. Less effective than imidazoles and triazoles. PO: large doses give occasional GI distress and diarrhea.

* From 2002 DRUG TOPICS RED BOOK, Medical Economics Data and Hospital Formulary Pricing Guide. **Price is average wholesale price (AWP)**.
All dosage recommendations are for adults (unless otherwise indicated) and assume normal renal function

TABLE 10B (3)

DRUG NAME, GENERIC (TRADE)/ USUAL DOSAGE/COST*	ADVERSE EFFECTS/COMMENTS
Terbinafine (Lamisil) 250 mg tab $8.33	Rare cases (B) of idiosyncratic & symptomatic hepatic injury and more rarely liver failure leading to death or liver transplantation reported in pts receiving terbinafine for onychomycosis. Non-concomitant hepatotoxicity. Therefore, the drug is **not recommended** for pts with **chronic or active liver disease** although hepatotoxicity may occur in pts with or without pre-existing disease. Pretreatment screening of serum transaminases (ALT & AST) is advised & alternate rx used for those with abnormal levels. Pts started on terbinafine should be warned about symptoms suggesting liver dysfunction (persistent nausea, anorexia, fatigue, vomiting, RUQ pain, jaundice, dark urine or pale stools). If symptoms develop, drug should be discontinued & liver function immediately evaluated. In controlled trials, changes in ocular lens and retina reported—clinical significance unknown. Major drug-drug interaction is 100% ↑ in rate of clearance by rifampin. AEs: usually mild, transient and rarely caused discontinuation of rx. % with AE, terbinafine vs placebo: nausea/diarrhea 2.6–5.6 vs 2.9; rash 5.6 vs 2.2; taste abnormality 2.8 vs 0.7. Inhibits CYP2D6 enzymes (see *Table 21*).
Voriconazole (Vfend) IV: **Loading dose 6 mg/kg q12h IV** × 1 d. IV, then **Maintenance dose 4 mg/kg q12h IV** for invasive aspergillus & serious mold infections; **3 mg/kg q12h IV** for serious candida infections Oral: **>40 kg body weight:** 400 mg po q12h × 1 d., then 200 mg po q12h **<40 kg body weight:** 200 mg po q12h × 1 d., then 100 mg po q12h. **Take oral dose 1 hour before or 1 hour after eating.** Reduce to ½ maintenance dose for moderate hepatic insufficiency.	A unique triazole with enhanced activity against Aspergillus sp. (MIC 90 = 0.25–2 μg/ml), including Ampho resistant strains of A. terreus (*JCM 37:2343*, 1999) Candida sp. (MIC 0.03–2 μg/ml but may be higher for some more resistant sp.), Fusarium sp. (MIC 0.25–8) & various molds. Steady state serum levels reach 2.5–4 μg/ml. Effective in infections caused by C. krusei & in ≥50% of invasive aspergillus infections in pts with hematologic malignancies (*NEJM 347:408*, 2002). Toxicity similar to other azole/triazoles including uncommon serious hepatic toxicity (hepatitis, cholestasis & fulminant hepatic failure, 4 cases either likely or possibly related to voriconazole reported). Liver function tests should be monitored during rx & drug dic'd if abnormalities develop. Rash reported in up to 20%, occ. photosensitivity & rare Stevens-Johnson, hallucinations, & anaphylactoid infusion reactions with fever and hypertension (*Clin Exp Dermatol 26:648*, 2001). **Approx. 30% experience a transient visual disturbance** following both IV & po ("altered/enhanced visual perception", blurred or colored visual change or photophobia) within 30–60 minutes. Do not drive at night for outpatient rx. These changes resolve within 30–60 min. after administration & are attenuated with repeated doses. No persistence of effect reported. Cause unknown. In patients with ClCr <50 ml/min, the drug should be given orally, not IV, since the intravenous vehicle (SBECD-sulfobutylether-B-cyclodextrin) may accumulate.

---

* From 2002 DRUG TOPICS RED BOOK, Medical Economics Data and Hospital Formulary Pricing Guide. **Price is average wholesale price (AWP).** *All dosage recommendations are for adults (unless otherwise indicated) and assume normal renal function*

TABLE 11A: TREATMENT OF MYCOBACTERIAL INFECTIONS*

Tuberculin skin test (abbreviation TST). The standard is the Mantoux test, 5 TU PPD in 0.1 ml diluent stabilized with Tween 80. Read at 48–72 hrs measuring maximum diameter of induration. A reaction of ≥5 mm is defined as + in the following: + HIV or risk factors, recent close contacts, CXR consistent with healed TBc; immunosuppressed & receiving ≥15 mg of prednisone (or equivalent corticosteroid) per day for ≥1 month. ≥10 mm is + in all others, including foreign-born in countries of high prevalence, injection drug users, low income populations, nursing home residents, pts with medical conditions which ↑ risk (see *IA* below); ≥15 mm = + only in patients at low risk in whom testing generally not indicated *(AJRCCM 161:S221, 2000; CID 34:365, 2002)* **Two-stage TST:** Those whose reactivity may diminish with age may have negative 1st test but have positive "booster" on second test done 1–3 wks later. Interpret as in recent converter. If TST first skin test negative but < 10 mm, repeat 5 TU in 1 week. If positive then = booster (+ positive reaction but is of a reaction of ≥10 mm in an adult who was vaccinated as a child and who is from a country with a high prevalence of TB should be attributed to M. tbc infection *(AJRCCM 161:S221, 2000)*. **BCG vaccination** (Ann IM 127:55, 1979) BCG may result in TST reaction ≥10 mm but a reaction of ≥10 mm in an adult who was vaccinated as a child and who is from a country with a high prevalence of TB should be attributed to M. tbc infection. Prior BCG may result in booster effect in 2-stage TST *(AIM 161:1760, 2001)*. For TST in children, see *Pediatrics 97:282, 1996*. Currently available PPD preparations are of comparable specificity *(JAMA 281:169, 1999)*. Routine anergy testing no longer recommended with HIV + *(MMWR 46:RR-5 1997)*. Newer assay recently approved by US FDA uses blood & diagnostic test for TB, but data on its sensitivity & specificity are conflicting *(JAMA 286:1740, 2001; CID 34:1449 & 1457, 2002)*. Overall recommendations for USA *NEJM 345:189, 2001; MMWR 51(RR-5), 2002*

I. Mycobacterium tuberculosis

CAUSATIVE AGENT/DISEASE	MODIFYING CIRCUMSTANCES	INITIAL THERAPY	SUGGESTED REGIMENS CONTINUATION PHASE OF THERAPY
I. Mycobacterium tuberculosis exposure but TST negative (household members & other close contacts of potentially infectious cases)	Neonate—Rx essential	INH (10 mg/kg/day for 3 months)	Repeat tuberculin skin test (TST) in 3 mos. If mother's smear negative & infant's TST negative & chest x-ray (CXR) normal, stop INH. In USA, BCG is then given *(Ln 2, 1479, 1990)*, unless mother HIV+. If infant's repeat TST positive &/or CXR abnormal (see *Category I) below*).
	Children <5 years of age– Rx indicated	As for neonate for 1st 3 months	If mother is being rx, separation of infant from mother not indicated.
	Older children and adults—Risk 2–4% 1st year	No rx	If repeat TST at 3 mos. is negative, stop. If repeat TST positive, continue INH for total of 9 months. If INH not given initially, repeat TST at 3 mos., if positive rx with INH x 9 mos. (see *Category I) below*).

II. Treatment of latent infection with M. tuberculosis, formerly known as "prophylaxis" *(AJRCCM 161: S221, 2000)*

CAUSATIVE AGENT/DISEASE	MODIFYING CIRCUMSTANCES	INITIAL THERAPY	SUGGESTED REGIMENS AND/OR MMWR
II. Treatment of latent infection with M. tuberculosis, formerly known as "prophylaxis" *(AJRCCM 161: S221, 2000)* **A. Not indicated due to high-risk.** Assumes INH susceptibility likely. INH 54–88% effective in preventing active TB for ≥20 years.	(1) + tuberculin reactor & HIV+ (risk of active disease 10%/yr, AIDS 170x †, HIV+ 113x †)*	INH (5 mg/kg/day, maximum 300 mg/d for adults; 10 mg/kg/d for children) Optional duration 9 mos. (includes children, HIV-, HIV+, old fibrotic lesions on chest x-ray). In some cases, 6 mos. may be given for cost-effectiveness *(AJRCCM 161: S221, 2000)*. Do not use 6 mo. regimen in HIV+ persons or with (2) or those with fibrotic lesions on chest film *(NEJM 345:189, 2001)*.	If compliance problem: INH by DOT† 15 mg/kg 2x/wk x9 mos. or **RIF** 600 mg/d po + PZA† 15–20 mg/kg/d po) for 2 mos. or **(RIF + PZA** 50 mg/kg 2x/wk) for 2–3 mos. or **RIF + PZA** x2 mos. *(JAMA 283:1445, 2000)*. RIF + PZA appears safe in HIV+ pts but there are recent descriptions of severe & fatal hepatitis in pts on RIF + PZA *(MMWR 50:289, 2001)*. Therefore, regimen should be avoided in HIV-neg. pts with underlying liver disease or alcoholism & in pts on concomitant hepatotoxic agents. If used, monitor LFTs & clinical status q2 wks *(MMWR 50:733, 2001)*. (HIV– and HIV+) **RIF** 600 mg/d po for 4 mos. (HIV– and HIV+)
	(2) Newly infected persons (TST conversion in past 2 yrs — risk 3.3%, 1st yr)		
	(3) Past tuberculosis, not rx with adequate chemotherapy (INH, RIF, or alternatives)		
	(4) + tuberculin reactors with CXR consistent with non-progressive tuberculous disease (risk 0.5–5.0%/yr)		
	(5) + tuberculin reactors with specific predisposing conditions: illicit intravenous drug use *(MMWR 38:236, 1989)*, silicosis, diabetes mellitus, prolonged adrenocortical rx (>15 mg prednisone/day), immunosuppressive rx, hematologic diseases (Hodgkin's, leukemia), end-stage renal disease, clinical weight loss or chronic under-nutrition, previous gastrectomy *(AARD 134:355, 1986)*.		

NOTE: For HIV, see SANFORD Guide to HIV/AIDS THERAPY and/or MMWR 48:RR-10, 1999

B. TST positive (organisms likely to be INH-susceptible)

CAUSATIVE AGENT/DISEASE	MODIFYING CIRCUMSTANCES	INITIAL THERAPY SUGGESTED REGIMENS	
B. TST positive (organisms likely to be INH-susceptible)	Age no longer considered modifying factor (see Comments)	INH (5 mg/kg/day, max 300 mg/d for adults; 10 mg/kg/d for children) Results with 6 mos. rx not as effective as 12 mos. (65% vs 75% reduction in current recommendation. See *IIA above* for details and alternate rx	COMMENTS Meta-analysis of earlier studies favors INH prophylaxis (if INH related hepatic case fatality <1% and INH prophylaxis appears to be the case) *(AIM 127:1051, 1997)*. Recent data suggest INH prophylaxis has positive risk-benefit ratio in pts ≥35 if monitored for hepatotoxicity 0.1–0.15% *(JAMA 281:1014, 1999)*. Overall risk of hepatotoxicity 0.1–0.15% *(JAMA 127: 1051, 1997)*.
	Any risk factors (IIA above)	Treat with INH as above. For women at risk for progression of latent TB to active disease, rx should not be delayed even during the first trimester.	Risk of INH hepatitis may be † *(Ln 346:199, 1995)*
	Pregnancy—Any risk factors (IIA above)		
	Pregnancy—No risk factors	No initial rx (see Comment)	Risk of INH hepatitis may be † *(Ln 346:199, 1995)* [Delay rx until 6 mos. after delivery *(AJRCCM 149:1359, 1994)*]

See pages 87 & 89 for all footnotes and abbreviations

* Dosages are for adults (unless otherwise indicated) and assume normal renal function   † DOT = directly observed therapy

TABLE 11A (2)

CAUSATIVE AGENT/DISEASE	MODIFYING CIRCUMSTANCES	SUGGESTED REGIMENS INITIAL THERAPY	ALTERNATIVE	COMMENTS
II. Treatment of latent infection with M. tuberculosis				
C. TST positive & drug resistance likely (For data on worldwide prevalence of drug resistance, see NEJM 344:1294, 2001; JID 185:1197, 2002)	INH-resistant (or adverse reaction to INH), RIF-sensitive organisms likely	**Prophylaxis "("prophylaxis")** (continued) **RIF** 600 mg/d po for 2 mos (HIV+ or HIV−) or **RIF** 600 mg po for 4 mos (HIV+ or HIV−)		See Comments in Section II.A re: RIF + PZA regimen. IDSA guideline lists rifabutin in 600 mg/d dose as another alternative; however, current recommended max. dose of rifabutin is 300 mg/d. Estimate RIF alone has protective effect of 56%; 26% of pts stopped therapy due to adverse effects (only 2/157 did not complete 6 mos. rx) (AJRCCM 155:1735, 1997). PZA + ofloxo has been associated with asymptomatic hepatitis (CID 21:1264, 1997).
	INH- and RIF-resistant organisms likely	Efficacy of all regimens unproven. (**PZA** 25–30 mg/kg/d to max. of 2 gm/d + **ETB** 15–25 mg/kg po) x6–12 mos.	[(**PZA** 25 mg/kg/d to max. of 2.0 gm/d + (**levoflox** 500 mg/d or **oflox** 400 mg bid), all x6, x6–12 mos.	

CAUSATIVE AGENT/DISEASE	MODIFYING CIRCUMSTANCES	SUGGESTED REGIMENS FOR DOSAGE AND DIRECTLY OBSERVED THERAPY (DOT) REGIMENS SEE COMMENTS FOR DOSAGE AND DIRECTLY OBSERVED THERAPY (DOT) REGIMENS INITIAL THERAPY	CONTINUATION PHASE OF THERAPY (in vitro susceptibility known)	
III. Mycobacterium tuberculosis **A. Pulmonary TB** (General reference on rx in adults & children: MMWR 52(RR-9), 2003; CID 28:130, 1999) Isolation essential! Pts with active TB should be isolated in single rooms, not cohorted. Older observations on infectivity of susceptible & resistant M. tbc before & after rx (ARRD 85:511, 1962) may not be applicable to MDR M. tbc or to HIV + individual. Extended isolation may be appropriate.	Rate of INH resistance known to be < 4%	**INH** + **RIF** (or **RFB**) + **PZA** daily x2 mos.	**INH** + **RIF** (or **RFB**) daily x4 mos. (total 6 mos.)	
	Rate of INH resistance not known or ≥4% —Compliant pt	**INH** + **RIF** (or **RFB**) + **PZA** + either **SM** or **ETB** daily until susc. data available. Even if susc., INH + RIF (or **RFB**) for total of 2 mos.	Authors add **pyridoxine** 25–50 mg po daily to any regimen that includes **INH** NOTE: For pts with cavitary pulm. or AFB pos. after 2 mos. of therapy, and longer for cavitary/laryngeal tbc: **INH** + **RIF** (or **RFB**) daily to complete 6 months of therapy. (Failure rates up to 10% in some areas with multiresistant TB (JAMA 283:2537, 2000].	
	—Non-compliant or unreliable pt	Directly observed therapy (DOT): 1. **INH** + **RIF** (or **RFB**) + **PZA** + either **SM** or **ETB** daily for 2 wks and then 2–3x/wk for 6 wks OR 2. **INH** + **RIF** (or **RFB**) + **PZA** + either **SM** or **ETB** 3x/wk for 6 months.	**INH** + **RIF** (or **RFB**) 2–3x/wk to complete 6 months of therapy in pts who are HIV-neg. without cavitation on chest film or rifapentine 600 mg/wk + INH 900 mg/wk appears as effective as INH given 2x/weeks (Ln 360:528, 2002).	
	Known resistance (or intolerance) to INH	DOT recommended for all drug-resistant tuberculosis: RIF (or RFB) + ETB + PZA daily x18 months (≥12 months post-negative sputum cultures). DOT may		
	Resistance (or intolerance) to RIF	**INH** + **ETB** + **PZA** daily x18 months (≥12 months post-negative sputum cultures)		

DOT regimens recommended if possible (JAMA 279:943, 1998)

(continued on next page)

Regimen	Dose in mg/kg (max. daily dose)				
	INH	RIF	PZA	ETB	SM	RFB
Daily						
Child	10–20 (300)	10–20 (600)	15–30 (2000)	15–25	15–25	10–20 (300)
Adult	5 (300)	10 (600)	15–30 (2000)	15–25	15	5 (300)
2x/wk (DOT):						
Child	20–40 (900)	10–20 (600)	50–70 (4000)	50	25–30 (1000)	10–20 (300)
Adult	15 (900)	10 (600)	50–70 (4000)	50	25–30 (1500)	5 (300)
3x/wk (DOT):						
Child	20–40 (900)	10–20 (600)	50–70 (3000)	25–30	25–30 (1500)	NA
Adult	15 (900)	10 (600)	50–70 (3000)	25–30	25–30 (1500)	NA

Second-line anti-TB agents can be dosed as follows to facilitate DOT:
Ethionamide 500–750 mg qd (5x/wk) po
Kanamycin or capreomycin 15 mg/kg qd (3–5x/wk) IM/IV
Cycloserine 750–1000 mg qd (5x/wk) po
Ciprofloxacin 750 mg qd (5x/wk) po
Ofloxacin 600–800 mg qd (5x/wk) po
Levofloxacin 750 mg qd (5x/wk) po

Risk factors for drug-resistant TB: Recent immigrant from Latin America or Asia (or the area of >4% resistance [24%] or previous rx without RIF: exposure to known MDR-TB. Incidence of INH-resistant TB in U.S. is established and is not decreasing. In early 1990s (JAMA 276:833, 1997). Incidence of primary drug resistance is particularly high (>25%) in parts of China, Thailand, Estonia & Latvia (NEJM 344:1294, 2001).

(continued on next page)

* Dosages are for adults (unless otherwise indicated) and assume normal renal function   † DOT = directly observed therapy

See pages 87 & 89 for all footnotes and abbreviations

TABLE 11A (3)

CAUSATIVE AGENT/DISEASE	MODIFYING CIRCUMSTANCES	SUGGESTED REGIMENS		COMMENTS
		INITIAL THERAPY	**CONTINUATION PHASE OF THERAPY (in vitro susceptibility known)**	
III. Mycobacterium tuberculosis/A. Pulmonary TB *(continued)* (continued from previous page) REFERENCE: CID 22:683. **Multidrug-Resistant Tuberculosis (MDR TB):** Defined as resistant to at least 2 drugs. Pt clusters with high mortality (AJHM 118:17, 1993)	• Resistance to both INH and RIF = multiple drug-resistant tuberculosis (MDR TB)	Want ≥3 drugs active vs MDR TB: **RIF (or RFB) + PZA + ETB or SM** + additional second-line drug (**AMK**) + quinolone (**CIP** or **levofloxacin** or **gatifloxacin**)	Continue ≥3 drugs shown active in vitro vs MDR TB. Appropriate duration of therapy is not known. ↑ Less effective and intensive regimens have ↑ failure rates (*Ln 353:969, 1999*).	*(continued from previous page)* For MDR TB, consider rifabutin (~30% RIF-resistant strains are susceptible to rifabutin). Gatifloxacin in multidrug regimen for susceptible TB (*CID 22:287, 1996*). Gatifloxacin and levofloxacin have enhanced activity compared with CIP against M. tuberculosis (*AAC 46:1022, 2002*). Mortality reviewed (*AJRCCM 159:3467-71, 1997*. Rapid (24-hr) diagnostic tests for M. tuberculosis: (1) the Amplified Mycobacterium tuberculosis Direct Test amplifies and detects M. tuberculosis ribosomal RNA. (2) the AMPLICOR Mycobacterium tuberculosis Test amplifies and detects M. tuberculosis DNA. Both tests have sensitivities and specificities >95% in sputum samples that are AFB-positive; in negative smears, specificity remains >95% but sensitivity is 40-77% (*4th J Clin Care Med 155:1497, 1997*).

CAUSATIVE AGENT/DISEASE: MODIFYING CIRCUMSTANCES	SUGGESTED REGIMENS		COMMENTS
	INITIAL THERAPY	**CONTINUATION PHASE OF THERAPY (in vitro susceptibility known)**	
III. Mycobacterium tuberculosis *(con't)* **B. Extrapulmonary TB**	**INH + RIF + PZA** daily x2 months. Authors add **pyridoxine** 25-50 mg po daily to regimens that include INH	**INH + RIF (or RFB)** daily x4-10 months (total 6-12 months)	6-month regimens probably effective. Most experience with 9-12 month regimens. Am Acad Ped (1994) recommends 6 mos. rx for isolated cervical adenitis, renal and 12 mos. for miliary, bone/joint. DOT useful here as well as for pulmonary tuberculosis.
C. Tuberculous meningitis For critical appraisal of adjunctive steroids: *CID 25:872, 1997*	**INH + RIF + ETB + PZA**	May add INH when susceptibility to INH and RIF is established. Treat total of 12 months. See Table 8C, page 59, for CSF drug clearance.	3 drugs often recommended for initial rx, we prefer 4. May substitute ethionamide for ETB because of its good CNS penetration. Steroids reduce long-term complications (*Pediatrics 99:226, 1997*). PCR of CSF markedly increases diagnostic sensitivity and provides rapid dx (*Neurol 45:2228, 1995; Arch Neurol 53:771, 1996*).
D. Tuberculosis during pregnancy	**INH + RIF + ETB** for 9 months		PZA not recommended: teratogenicity data inadequate. Because of potential ototoxicity to fetus throughout gestation (16%), SM should not be used unless other drugs contraindicated.
E. Treatment failure or relapse: Usually due to poor compliance or resistant organisms (*AJM 102:164, 1997*)	Directly observed therapy (DOT). Check susceptibilities. *(See section III.A, pages 83, 84)*	PZA not recommended... patients whose sputum has not converted after 5-6 mos. Non-compliance common, therefore institute DOT. If isolates show resistance, modify regimen to include at least 2 effective agents, preferably ones which patient has not received. Surgery may be necessary	Failures may be due to non-compliance. Check susceptibility on current isolates and obtain susceptibility on current isolates...
F. HIV infection or AIDS—pulmonary or extrapulmonary (NOTE: 60-70% of HIV+ pts with TB have extrapulmonary disease)	**INH + RIF (or RFB) + PZA** daily x2 months. (Authors add **pyridoxine** 25-50 mg po daily to regimens that include INH)	**INH + RIF (or RFB)** daily x4 months (total 6 mos.). May treat up to 9 mos. in pts with delayed response.	1. Because of the possibility of developing resistance to RfB in pts with low CD4 cell counts who receive weekly or biweekly doses of RfB, it is recomm. that such pts receive daily (or minimally 3x/weekly) doses of RFB for initiation & continuation phase of rx (*MMWR 51:214, 2002*) 2. Clinical and microbiological response same as in HIV-negative although there is considerable variability in outcomes among currently available studies (*CID 32:623, 2001*). 3. Post-treatment suppression not necessary for drug-susceptible strains. 4. Rate of INH resistance known to be <4% (for ↑ rates of resistance, see *Section III.A*) 5. For more information, see *MMWR 47(RR-20):1, 1998 & CID 28:139, 1999.* 6. May use partially intermittent therapy: 1 dose/day for 2 weeks followed by 2-3 doses/week for 24 weeks (*MMWR 47(RR-20), 1998*)

Dosages are for adults (unless otherwise indicated) and assume normal renal/renal function   †DOT = directly observed therapy

See pages 87 & 89 for all footnotes and abbreviations

TABLE 11A (4)

CAUSATIVE AGENT/DISEASE	MODIFYING CIRCUMSTANCES	SUGGESTED REGIMENS PRIMARY	ALTERNATIVE	COMMENTS
III. Mycobacterium tuberculosis (continued) **F. HIV infection and AIDS—pulmonary or extrapulmonary** (continued) Concomitant protease inhibitor (PI) therapy (Modified from MMWR 49:185, 2000)		**Initial & cont. therapy:** Use indinavir 1250 mg bid) or (indinavir 800 mg q8h) as the PI component of antiretroviral rx. (INH 300 mg + rifabutin 150 mg + PZA 25 mg/kg + ETB 15 mg/kg) qd daily for 2 mos., then INH + rifabutin for 4–7 mos.	**Alternative regimen:** INH + SM + PZA + ETB x2 mos. (then INH + SM + PZA + ETB 2–3 times/ wk for 7 mos. May be used with any PI regimen. May be used in pts with delayed response.	**Comments:** Rifamycins induce cytochrome CYP450 enzymes (RIF -> RFP > RFB) & reduce serum levels of concomitantly administered PIs (conversely, PIs (ritonavir > amprenavir > indinavir > nelfinavir > saquinavir) inhibit CYP450 & cause ↑ serum levels of RIF, RFP & RFB. If dose of RFB is not reduced, toxicity↑. **Do not use RIF + PI.** RFB/PI combinations are therapeutically effective (CID 30:779, 2000). RFB has no effect on nelfinavir levels at dose of 1250 mg bid (Can JID 10:21B, 1999).
IV. Other Mycobacterial Disease ("Atypical") (See ATS Consensus; AJRCCM 152:51, 1997; IDC No. Amer. March 2002)) **A. M. bovis**		(then INH + rifabutin for 4–7 mos.)	The M. tuberculosis complex includes M. bovis. All isolates resistant to PZA. 9–12 months of rx used by some authorities. Isolation not required.	
B. Bacillus Calmette-Guerin (BCG) (derived from M. bovis)	Only for rx (>38.5°C) for 12–24 hrs. Systemic illness or sepsis	INH 300 mg qd x3 months (INH 300 mg) + (RIF 600 mg) + (ETB 1200 mg) po x6 mos.	Intravesical BCG effective in superficial bladder tumors and carcinoma in situ. Adverse effects: fever 2.9%, granulomatosis, pneumonitis, hepatitis 0.7%, sepsis 0.4% (J Urol 147:596, 1992). With sepsis, consider initial adjunctive prednisolone. Resistant to PZA.	
C. M. avium–intracellulare complex (MAC, MAI or Battey bacillus) [Excellent rev (AJM 102 (5C), 1997)] ATS Consensus Statement: AJRCCM 156:51, 1997	**Immunocompetent patients** with chronic pulmonary, disseminated disease (subcutaneous, bone)	**Clarithro** 500 mg po bid or **azithro** 600 mg po qd + **ETB** 25 mg/kg po x2 mos, then 15 mg/kg po qd + **RIF** 600 mg po qd (or **RFB** 300 mg po qd). May also add **CLO** 100–200 mg po qd or **AMK** 15 mg/kg iv for 2–6 mos. for severe disease. Rx until culture neg. x1 yr. Alternative: **Clarithro** 500 mg po bid + **ETB** 15–25 mg/kg po qd + **RFB** 300 mg po qd for up to 24 mos. (Curr Inf Dis Repts 2:193, 2000; CID 32:1547, 2001). Regimens dosing azithro 600 mg tiw also effective (CID 32:1547, 2001).	"Classic" pulmonary MAC: Men 50–75, smokers, COPD. "New" pulmonary MAC: Women 30–70, scoliosis, mitral valve prolapse, (bronchiectasis), pectus excavatum. Susceptibility testing of MAC not recommended except clarithro isolates from pts who have failed prior clarithro rx. Preliminary studies suggest 3x/wk azithro (600 mg po), ETB (25 mg/kg po), RFB (600 mg po), and initial 2x/wk SM may be effective in immunocompromised patients (JID 178:121, 1998). Late "relapses" (following completion of therapy) after treatment with clarithro or azithro in pts with nodular bronchiectasis usually represent reinfection, not failure of therapy (JID 185:266, 2002).
	Immunocompromised pts. **Primary prophylaxis** Pts with CD4 count <50–100/mm³ Discontinue when CD4 count >100/mm³ in response to HAART (NEJM 342:1085, 2000) Guideline: AnIM 137:435, 2002	**PRIMARY** **Azithro** 1200 mg po q week OR **Clarithro** 500 mg po bid	**ALTERNATIVE** **RFB** 300 mg po qd OR **Azithro** 1200 mg po q weekly + **RIF** 300 mg qd	RFB reduces MAC infection rate by 55% (no survival benefit); clarithro by 69% (30% survival benefit); azithro by 59% (RFB + azithro reduces infection rate by 72% more effective than either alone but not as well tolerated (NEJM 335:392, 1996). Many drug-drug interactions, see Table 21, pages 138, 139, 140. RFB metabolism and ↓ZDV with 32% ↓ in AUC. Clarithro ↑ blood levels of non-sedating antihistamines when taking clarithro prophylaxis & in 11% of those on azithro but had not been observed with RFB prophylaxis (J Inf 38:6, 1999). Clarithro resistance more likely to be seen in pts with extremely low CD4 counts at initiation (CID 27:807, 1998). Need to be sure no active M. tbc. RFB used for prophylaxis may promote selection of rifamycin-resistant M. tbc (NEJM 335:384 & 428, 1996).

See pages 87 & 89 for all footnotes and abbreviations

Dosages are for adults (unless otherwise indicated) and assume normal renal function   *Dosages are for adults (unless otherwise indicated)*   † DOT = directly observed therapy

TABLE 11A (5)

CAUSATIVE AGENT/DISEASE	MODIFYING CIRCUMSTANCES	SUGGESTED REGIMENS		COMMENTS
		PRIMARY/ALTERNATIVE		
IV. Other Mycobacterial Disease ("Atypical") (continued)				
M. avium-intracellulare complex (continued)	**Immunocompromised pts** (continued) **Treatment** Either presumptive dx or after culture dx of blood, bone marrow or other usually sterile body fluids, e.g. liver	Clarithro 500 mg* po bid or azithro 600 mg po qd **+** ETB 15-25 mg/kg/d **+** RFB 300 mg po qd *Higher doses of clari (1000 mg bid) may be associated with ↑ mortality (CID 29:125, 1999)	Clarithro + ETB + RFB + one or more of: CIP 750 mg po bid or Ofloxo 400 mg po bid or Amikacin 7.5-15 mg/kg/d In pts receiving protease inhibitors can use clarithro 500 mg bid (or azithro 600 mg qd) + ETB 15-25 mg/kg/d] if the pt has not had previous prophylaxis with a neo- macrolide (Johns Hopkins AIDS Report 9:2, 1997)	Median time to neg. blood culture: clarithro + ETB 4.4 wks vs azithro + ETB >16 wks. At 16 wks, clearance of bacteremia seen in 37.5% of clarithro-treated pts (CID 27:1278, 1998). More recent study suggests similar clearance rates for azithro (46%) vs clarithro (56%) at 24 wks when combined with ETB (CID 31:1245, 2000). Azithro 250 mg po qd not effective, but azithro 600 mg po qd as effective as 1200 mg/wk. Adding RFB to clarithro + ETB did not improve survival or response to therapy & emergence of resistance to clari but had no effect on response or survival (CID 28:1080, 1999). Data on clofazimine difficult to assess. Earlier study suggested adding CLO of no value (CID 25:621, 1997). More recent study suggests it may be as effective as RFB in 3 drug regimens containing clari & RFB (CID 29:125, 1999) although it may not be as effective as RFB at preventing clari resistance (CID 28:136, 1999). Thus, pending more data, we still do not recommend CLO of MAI in HIV+ pts. Drug toxicity: With clarithro, 23% pts had to stop drug 2° to dose-limiting adverse reaction (AnIM 121:905, 1994). Combination of clarithro, ETB and RFB led to uveitis and pseudojaundice (NEJM 330:438, 1994); result is reduction in max. dose of RFB to 300 mg. Treatment failure rate is high. Reasons: drug toxicity, development of drug resistance, & inadequate serum levels. Serum levels of clarithro ↓ in pts also given RIF or RFB (JID 171:747, 1995). If pt not responding to initial regimen after 2-4 weeks, add one or more drugs. Several anecdotal reports of pts not responding to usual primary regimen who gained weight and became afebrile with dexamethasone 2-4 mg/d (AnIM 132:215, 1994; CID 26:682, 1998).
	Chronic post-treatment suppression—secondary prophylaxis	Always necessary. Clarithro or azithro + ETB (dosage above)	Clarithro or azithro + ETB (lower dose to 15 mg/kg/d, dosage above)	Recurrences almost universal without chronic suppression. However, in patients on HAART with robust CD4 cell responses, it may be possible to discontinue chronic suppression (JID 178:1446, 1998; NEJM 340:1301, 1999).
D. Mycobacterium celatum	Treatment	Not defined. May be susceptible to clarithro; FQ (Clin Micro- biol Inf 3:582, 1997). Suggest rx "like MAI" but often resistant to RIF (JID 178:1571, 1998)		Isolated from pulmonary lesions and blood in AIDS patients (CID 24:144, 1997). Easily confused with M. xenopi (and MAC). Susceptibilities similar to MAC, but highly resistant to RIF (CID 24:1567, 1997).
E. Mycobacterium chelonae ssp. abscessus	Treatment. Surgical exci- sion may facilitate clarithro rx in subcutaneous abscess and is important adjunct to rx (CID 24:1147, 1997).	Clarithro 500 mg po bid x6 mos (AJR 119:482, 1993; CID 24:1147, 1997; EJCMID 19: 43, 2000)		M. abscessus susceptible to AMK (70%), clarithro (95%), cefoxitin (70%), CLO. cefmetazole. Single isolates of M. abscessus often not associated with disease (JCM 39:2745, 2001).
Mycobacterium chelonae ssp. chelonae		Clarithro 500 mg po bid x6 months		M. chelonae susceptible to AMK (80%), clarithro, azithro, tobramycin (100%), IMP (60%). Resistant to cefoxitin, FQ (CID 24:1147, 1997; AJRCCM 156:S1, 1997).
F. Mycobacterium fortuitum	Treatment; optimal regimen not defined. Surgical exci- sion of infected areas.	AMK + cefoxitin + probenecid 2-6 weeks, then po TMP/SMX or doxycycline 2-6 mos. (JID 152:500, 1985) Usually responds to 6-12 mos. of oral rx with 2 drugs to which it is susceptible (AJRCCM 156:S1, 1997)		**Resistant to all standard anti-TBc drugs.** Sensitive in vitro to doxycycline, minocycline, cefoxitin, IMP, AMK, TMP/SMX, CIP, ofIox, azithro, clarithro. Trials with neomacrolides (clarithro, azithro) indicated (AAC 36:180, 1992), but may be resistant to azithromycin, rifabutin (JAC 39:567, 1997).

CAUSATIVE AGENT/DISEASE; MODIFYING CIRCUMSTANCES	SUGGESTED REGIMENS		COMMENTS
	PRIMARY	ALTERNATIVE	
G. Mycobacterium haemophilum	Regimen(s) not defined. In animal model: clarithro + rifabutin effective (AAC 39:2316, 1995). In humans: CIP or RFB + clarithro or RFB + clarithro effective but clinical experience limited (CMR 9:435, 1996). Surgical debridement may be necessary (CID 26:505, 1998).		Clinical: Ulcerating skin lesions, synovitis, osteomyelitis. Resistant to: INH, ETB, PZA (AnIM 120:118, 1994). Sensitive in vitro to: CIP, cycloserine, rifabutin. Over ½ resistant to RIF.
H. Mycobacterium genavense	Regimens used include ≥2 drugs: ETB, RIF, RFB, CLO, clarithro. In animal model: clarithro & RFB (& to lesser extent amikacin) ↓ bacterial counts. CIP not effective (JAC 42:483, 1998).		Clinical: CD4 <50. Symptoms of fever, weight loss, diarrhea. Lab: Growth in BACTEC vials slow (mean 42 days). Subcultures grow only on Middlebrook 7H11 agar containing 2 mg/ml of mycobactin J and incubated for >8 weeks (RID 18:1379, 1996; AnIM 117:586, 1992). Survival ↑ from 81 to 263 days in pts treated with ≥2 drugs (Arch Int Med 155:400, 1995).

See pages 87 & 89 for all footnotes and abbreviations

*Dosages are for adults (unless otherwise indicated) and assume normal renal function

DOT = directly observed therapy

TABLE 11A (6)

CAUSATIVE AGENT/DISEASE; MODIFYING CIRCUMSTANCES	SUGGESTED REGIMENS		COMMENTS
	PRIMARY	ALTERNATIVE	
IV. Other Mycobacterial Disease ("Atypical") (continued)			
I. Mycobacterium gordonae	Regimen(s) not defined, but consider **RIF** + **ETB** + **KM** or **CIP** (Jnt 38; DJH, 1999)		In vitro, sensitive to ETB, RIF, AMK, CIP, clarithro. Resistant to INH (CID 14:1229, 1992). Surgical excision.
J. Mycobacterium kansasii	**INH** po (300 mg) + **RIF** (600 mg) + **ETB** (25 mg/kg x2 mos., then 15 mg/kg) x 18 mos. (until culture-neg sputum x12 mos, 15 mos. if HIV+ pt) (See Comment)	If RIF-resistant, daily po: **INH** (900 mg) + **pyridoxine** (50 mg) + **ETB** (25 mg/kg) + **sulfamethoxazole** (1.0 gm tid). Rx until pt culture-neg x12-15 mos. (See Comment)	Susceptibility testing. Test only RIF. Testing INH and streptomycin give misleading results. **All isolates are resistant to PZA.** Rifapentine, azithro, ETB shown effective alone or in combination in arhymic mice (AAC 42:477, 2001). If HIV+ pt taking protease inhibitor, substitute either clarithromycin (500 mg bid) or rifabutin (150 mg/d) for INH (See CID 25:S1, 1997). Because of variable susceptibility to INH, some would substitute clarithromycin (500-750 mg bid) or rifabutin (300-450 mg/d) for INH. However, resistance to clarithromycin has been reported (DMID 31:369, 1998).
K. Mycobacterium marinum	(**Clarithro** 500 mg bid) or (**minocycline** 100-200 mg qd) or (**doxycycline** 100-200 mg qd), or (**TMP/SMX** 160/800 mg po bid), or **RIF** + **ETB**) x 3 mos. (AJRCCM 156:S1, 1997). Surgical excision.		Resistant to INH and PZA (AJRCCM 156:S1, 1997). Also susceptible in vitro to linezolid (CIP, gatifloxacin, moxifloxacin also show moderate in vitro activity (AAC 46:1114, 2002).
L. Mycobacterium scrofulaceum	Surgical excision. Chemotherapy seldom indicated. Although regimen(s) not defined, **clarithro** + **CLO** with or **without ETB**, **INH**, **RIF**, **strep** + **cycloserine** have also been used.		In vitro resistant to INH, RIF, ETB, PZA, AMK, CIP (CID 20:549, 1995). Susceptible to clarithro, strep, erythromycin.
M. Mycobacterium simiae	Regimen(s) not defined. Start 4 drugs as for disseminated MAI.		Most isolates resistant to all 1st-line anti-tbc drugs. Isolates often not clinically significant (CID 26:625, 1998).
N. Mycobacterium ulcerans (Buruli ulcer)	[**RIF** + **AMK** (7.5 mg/kg IM bid)] or [**ETB** + **TMP/SMX** (160/800 mg po bid)] for 4-6 weeks. Surgical excision.		Susceptible in vitro to RIF, strep, CLO, clarithro, ofloxacin, sparflox, ofloxacin, amikacin (AAC 42:2070, 1998; AAC 45:231, 2000). Treatment generally disappointing—see review. Ln 354:1013, 1999. RIF + dapsone only slightly better (82% improved) than placebo (75%) in small study (LID 6:60, 2002).
O. Mycobacterium xenopi	Regimen(s) not defined (CID 24:226 & 233, 1997). Some recommend a macrolide + (**RIF** or **rifabutin**) + **ETB** + **SM** (AJRCCM 156:S1, 1997).		In vitro, sensitive to clarithro (AAC 36:2841, 1992) and rifabutin (AAC 39:567, 1997) and many standard antimycobacterial drugs. Clarithro-containing regimens more effective than RIF/INH/ETB regimens in mice (AAC 45:3229, 2001).
Mycobacterium leprae(leprosy) Paucibacillary (tuberculoid or indeterminate) **See Comment for erythema nodosum leprosum**	**Dapsone** 100 mg daily unsupervised + **RIF** 600 mg po 1x/month supervised for 6 months		Side-effects overall 0.4%. Single lesion paucibacillary disease may be treated with single-dose rx [RIF 600 mg + ofloxacin 400 mg + minocycline 100 mg] (Ln 353:655, 1999).
Multibacillary (lepromatous or borderline)	**Dapsone** 100 mg daily + **CLO** 50 mg daily unsupervised + [**RIF** 600 mg + **CLO** 300 mg 1x/month supervised] daily may be substituted for CLO	**Ethionamide** (250 mg daily) or **prothionamide** (375 mg daily) may be substituted for CLO	For erythema nodosum leprosum: prednisone 60–80 mg/d or thalidomide 300 mg/d (BMJ i:4 775, 1988; AJM 108:487, 2000). CLO available from Ciba-Geigy (908) 277-3572). *Pefloxacin 800 mg po, ofloxacin 400 mg po, sparfloxacin 200 mg po bactericidal and effective clinically with 4 log ↓ in organisms in small trials (Int J Lepr 58:281, 1990; AAC 38:662, 1994; AAC 38:515, 1994). Clarithro also rapidly bactericidal (AAC 38:515, 1994) (Good reference: AAC 40:S45, 1991.) 1 recent study suggests dapsone monotherapy as effective as combination rx for multibacillary leprosy (AAC 38:2249, 1994). Regimens incorporating clarithro, minocycline, RIF and/or ofloxacin also show promise (AAC 41:1618, 1997). High relapse rate in pts treated with daily RIF + ofloxacin for 4 wks (AAC 41:1953, 1997). Resistance to dapsone. RIF & ofloxacin reported (Ln 349:103, 1997). Dapsone or acetadapsone[notwork] effective for prophylaxis (Int 41:27, 2000).

Abbreviations: **AMK** = amikacin; **ATS** = American Thoracic Society; **Azithro** = azithromycin; **BL/BLI** = β-lactam/β-lactamase inhibitors; **CIP** = ciprofloxacin; **Clarithro** = clarithromycin; **CLO** = clofazamine; **CXR** = chest x-ray; **dc** = discontinue; **ddC** = zalcitabine; **DOT** = directly observed therapy; **ETB** = ethambutol; **FQ** = fluoroquinolones; **IDSA** = Infectious Diseases Society of America; **IMP** = imipenem cilastatin; **INH** = isoniazid; **INH-CR** = complete INH resistance; **KM** = kanamycin; **Neomacrolides** = azithromycin, clarithromycin, roxithromycin; **NUS** = not available in the U.S.; **Oflox** = ofloxacin; **pts** = patients; **PZA** = pyrazinamide; **RFB** = rifabutin; **RFP** = rifapentine; **RIF** = rifampin; **rx** = treatment; **sens** = sensitive; **SM** = streptomycin; **TBc** = tuberculosis; **TMP/SMX** = trimethoprim/sulfamethoxazole

See pages 87 & 89 for all footnotes and abbreviations

* *Dosages are for adults (unless otherwise indicated) and assume normal renal function*   † *DOT = directly observed therapy*

TABLE 11B: DOSAGE, PRICE AND SELECTED ADVERSE EFFECTS OF ANTIMYCOBACTERIAL DRUGS[1]

AGENT (TRADE NAME)	USUAL DOSAGE	ROUTE[1]* DRUG RESISTANCE (RES) US/COST[2]	SIDE-EFFECTS, TOXICITY AND PRECAUTIONS	SURVEILLANCE
FIRST LINE DRUGS				
Ethambutol (Myambutol)	25 mg/kg/day for 2 months & then 15 mg/kg qd as 1 dose (<10% protein binding) [Bacteriostatic to both extracellular & intracellular organisms]	po RES: 0.3% (0–0.7%) 400 mg tab $2.00	Optic neuritis with decreased visual acuity, central scotomata, and loss of green and red perception, peripheral neuropathy and headache (<1%), rashes (rare), arthralgia (rare), hyperuricemia (rare). Anaphylactoid reaction (rare). Comment: Primarily used to delay resistance. Disrupts outer cell membrane in M. avium with [1] activity to other drugs.	Monthly visual acuity & red/green with dose >15 mg/day. ≥10% loss considered significant. Usually reversible if drug discontinued.
Isoniazid (INH) (Nydrazid, Laniazid, Teebaconin)	Daily dose: 5–10 mg/kg/day up to 300 mg/day as 1 dose. Twice weekly dose: 15 mg/kg (900 mg maximum dose) (<10% protein binding) [Bactericidal to both extracellular and intracellular organisms]	po RES: 4.1% (2.6–8.5%) 300 mg tab $0.02 [IV (IM route not FDA-approved but has been used, esp. in AIDS)] 100 mg/ml in 10 ml vials (IM) $16.64	Overall ~1%. Liver Hepatitis (children 10% mild [1] SGOT, normalizes with continued rx; age <20 years rare, 20–34 years 1.2%, ≥50 years 2.3%) (also [1] with daily dose). May be fatal. With prodromal sx, discontinue rx. [1] incidence with alcohol. Peripheral neuropathy (17% at 6 mg/kg, less on 300 mg, incidence [1] in slow acetylators), syndrome (B6 [1]) with malnutrition, other neurologic sequelae: convulsions, optic neuritis, toxic encephalopathy, psychosis, muscle twitching, dizziness, coma (all rare); allergic skin rashes; fever, minor disulfiram-like reaction, flushing after Swiss cheese; blood dyscrasias (rare); + antinuclear (20%). **Drug-drug interactions common, see Table 21.**	Pre-rx liver functions. Repeat if symptoms (fatigue, weakness, malaise, anorexia, nausea or vomiting) >3 days (AJRCCM 152: 1705, 1995). Some recommend SGOT at 2, 4, 6 months esp. if age >50 years. Clinical evaluation every month.
Pyrazinamide	25 mg/kg/day (maximum 2.5 gm/d) qd as 1 dose [Bactericidal for intra-cellular organisms]	po 500 mg tab $1.04	**Arthralgia; hyperuricemia** (with or without symptoms); hepatitis (not over 2% if recommended dose not exceeded); gastric irritation, photosensitivity (rare)	Pre-rx liver functions. Monthly SGOT, uric acid. Measure serum uric acid if symptomatic gouty attack occurs.
Rifamate[R] combination tablet	2 tablets single dose qd	po (1 hr before meal) 1 tablet contains 150 mg INH, 300 mg RIF		As with individual drugs
Rifampin (Rifadin, Rimactane, Rifocin)	10.0 mg/kg/day up to 600 mg/day as 1 dose (60–90% protein binding) [Bactericidal to all populations of organisms]	po RES: 3.9% (2.7–7.6%) 300 mg tab $1.90 [IV available, Merrell-Dow] $84.14]	INH-RIF and/or ~3% for toxicity, gastrointestinal irritation, antibiotic-associated colitis, drug fever (1%), pruritus with or without skin rash (1%), anaphylactoid reactions in HIV+ pts, mental confusion, thrombocytopenia (1%), leucopenia (1%), hemolytic anemia, transient **abnormalities in liver function.** "**Flu syndrome**" (fever, chills, headache, bone pain, shortness of breath) seen if RIF taken irregularly or if daily dose restarted after an interval of no rx. **Discolors urine, tears, sweat, contact lens an orange-brown color.** May cause drug-induced lupus erythematosus (Ln 349:1521, 1977).	Pre-rx liver function. Repeat if symptoms. **Multiple significant drug-drug interactions, see Table 21.**
Rifater[R] combination tablet (See Side-Effects)	Wt ≥55 kg, 6 tablets single dose qd	po (1 hr before meal) 1 tab $1.91	1 tablet contains 50 mg INH, 120 mg RIF, 300 mg PZA. Used in 1st 2 months of rx (if >55 kg). For pts to improve convenience in dosing, compliance (AnM 122: 951, 1995) but cost 1.58 more. Side-effects = individual drugs.	As with individual drugs. PZA 25 mg/kg
Streptomycin	15 mg/kg IM qd, 0.75–1.0 gm/day initially for 60–90 days, then 1.0 gm 2–3 times/week (15 mg/kg) qd as 1 dose	IM (or IV) RES: 3.9% (2.7–7.6%) 500 mg NB $6.45	Overall 8%. Ototoxicity vestibular dysfunction (vertigo); paresthesias; dizziness & nausea (all less in pts receiving 2–3 doses/week); tinnitus and high frequency loss (1%); nephrotoxicity (rare); peripheral neuropathy (rare); allergic skin rashes (4–5%); drug fever. Available at no charge for treatment of new pts with labelled use from Pfizer/Roerig 1-800-254-4445. Reference IV→CID 171150, 1994	Monthly audiogram. In older pts, serum creatinine or BUN at start of rx and weekly if pt stable
SECOND LINE DRUGS (more difficult to use and/or less effective than first line drugs)				
Amikacin (Amikin)	7.5–10.0 mg/kg qd [Bactericidal for extracellular organisms]	IV or IM RES: (est. 0.1%) 500 mg NB $33, G $18.70	See Table 9, pages 60 & 70	Monthly audiogram. Serum creatinine or BUN weekly if pt stable

[1] Note: Malabsorption of antimycobacterial drugs may occur in patients with AIDS enteropathy.
[2] RES = % resistance of M. tuberculosis.

See pages 87, 88 & 89 for all footnotes and abbreviations.

* Dosages are for adults (unless otherwise indicated) and assume normal renal function   [1] DOT = directly observed therapy

TABLE 11B (2)

SECOND LINE DRUGS *(more difficult to use and/or less effective than first line drugs)* *(continued)*

Drug	Dosage*	Route/RES/Cost**	Adverse Effects/Comments	Monitoring
Capreomycin sulfate (Capastat sulfate)	1 gm/day (15 mg/kg/day) qd as 1 dose	IM or IV RES: 0.1% (0-0.9%) 1 gm $25.54	Nephrotoxicity (36%), ototoxicity (auditory 11%), eosinophilia, leucopenia, skin rash, fever, hypokalemia, neuromuscular blockade.	Monthly audiogram, biweekly serum creatinine or BUN
Ciprofloxacin (Cipro)	750 mg bid	IM or IV 750 mg (po) $4.32	TB not an FDA-approved indication for CIP. Desired CIP serum levels 4-6 μg/ml requires median dose 800 mg (AJRCCM 151:2006, 1995). Discontinuation rates 6-7%. CIP well tolerated (AJRCCM 151:1148, 1996, 1995). FQ-resistant M. Tb identified in New York (Ln 345:1148, 1995). See Table 9, pages 62 & 67 for adverse effects.	None
Clofazimine (Lamprene)	50 mg/d (unsupervised) + 300 mg 1x/month supervised or 100 mg/d	po (with meals) 50 mg $0.13	Skin: **pigmentation (pink-brownish black)** 75-100%, dryness 20%, pruritus 5%. GI: abdominal pain 50% (rarely severe leading to exploratory laparoscopy), splenic infarction (VR), bowel obstruction (VR), GI bleeding (VR). Eye: conjunctival irritation, retinal crystal deposits.	None
Cycloserine (Seromycin)	750-1000 mg/day (15 mg/kg/day) 2-4 doses/day [Bacteriostatic for both extracellular & intracellular organisms]	po RES: 0.1% (0-0.3%) 250 mg cap $4.00	Convulsions, **psychoses** (5-10% of those receiving 1.0 gm/day); headache; somnolence; hyperreflexia; increased CSF protein and pressure; **peripheral neuropathy**. 100 mg pyridoxine (or more) daily should be given concomitantly. Contraindicated in epileptics	None
Dapsone	100 mg/day	po 100 mg $0.20	Blood: ↓ hemoglobin (1-2 gm) & ↑ retics (2-12%), in most pts. Hemolysis in G6PD deficiency. **Methemoglobinemia**. CNS: peripheral neuropathy (rare). GI: nausea, vomiting. Renal: albuminuria, nephrotic syndrome. Peripheral neuropathy in pts rx for leprosy (1% pts 1st year)	None
Ethionamide (Trecator-SC)	500-1000 mg/day (10-15 mg/kg/day) 1-3 doses/day [Bacteriostatic for extracellular organisms only]	po RES: 0.8% (0-1.5%) 250 mg tab $2.19	**Gastrointestinal irritation** (up to 50% on large dose); goiter; peripheral neuropathy (rare); convulsions (rare); changes in affect (rare); difficulty in diabetes control; rashes; hepatitis; purpura; stomatitis; gynecomastia; menstrual irregularity. Give drug with meals or antacids, 50-100 mg pyridoxine per day concomitantly; SGOT monthly. Possibly teratogenic.	Liver functions monthly
Ofloxacin (Floxin)	400 mg bid	po, IV 400 mg (po) $4.54	Not an FDA-approved indication. Overall adverse effects 11%, 4% discontinued due to side-effects. GI: nausea 3%, diarrhea 1%. **CNS**: insomnia 3%, headache 1%, dizziness 1%	None
Para-aminosalicylic acid (PAS, Paser) (Na⁺ or K⁺ salt)	4-6 gm bid (200 mg/kg/day) [Bacteriostatic for extracellular organisms only]	po RES: 0.8% (0-1.5%) 450 mg tab $0.08 (see Comment)	**Gastrointestinal irritation** (10-15%); goitrogenic action (rare); depressed prothrombin (rare); ↓ K⁺ (rare); G6PD-mediated hemolytic anemia (rare); drug fever; rashes; hepatitis, myalgia, arthralgia. Retards hepatic enzyme induction, may ↓ INH hepatotoxicity. Available from CDC, (404) 639-3670, Jacobus Pharm. Co. (609) 921-7447.	None
Rifabutin (Mycobutin)	300 mg/day (prophylaxis or treatment)	po 150 mg $4.54	Polymyalgia, polyarthralgia, leucopenia, granulocytopenia. Anterior uveitis when given with concomitant clarithromycin; avoid 600 mg dose (NEJM 330:438, 1994). Uveitis reported with 300 mg/d (AnIM 12:510, 1994). Reddish urine, orange skin.	None
Rifapentine (Priftin)	600 mg twice weekly for 1st 2 mos., then 600 mg q week	po 150 mg $2.91	Similar to other rifabutins. (See RIF, RFB.) Hyperuricemia seen in 21%. Causes red-orange discoloration of body fluids. Note ↑ prevalence of RIF resistance in pts on once-a-day rx.	None
Thalidomide (Thalomid)	100-300 mg po qd (may use up to 400 mg po qd for severe erythema nodosum leprosum)	po 50 mg $11.46	**Contraindicated in pregnancy. Causes severe life-threatening birth defects. Both male and female patients must use barrier contraceptive methods (Pregnancy Category X). Frequently causes drowsiness or somnolence. May cause peripheral neuropathy.**	Available only through pharmacists participating in System for Thalidomide Education and Prescribing Safety (S.T.E.P.S.)

* Adult dosage only; ** Average wholesale price according to 2002 DRUG TOPICS RED BOOK, Medical Economics
Abbreviations: VR = very rare; **esp** = especially; **dc** = discontinue; **RES** = % resistance to M. tuberculosis

* Dosages are for adults (unless otherwise indicated) and assume normal renal function † **DOT** = directly observed therapy

See pages 87 & 89 for all footnotes and abbreviations

TABLE 12A: TREATMENT OF PARASITIC INFECTIONS

Many of the drugs suggested are not licensed in the United States. The following are helpful resources through the Center for Disease Control and Prevention (CDC) in Atlanta. Website is www.cdc.gov. General advice for parasitic diseases other than malaria: (770) 488-7760 or (770) 488-7775.
For malaria: (770) 488-7788 (or) (770) 488-7100 (24 hrs/day; 8:00 a.m. - 4:30 p.m. EST; (404) 639-2888; fax: (404) 639-3717.
For malaria: Prophylaxis advice (770) 488-7788 or (877) 394-3228; treatment: (770) 488-7788; website: www.cdc.gov; fax (888) 232-3299
NOTE: All dosage regimens are for adults with normal renal function unless otherwise stated.
Occasionally, post-licensure data may alter dosage as compared to package inserts.
For abbreviations of journal titles, see Table 1, page 45. **Reference with pediatric dosages: Medical Letter on-line version: www.medletter.com (April 2002)**

INFECTING ORGANISM	SUGGESTED REGIMENS		COMMENTS
	PRIMARY	**ALTERNATIVE**	
PROTOZOA—INTESTINAL (non-pathogenic: E. hartmanni, E. dispar, E. coli, Iodamoeba butschlii, Endolimax nana, Chilomastix mesnili)			
Balantidium coli	**Tetracycline** 500 mg po qid x10 d.	**Metronidazole** 750 mg po tid x5 d.	See Table 9B for side-effects.
Blastocystis hominis	Role as pathogen supported random. trial: metro vs placebo	**Metronidazole** 750 mg po tid x10 d. **High dose** increases risk of adverse effects. Metro resist. reported (Trop Med Int Health 4:274, 1999)	
Cryptosporidium parvum Treatment is unsatisfactory. Ref.: NEJM 346:1723, 2002	**Immunocompetent pt:** No specific therapy. Hydration only. **Pts with AIDS:** Restore immune function with active antiretroviral therapy; if anti-HIV rx fails, the try antidiarrheal + **nitazoxanide** or (**paromomycin** + **azithro**)—see Alternative Regimens	If HAART fails: (1) **Nitazoxanide (Cryptaz)** 0.5–1.0 gm po bid. Contact: Remark Labs 813-282-8544. OR (2) **Paromomycin** 1.0 gm po 2x/d. + **azithro** 600 mg po qid	Supplemental benefit from Imodium, diphenoxylate, or tincture of opium (may help in combination). Octreotide (Sandostatin) may help, but expensive.
Cyclospora cayetanensis	**Immunocompetent pts: TMP/SMX-DS** tab 1 po qid x10 d.; then 1 po 3x/week	AIDS pts. **TMP/SMX-DS** tab 1 po qid x10 d.; tab 1 po 3x/week	Ref.: CID 23:429, 1996
Dientamoeba fragilis	**Iodoquinol** 650 mg po tid x20 d.	Other alternatives: **doxy** 100 mg po bid x10 d.; **paromomycin** 500 mg po tid x7 d.	
Entamoeba histolytica; amebiasis: Distinguish from non-pathogenic E. histolytica and non-pathogenic E. dispar (CID 29:1117, 1999)			
Asymptomatic cyst passer	**Paromomycin** (aminosidin in U.K.) 500 mg po tid x7 d. OR **iodoquinol** 650 mg po tid x20 d.	**Diloxanide furoate**[NUS] (Furamide) 500 mg po tid x10 d. Manufacturer: Boots, United Kingdom.	Metronidazole not effective vs cysts.
Patient with diarrhea/dysentery; mild/moderate disease. Oral rx possible	**Metronidazole** 500–750 mg po tid x10 d., followed by: Either [**paromomycin** 500 mg po tid x7 d.] or [**iodoquinol** 650 mg po tid x20 d]	[**Tinidazole**[NUS] 2.0 gm po qd x3 d.] or [**ornidazole**[NUS] 500 mg po q12h x3 d.] followed by:	Drug side-effects in Table 9B. Colitis can mimic ulcerative colitis; ameboma can mimic adenocarcinoma of colon. Dx: trophs or cysts in stool. Watch out for non-pathogenic but morphologically identical E. dispar (Ln 351:1672, 1998).
Severe or extraintestinal infection, e.g., hepatic abscess	**Metronidazole** 750 mg **IV** to **PO** tid x10 d. followed by **paromomycin** 500 mg po tid x7 d. Outside U.S. may substitute **tinidazole** (600 mg bid or 800 mg tid) po x5 d. for metro.		**Serology positive (antibody present) with extraintestinal disease.**
Giardia lamblia; giardiasis Ref.: MMWR 49:SS-7, 2000	**Metronidazole** 250 mg po tid x5 d. OR **furazolidone** 100 mg qid x7 d.	**Tinidazole**[NUS] 2.0 gm po x1 OR [**quinacrine 100 mg po tid** (with meals) x5 d.] See comment Rx if pregnant: **Paromomycin** 500 mg tid x5–10 d.	Refractory pts: (metro **750 mg po + quinacrine 100 mg po bid** x14 d. (Ref. CID 33:22, 2001). Another option for AIDS pts: **Nitazoxanide** 1.5 gm po bid x30 d. (Contact: Romark Labs 813-282-8544.
Isospora belli	**TMP/SMX-DS** tab 1 po bid x28 d. If AIDS pt, TMP/SMX-DS qid x10 d. & then bid x3 wks.	**Pyrimethamine** 75 mg/d po + **folinic acid** 10 mg/d po x14 d. OR **CIP** 500 mg po bid x7 d.—87% responses (AnIM 132:885, 2000).	Chronic suppression in AIDS pts: either 1 TMP/SMX-DS tab 3x/wk OR (pyrimethamine 25 mg/d po + folinic acid 5 mg/d po)

---

[1] **Drugs available from CDC Drug Service: 404-639-2888 or -3670: Bithionol, dehydroemetine, diethylcarbamazine, melarsoprol, nifurtimox, stibogluconate (Pentostam), suramin.**
[2] Both quinacrine and tinidazole available from Panorama Compounding Pharmacy, (800) 247-9767; (818) 988-7979.
* All doses are for adults (unless otherwise indicated) and assume normal renal function. See page 101 for abbreviations.

TABLE 12A (2)

INFECTING ORGANISM	SUGGESTED REGIMENS		COMMENTS
	PRIMARY	ALTERNATIVE	
PROTOZOA—INTESTINAL (continued)			
Microsporidiosis (Ref.: CID 27:1, 1998)			
Ocular: Encephalitozoon hellum or cuniculi, Vittaforma corneae (Nosema sp.)	Albendazole 400 mg po bid x3 weeks	In HIV+ pts, reports of response of E. hellum to **fumagillin** eyedrops (see Comment). For V. corneae, may need keratoplasty	To obtain fumagillin: 1-800-547-1392. Thrombocytopenia when fumagillin used to rx E. bieneusi. Dx: Most labs use modified trichrome stain. Need electron micrographs for species identification. FA and PCR methods in development.
Intestinal (diarrhea): Enterocytozoon bieneusi, Encephalitozoon (Septata) intestinalis	Albendazole 400 mg po bid x3 weeks	Oral **fumagillin** reported effective for E. bieneusi (NEJM 346:1963, 2002)—see Comment	
Disseminated: E. hellum, cuniculi or intestinalis, Pleistophora sp.	Albendazole 400 mg po bid x3 weeks	No established rx for Pleistophora sp.	Other species reported pathogenic: Trachipleistophora sp., Brachiola vesicularum.
PROTOZOA—EXTRAINTESTINAL			
Amebic meningoencephalitis			
Acanthamoeba sp.— no proven rx	Success with IV **pentamidine**, topical **chlorhexidine** & 2% **ketoconazole** cream & then po **itra** (NEJM 331:85, 1994). 2 children responded to po rx: **TMP/SMX** + **rifampin** + **keto** (PIDJ 20:623, 2001).		For treatment of keratitis, see Table 1, page 9
Balamuthia mandrillaris	Pentamidine amebastatic in vitro	One pt responded to **clarithro** + **flucon** + **sulfadiazine** + **flucytosine**	A cause of chronic granulomatous meningitis
Naegleria fowleri: >95% mortality. Sappinia diploidea	**Ampho B** 1 mg/kg/d IV + 0.1-1.0 mg into lateral ventricle via an Ommaya reservoir. Duration? (JAMA 285:2450, 2001)	**Azithro** + **pentamidine** + **itra** + **flucytosine**	Case report: Ampho, miconazole, & RiF (NEJM 306:346, 1982).
Babesia microti; babesiosis (CID 22:1117, 2001)	**Atovaquone** 750 mg bid po x7-10 d. + **azithro** 500 mg po x1 d. then 250 mg/d. x7 d. (NEJM 343:1454, 2000).	(**Clindamycin** 600 mg po tid) + (**quinine** 650 mg po bid) x7 d. For adults, can give **clinda** IV as 1.2 gm bid	Can cause overwhelming infection in asplenic patients.
Ehrlichiosis—See Table 1, pages 38-39			
Leishmaniasis (see AAC 45:2185, 2001 & Ln Inf Dis 2:494, 2002). **NOTE:** Responses of various species differ—see references.			
Visceral—Kala-azar L. donovani: India/Africa L. infantum: Mediterranean L. chagasi: New World **WARNING: Avoid combined antimony & ampho B** (Ln 351:1928, 1998)	**Antimony** (**stibogluconate** or **meglumine antimoniate**) 20 mg/kg/d of antimony (Sb) (in 2 div. doses) IM or IV x28 d. Not marketed by US. Contact CDC Drug Service: (404) 639-3670.	[**AmB** IV (1.0 mg/kg x20 d.) or 0.5 mg/kg qod x8 weeks)] or (**AmB** IV 3 mg/kg/d on days 1-5 & 14 & 21) or (**ABCD** (IV 2 mg/kg/d x10 d.) or (**ABLC** (IV 3 mg/kg qod x5 doses) Refs: CID 28:42 & 49, 1999; Ann Trop Med Parasit 92:755, 1998 Other alternative regimens with approx. cure rate (%): 1. **Pentamidine** 4 mg/kg IV 3x/wk x15-25 doses (75) 2. **Paromomycin** 15 mg/kg/d IV x20 d. (80) when antimony-resistant 3. **Interferon gamma** 100 μg/M² qod IV + antimony as in primary rx (90) 4. **Miltefosine**[NUS] 50 mg bid po x21 d. **Pregnancy—No** (CID 31:1110, 2001). Vomiting in >50% of pts.	Antimony resistance a problem in India (JID 180:564, 1999); an ampho B regimen should be used.
Mucosal—L. braziliensis	**Antimony**, as for Visceral		Approx. cure rates: antimony 60%, AmB >75%
Cutaneous— **Most resolve spontaneously; Rx to prevent mucosal in New World:** L. mexicana and L. braziliensis in New World L. tropica and L. major in Old World	**Fluconazole** 200 mg po once daily x6 wks. Effective vs L. major (NEJM 346:891, 2002)	**Miltefosine**[NUS] 2.25 mg/kg once daily po x3-4 wks. Cure in 94% (CID 33:657, 2001). Contact Astra Medica, Ger. Poor balance & GI "unease" in 40% of pts.	Other options as IV: **Antimony** as for visceral, or **Pentamidine** 2-4 mg/kg qd or q2 days IV x15 doses

---

[1] AmB = amphotericin B; L-AmB = liposomal ampho B; ABCD = ampho B colloidal dispersion; ABLC = ampho B lipid complex
NOTE: All dosage recommendations are for adults (unless otherwise indicated) and assume normal renal function. See page 101 for abbreviations.

TABLE 12A (3)

INFECTING ORGANISM	SUGGESTED REGIMENS		COMMENTS
	PRIMARY	ALTERNATIVE	

PROTOZOA—EXTRAINTESTINAL (*continued*)

Malaria (Plasmodium species)—NOTE: CDC Malaria info—prophylaxis (888) 394-8747; treatment (770) 488-7788. Websites: www.cdc.gov/ncidod/dpd/parasites/malaria/default.htm; www.who.int/health-topics/malaria.htm.

INFECTING ORGANISM	PRIMARY	ALTERNATIVE	COMMENTS
Prophylaxis—Drugs plus personal protection: screens, nets, 30–35% DEET skin repellent (avoid 95% products in children), permethrin spray on clothing and nets (*AnIM 128:931, 1998*)			
For areas free of chloroquine (CQ)-resistant *P. falciparum*: Haiti, Central Dominican Republic, Central America west and north of the Panama Canal, and parts of the Middle East. For areas with CQ-**resistant P. falciparum**:	**CQ**[1] 500 mg (300 mg base) po per week starting 1–2 wks before travel, during travel, & 4 wks post-travel	**Doxycycline** 100 mg po daily for adults & children >7 years of age[3] OR **Atovaquone**/**proguanil** 100 mg (Malarone) comb. tablet, 1/day with food 1–2 d. prior to, during, & 7 d. post-travel. Peds dose in footnote.[3] (*Ref: Med Lett 42:109, 2000*)	The areas free of CQ-resistant *falciparum* malaria continue to shrink: Central America and Middle East/Africa should be CQ-resistant falciparum malaria reported from Saudi Arabia, Yemen, Oman, & Iran.
CDC voice info on prophylaxis at (888) 232-3228 or website: www.cdc.gov Ref: *JAMA 278:1767, 1997*	**Mefloquine (MQ)** 250 mg (228 mg base) po per wk, 1 wk. before, during, and for 4 wks after travel. Peds dose in footnote.[3] MQ outside U.S.: 275 mg tab, contains 250 mg of base. Another option for adults: **primaquine (PQ)** 30 mg base po daily x14 d. Check for severe G6PD deficiency before tx.	**Doxycycline** 100 mg po daily for adults & children >7 years of age[3] OR **Atovaquone**/**proguanil** 100 mg (Malarone) comb. tablet, 1/day with food 1–2 d. prior to, during, & 7 d. post-travel. Peds dose in footnote.[3] (*Ref: Med Lett 42:109, 2000*)	**Pregnancy: MQ current best option.** Insufficient data with Malarone. **Avoid doxycycline and primaquine.** Primaquine: Used only if prolonged exposure to endemic area (e.g., Peace Corps). **Can cause hemolytic anemia if G6PD deficiency present.** MQ not recommended if cardiac conduction abnormalities, seizures, or psychiatric disorders.
Treatment (*NEJM 335:800, 1996*) (*P. falciparum*, *P. malariae*, *P. ovale*) (*P. vivax &/or P. ovale* For chloroquine (CQ)-sensitive plasmodia:	**CQ** [1.0 gm (=600 mg base) po, 0.5 gm in 6 hrs, then 0.5 gm daily x2 d]	Travelers 98% protective vs P. falciparum & >92% vs. P. vivax (*Clin 33:1990, 2001*)	
Blood smear consistent with P. vivax &/or P. ovale		**[Quinine sulfate (QS)** 650 mg po qid x3–7 d. + **doxycycline** 100 mg po bid x7 d. OR **mefloquine** 750 mg po, then 500 mg 12 hrs later OR **halofantrine** 500 mg po q6h x3 doses.	**CQ-resistant P. vivax** reported from Oceania and South America. Rx as CQ-resistant P. falciparum. Pregnancy: CQ safe all trimesters. No PQ in pregnancy or in newborns—risk of hemolytic anemia. For CQ 10 mg of base per kg po, then 5 mg base/kg/d x14
CDC: Malaria treatment— (770) 488-7788 or website: www.cdc.gov	**Primaquine (PQ)** 26.3 mg (15 mg base) po daily x14 d. OR 79 mg (45 mg base) po q wk x8 doses	To prevent relapses, give PQ 26.3 mg (15 mg base) 1 tab po daily x14 d.; screen for G6PD def. to avoid severe hemolysis.	For PQ use 0.3 mg base/kg/d x14
		Vigenol prolonged time to clear parasitemia (*Lin 350:704, 1997*)	
Blood smear consistent with P. falciparum or P. malariae	**[Chloroquine (CQ)** as for CQ-sensitive **primaquine** (CQ) P. falciparum; see below.	Assumes P. falciparum CQ-sensitive, i.e. acquired in Central America (west of Panama Canal), Haiti, and most of Middle East	
Blood smear shows P. falciparum assumed CQ-resistant OR Rx therapy not possible.	**Quinine sulfate (QS)** 325 mg [=250mg base]. Give 650 mg po tid x7 d. + **(doxycycline** 100 mg po bid x7 d.)	Areas of drug resistance, e.g. NW Thailand. (**Artesunate** 4 mg/kg/d po x3 d. & then **mefloquine** 750 mg po & then 500 mg 12 hrs later)	**Other rx alternatives:** (1) MQ: 750 mg, then 500 mg 12 hrs later (peds & adults). Resistance reported (*JID 180:2077, 1999*). (2) **Halofantrine**, ages >8–12 yrs: 2 mg/kg/d up to 100 mg/day
Ref: *NEJM 335:800, 1996* Rx same for CQ-resistant P. vivax	Peds. **QS** x3 d. + **Fansidar** x1 day of QS (*dosage in footnote*[3]) OR **Atovaquone/proguanil** 1 gm/400 mg (4 adult tabs) po 1x/day for 3 days, with food. Peds dose in footnote.[3]	Peds: 25 mg/kg po div q8h x3 d. + a single po dose of **Fansidar** (pyrimethamine sulfadoxine) given on last day of quinine. Fansidar single dose by age (yr.) of child by weight: 11–20 kg ½250/100 mg, 21–30 kg ½250/100 mg, 31–40 kg 750/300 mg, >40	**Pregnancy:** Possible concerns of potential fetal toxicity, use **quinine** or **IV quinidine** followed by **Fansidar** (sulfadoxine-pyrimethamine). 3 tablets (each tab 25/500 mg) or 1500 mg **sulfadoxine + 75 mg pyrimethamine**, single dose. Alternatives: (quinine + **doxycycline** (despite fetal concerns)) OR (quinine + clindamycin (*AAC 46:2315, 2002*))

TABLE 12A (4)

INFECTING ORGANISM	SUGGESTED REGIMENS		COMMENTS
	PRIMARY	**ALTERNATIVE**	
PROTOZOA—EXTRAINTESTINAL/Malaria/Treatment (continued)			
Blood smear consistent with *P. falciparum* **Pt too ill for initial po therapy** **NOTE:** Steroids are harmful in cerebral malaria. *Drug resistance ref.: Ln Inf Dis 2:209, 2002*	In U.S.: **Quinine dihydrochloride**[NUS] in 5% saline (10 mg/kg IV over 1 hr, then 0.02 mg/kg/min. (monitor EKG) x72 hrs] OR [15 mg/kg IV over 4 hrs, then 7.5 mg/kg IV over 4 hrs q8h x72 hrs) OR until patient can take po meds.	Outside U.S.: **Quinine dihydrochloride**[NUS] in 5% dextrose 20 mg/kg IV over 4 hrs, then 10 mg/kg over 2–8 hrs q8h x72 hrs OR **Artesunate**[NUS] 3.2 mg/kg IM, then 1.6 mg/kg IM, daily For both, switch to po regimen when possible to finish 7 days of rx.	May be manifest as cerebral malaria, renal failure, or ARDS. **Monitor parasitemia!** If rx effective, expect >75% x parasite count after 48 hrs of rx. If parasitemia exceeds 15%, consider exchange transfusion; efficacy unclear (*CID 34:1192, 2002*). CDC: Malaria info (770) 488-7788 **Pregnancy:** See *Comment, po therapy, bottom of page 92*
Microsporidia—systemic—see page 91			
Pneumocystis carinii Pneumonia (PCP). **Not acutely ill, po rx not possible. PaO₂ >70 mmHg**	Official new name is **Pneumocystis jiroveci** (yee-row-vet-zee). *EID 8:891, 2002.* Resistance to **(TMP/SMX-DS** 2 tabs po q8h x21 d.) OR **(Dapsone** 100 mg po q8h + **trimethoprim** 5 mg/kg po bid x21 d.]	(vee-row-vet-zee). *EID 8:891, 2002.* Resistance to **(Clindamycin** 300–450 mg po q6h + **primaquine** 15 mg base po qd x21 d.) OR **Atovaquone** suspension 750 mg po bid with food x21 d.	TMP/SMX and atovaquone may emerge (*JAMA 286:2450, 2001*) DAP/TMP, TMP/SMX, clinda/prima regimens equally effective. Rash/fever 10% with DAP/TMP, 19% with TMP/SMX, 21% with clinda/prima. Ref. clindamycin vs TMP/SMX: *CID 27:524, 1998.* Dapsone ref.: *CID 27:191, 1998.* **After 21 days, chronic suppression in AIDS pts (see below)**
	NOTE: Concomitant use of corticosteroids usually reserved for sicker pts with PaO₂ <70 (see below).		
Acutely ill, po rx not possible. PaO₂ <70 mmHg	**(TMP/SMX** (15–30 min. before TMP/SMX): 40 mg po bid x5 d., then 40 mg po qd x5 d., then 20 mg po qd x11 d.) + **TMP/SMX** [15 mg of TMP component/kg/d] IV div. q6–8h x21 d.]	**Prednisone** as in primary rx, PLUS **(Clinda** 600 mg IV q8h) + **primaquine** 30 mg base po qd] x21 d. OR **Pentamidine** 4 mg/kg IV x21 d.	**After 21 days, chronic suppression in AIDS pts (see below).** **PCP can occur in absence of HIV infection and steroids (*CID 25:215 & 219, 1997*).**
	Can substitute IV prednisolone [reduce dose 25%] for prednisone		
Primary prophylaxis and post-treatment suppression *(Reference: MMWR 51(RR-8), 6/14/2002; AnIM 137:435, 2002)*	**(TMP/SMX-DS** or **-SS**, 1 tab po qd or 1 DS 3x/wk) OR **(dapsone** 100 mg po qd). DC if CD4 >200 x3 mos. (*NEJM 344:159, 2001*).	**[Pentamidine** 300 mg in 6 ml sterile water by aerosol q4 wks) OR **(dapsone** 200 mg po + **pyrimethamine** 75 mg po weekly) OR **(dapsone** 50 mg po qd + **pyri 50 mg + leucovorin** 25 mg po—all once a week) OR **atovaquone** 1500 mg po qd with food.	TMP/SMX-DS regimen provides cross-protection vs toxo and other bacterial infections. Dapsone + Pyrimethamine protects vs toxo. Atovaquone suspension 1500 mg/day as effective as daily dapsone (*NEJM 339:1889, 1998*) & inhaled pentamidine (*JID 180:369, 1999*).
Toxoplasma gondii. (Reference: Remington and McLeod in INFECTIOUS DISEASES, Gorbach et al., Eds., 2nd Ed., 1997, pp 1620–40)			
Immunologically normal patients (For pediatric doses, see reference) Acute illness with lymphadenopathy	No specific rx unless severe/persistent symptoms or evidence of vital organ damage.		
Acquired via transfusion (lab accident)	[Treat as for active chorioretinitis]		
Active chorioretinitis: meningitis; lowered resistance due to steroids or cytotoxic drugs	**[Pyrimethamine (pyri)** 200 mg po x1, then 75 mg po bid x3 d., then 25 mg po qd + **sulfadiazine** (footnote¹) 1–1.5 gm po qid + **leucovorin (folinic acid)** 10 mg po q6h x3–6 wks. Treat 1–2 wks beyond resolution of signs/symptoms; continue leucovorin 1 wk after stopping pyri.		For congenital toxo, toxo meningitis in adults, and chorioretinitis, add **prednisone 1 mg/kg/d in 2 div. doses** until CSF protein conc. falls or vision-threatening inflammation has subsided. Adjust folinic acid dose by following CBC results.
Pregnancy: 1st 18 weeks of gestation, or to term if fetus not infected	**Spiramycin** [From FDA, call (301) 827-2336] 1.0 gm po q8h x3–4 wks. NOTE: Use caution in interpretation of commercial tests for toxoplasma IgM antibody; for help, FDA Advisory (301) 594-3060 or Toxoplasma Serology Lab of Palo Alto Med. Found. (650) 853-4828		IgG avidity test of help in 1st trimester (*JID 183:1248, 2001*).

---

¹ Sulfonamides for toxo. Sulfadiazine now commercially available. Sulfisoxazole much less effective.
NOTE: All dosage recommendations are for adults (unless otherwise indicated) and assume normal renal/renal function. See page 101 for abbreviations.

TABLE 12A (5)

INFECTING ORGANISM	SUGGESTED REGIMENS		COMMENTS
	PRIMARY	**ALTERNATIVE**	
PROTOZOA—EXTRAINTESTINAL/Toxoplasma gondii (continued)			
Acquired immunodeficiency syndrome (AIDS)			
Cerebral toxoplasmosis Ref.: See Remington & McLeod ref., above	[Pyrimethamine (pyri) 200 mg x1 po, then 75–100 mg/d po] + (sulfadiazine 1.0–1.5 gm po q6h) + (folinic acid 10–15 mg/d po) x3–6 wks and then suppressive rx (see below) OR TMP/SMX 10/50 mg/kg/d (IV or po) in IV div q12h x30 d. (AAC 42:1346, 1998)	[Pyri + folinic acid (as in primary regimen)] + 1 of the following: (1) Clinda 600 mg po/IV q6h or (2) clarithro 1.0 gm po bid or (3) azithro 1.2–1.5 gm po qd or (4) dapsone 100 mg po qd. Treat 3–6 wks, then suppression.	Use alternative regimen for pts with severe sulfa allergy. If multiple ring-enhancing brain lesions (CT or MRI), >85% of pts respond to 7–10 days of empiric rx; if no response, suggest brain biopsy. IgG toxo antibody positive in approx. 84% (NEJM 327:1643, 1992)
Primary prophylaxis. AIDS pts—IgG toxo antibody + CD4 count <100/µl	TMP/SMX-DS, 1 tab po qd or (TMP/SMX-SS, 1 tab po qd)	[Dapsone 50 mg po qd + (pyri 50 mg po q week) + (folinic acid 25 mg po q week)] OR atovaquone 1500 mg po qd	Prophylaxis for pneumocystis also effective in approx. 50% of pts. Refs: MMWR 51(RR-8), 6/14/2002; AnIM 137:435, 2002
Suppression after rx of cerebral toxo	(Sulfadiazine 500–1000 mg po q6h) + pyri 25–50 mg po qd) + (folinic acid 10–25 mg po qd)	[(Clinda 300–450 mg po q6-8h) + (pyri 25–50 mg po qd) + folinic acid 10–25 mg po qd)] OR atovaquone 750 mg po q6-12h	[Pyri + sulfa] prevents PCP and toxo; (clinda + pyri) prevents toxo only.
Trichomonas vaginalis	See Vaginitis, Table 1, page 17		
Trypanosomiasis Ref.: Ln Inf Dis 2:437, 2002			
T. brucei gambiense or T. brucei rhodesiense: African sleeping sickness	Pentamidine isethionate 4 mg/kg IM daily x10 days	(Suramin[20CI] test dose of 0.2 gm IV, then 20 mg/kg, IV on days 1, 3, 7, 14 & 21. Children: 20 mg/kg on same schedule)	CSF abnormal if 5 cells/µl or ↑ protein concentration. Melarsoprol-induced encephalopathy in 10% of pts. NOTE: T. brucei rhodesiense are resistant to nifurtimox and eflornithine.
Early infection with normal CSF			
Late infection with CNS symptoms and abnormal CSF →Prednisolone 1 mg/kg/d po may ↓ post-rx encephalopathy (see Comment)	Melarsoprol[2&3] 2-3.6 mg/kg IV x3 doses, repeat after 1 week and again after 10-21 days (active vs rhodesiense) See Peds dose in Table 12B, page 99	Eflornithine 100 mg/kg IV q6h IV x14 d. and then 75 mg/kg po x21–30 d. for gambiense but not rhodesiense! Peds: dose of eflornithine: 100 mg/kg IV q6h x2 wks, then 75 mg/kg po x3-4 wks.	
T. brucei gambiense relapse post-rx with melarsoprol	Eflornithine 100 mg/kg IV x14 d., then 75 mg/kg po q6h x21-30 d.		Under study as facial cream (Vaniqa) to remove unwanted hair.
T. brucei rhodesiense prophylaxis	Pentamidine isethionate 3 mg/kg IM q6 months		Risk for casual visitor. Not effective for T. brucei rhodesiense.
T. cruzi—Chagas disease or acute American trypanosomiasis Ref.: Ln 357:797, 2001	Nifurtimox[20CI] 8-10 mg/kg/d po div. 4x/d, after meals x120 d. Ages 11–16 yrs: 12.5-15 mg/kg/d div. qid po x90 d. Children <11 yrs: 15–20 mg/kg/d div. qid po x90 d.	Benznidazole[3&5] 5–7 mg/kg/d po div. 2x/d x30–60 d. (AJTMH 63:111, 2000). NOTE: Avoid tetracycline and steroids.	Not for tourists Not for casual visitor. No benefit in chronic late disease. Nifurtimox reported 70–85% effective. Immunosuppression for heart transplant can reactivate chronic Chagas disease.
NEMATODES—INTESTINAL (Roundworms) For significance of eosinophilia, see CID 34:407, 2002			
Angiostrongylus cantonensis	Mebendazole 100 mg po bid x5 d.	Anthelminth therapy may worsen meningitis (NEJM 346:668).	For eosinophilic meningitis, corticosteroids of benefit (CID 31:660, 2000).
Angiostrongylus costaricensis	Mebendazole 200–400 mg po tid x10 d.	Thiabendazole 75 mg/kg/d in 3 div. doses (max. 3 gm/d.)	Can cause inflammatory mass that mimics appendicitis.

---

1 **CDC** = available from CDC Drug Service
2 **Melarsoprol** 2.2 mg/kg IV x10 d. as effective as standard regimen (Ln 355:1419, 2000).

NOTE: All dosage recommendations are for adults (unless otherwise indicated) and assume normal renal function. See page 101 for abbreviations.

TABLE 12A (6)

INFECTING ORGANISM	SUGGESTED REGIMENS		COMMENTS
	PRIMARY	**ALTERNATIVE**	
NEMATODES—INTESTINAL (Roundworms) *(continued)*			
Ascaris lumbricoides (**ascariasis**)	**Albendazole** 400 mg po x1 dose or **mebendazole** 100 mg po bid x3 d. or 500 mg po x1 dose	**Pyrantel pamoate** 11 mg/kg po x1 dose (max. dose 1.0 gm)	Can present with intestinal obstruction.
Capillaria philippinensis (**capillariasis**)	**Mebendazole** 200 mg po bid x20 d.	**Albendazole** 200 mg po bid x10 d.	
Enterobius vermicularis (**pinworm**)	**Albendazole** 400 mg po x1, repeat in 2 wks OR **mebendazole** 100 mg po x1, repeat in 2 wks	**Pyrantel pamoate** 11 mg/kg (to max. dose of 1.0 gm) po x1 dose; repeat every 2 wks x2.	Side-effects in Table 12B, pages 98, 100
Hookworm (Necator americanus and Ancylostoma duodenale)	**Albendazole** 400 mg po x1 or **mebendazole** 100 mg po bid x3 d.	**Pyrantel pamoate** 11 mg/kg (to max. dose of 1.0 gm) po x1 dose x3 d.	NOTE: Ivermectin not effective. Eosinophilia may be present or eggs detectable in stool.
Strongyloides stercoralis (**strongyloidiasis**)	**Ivermectin** 200 μg/kg/d. po x1–2 d.	**Thiabendazole** 25 mg/kg po bid (max. 3 gm/ d) x2 d. (7–10 d for hyperinfection syndrome)	Case report of ivermectin failure in pt with hypogamma-globulinemia (Am J Med Sci 371:178, 1996).
Trichostrongylus orientalis	**Albendazole** 400 mg po x1 dose	**Pyrantel pamoate** 11 mg/kg (max. 1.0 gm) po x1	**Mebendazole** 100 mg po bid x3 d.
Trichuris trichiura (**whipworm**)	**Albendazole** 400 mg po once daily x3 days	**Mebendazole** 100 mg po bid x3 d.	May need repeat rx if heavily infected.
NEMATODES—EXTRAINTESTINAL (Roundworms)			
Anisakis simplex (**anisakiasis**)	Physical removal: endoscope or surgery	Questionable response to albendazole (Ln 360:54, 2002)	Anisakiasis acquired by eating raw fish: herring, salmon, mackerel, cod, squid. Similar illness due to Pseudoterranova species acquired from cod, halibut, red snapper.
Ancylostoma braziliense causes **cutaneous larva migrans**	**Ivermectin** 200 μg/kg po x1 dose/d. x1–2 d	**Albendazole** 200 mg po bid x3 d.	Also called "creeping eruption," dog and cat hookworm. Ivermectin cure rate 77% (1 dose) to 97% (2–3 doses) (CID 31:493, 2000)
Dracunculus medinensis: **Guinea worm**	Surgical removal pre-emergent worm	**Metronidazole** 250 mg po tid x10 d. used to ↓ inflammatory response and facilitate removal. Immersion in warm water promotes worm emergence. Mebendazole 400–800 mg/d. x6 d. may kill worm.	
Filariasis			
Lymphatic (**Elephantiasis**): Wuchereria bancrofti or Brugia malayi or B. timori	**Ivermectin**[1] (see Comment) 100–440 μg/kg x1 dose OR Rx of children with both **ivermectin** 200–400 μg/kg and **albendazole** 400 mg, one dose of each (Ln 350:480, 1997)	**Diethylcarbamazine**[1] (DEC) po over 14 days: Day 1, 50 mg; day 2, 50 mg tid; day 3, 100 mg tid; days 4–14, 2 mg/kg tid. (See Comment)	DEC 300 mg/wk po over 6 weeks effective prophylaxis [ivermectin ↓ number of microfilariae in skin and impairs female worm fertility; does not kill adult worms (nothing does). Ivermectin OK in pregnancy.
Cutaneous Loiasis: **Loa loa**, eyeworm disease[3] Onchocerca volvulus[1] (**onchocerci-asis**)— river blindness (Ln 360:203, 2002)	**Diethylcarbamazine** (DEC).[1,3]—dose as for Wuchereria, except x30 d. **Ivermectin** 150 μg/kg po x1 dose, repeat q6 months to suppress dermal and ocular microfilariae. If eye involved, start **prednisone** 1 mg/kg/d po several days before ivermectin. NOTE: Worm survival requires symbiotic bacteria Wolbachia (Science 296:1365, 2002)	**Diethylcarbamazine**[1] as above for Wuchereria OR **ivermectin** 150 μg/kg x1	
Mansonella perstans (**dipetalonemiasis**)	**Mebendazole** 100 mg po bid x30 d. or **albendazole** 400 mg po bid x10 d.		Usually no or vague allergic symptoms + eosinophilia. Ivermectin has no activity against this species.
Mansonella streptocerca	**Diethylcarbamazine**[1] as above for Wuchereria OR **ivermectin** 150 μg/kg x1		Chronic pruritic hypopigmented lesions that may be confused with leprosy. Can be asymptomatic.
Mansonella ozzardi	**Ivermectin** 200 μg/kg x1 dose may be effective		Usually asymptomatic. Articular pain, pruritus, lymphadenopathy reported. May have allergic reaction from dying organisms.

[1] May need antihistamine or corticosteroid for allergic reaction from disintegrating organisms
[2] Diethylcarbamazine available from Wyeth-Ayerst (610) 971-5509
[3] Occasional serious reactions reported in pts with both loiasis and onchocerciasis given ivermectin (Ln 350:18, 1997)
NOTE: All dosage recommendations are for adults (unless otherwise indicated) and assume normal renal function. See page 101 for abbreviations.

TABLE 12A (7)

INFECTING ORGANISM	SUGGESTED REGIMENS		COMMENTS
	PRIMARY	ALTERNATIVE	
NEMATODES—Extraintestinal (Roundworms)/Filariasis/Body cavity (continued)			
Dirofilariasis: Heartworms	No effective drugs; surgical removal only option		Can lodge in pulmonary artery → coin lesion. Eosinophilia rare.
D. immitis, (dog heartworm. D. tenius (raccoon), D. ursi (bear), D. repens (dogs, cats)	No effective drugs		Worms migrate to conjunctivae, subcutaneous tissue, scrotum, breasts, extremities
Gnathostoma spinigerum: eosinophilic myeloencephalitis		**Ivermectin** 200 μg/kg/d	
Toxocariasis	Rx directed at relief of symptoms as infection self-limited, e.g., steroids & antihistamines; use of anthelminthic controversial.		
Visceral larval migrans	**Albendazole** 400 mg bid x5 d.	**Mebendazole** 100–200 mg po bid x5 days	Severe lung, heart or CNS disease may warrant steroids. Differential dx of larval migrans syndromes: Toxocara canis and catis, Ancylostoma spp., Gnathostoma spp., Spirometra spp.
Ocular larval migrans	First 4 wks of illness: (Oral **prednisone** 30-60 mg po qd + subtenon **triamcinolone** 40 mg weekly) x2 weeks		No added benefit of anthelminthic drugs. Rx of little effect after 4 wks.
Trichinella spiralis (**trichinosis**)—muscle infection	**Albendazole** 400 mg po bid x8–14 d. Concomitant **prednisone** 40-60 mg po qd	**Mebendazole** 200–400 mg po tid x3 d, then 400–500 mg po tid x10 d.	Use albendazole/mebendazole with caution during pregnancy.
TREMATODES (Flukes)			
Clonorchis sinensis (liver fluke)	**Praziquantel** 25 mg/kg po tid x1 day or **albendazole** 10 mg/kg/d po x7 d.		Same dose in children
Fasciola buski (intestinal fluke)	**Praziquantel** 25 mg/kg po tid x1 day		Same dose in children
Fasciola hepatica (sheep liver fluke)	**Triclabendazole**[CDC8] (Fasinex; Novartis Agribusiness) 10 mg/kg po x1 dose. Ref: CID 32:1, 2001	**Bithionol**[CDC8] Adults and children: 30–50 mg/kg (max. dose 2 gm/d) x10–15 doses	
Heterophyes heterophyes (intestinal fluke); Metagonimus yokogawai (intestinal fluke); Opisthorchis viverrini (liver fluke)	**Praziquantel** 25 mg/kg po tid x1 day		Same regimen for Metorchis conjunctus (North American liver fluke)
Paragonimus westermani (lung fluke)	**Praziquantel** 25 mg/kg po tid x2 days or **bithionol**[CDC8] 30–50 mg/kg po x1 qod x10 d.		Same dose in children
Schistosoma haematobium; GU bilharziasis	**Praziquantel** 20 mg/kg po bid x1 day (2 doses)		Same dose in children. Alternative: metrifonate 10 mg/kg/dose po q2 wks x 3 doses
Schistosoma intercalatum	**Praziquantel** 20 mg/kg po bid x1 day (2 doses)		Same dose in children
Schistosoma japonicum; Oriental schisto	**Praziquantel** 20 mg/kg po bid x1 day (3 doses)		Same dose in children
Schistosoma mansoni (intestinal bilharziasis) Possible praziquantel resistance	**Praziquantel** 20 mg/kg po bid x1 day (2 doses)	**Oxamniquine**[N.8] single dose of 15 mg/kg po once; in North and East Africa 20 mg/kg po daily x3 d.	Same dose for children. For neurological manifestations: CID 18:354, 1994
Schistosoma mekongi	**Praziquantel** 20 mg/kg po x1 day (3 doses)		Same dose for children
Toxemic schisto, Katayama fever	**Praziquantel** 20 mg/kg po q4h withfood x3 doses		Massive infection with either S. japonicum or S. mansoni
CESTODES (Tapeworms)			
Echinococcus granulosus (hydatid disease). Rx lowers cyst content non-infectious in 80–90% and cyst disappearance in 30% of pts. (Refs. NEJM 337:881, 1997; IDCP 6:759, 1997)	Combine percutaneous drainage with 3 or more cycles of po **albendazole**: **>60 kg**: 400 mg po bid with meals x28 days; **<60 kg**: 15 mg/kg/d (with meals, max daily dose 800 mg) x28 days, then 2-week rest period, then repeat, twice for 3 cycles. Repeat for 3 cycles. 28-day cycle, then 14 days no drug. Repeat for 3 cycles.	Another option: cyst puncture with ultrasound, content aspiration, injection 95% ethanol or hypertonic saline, re-aspirate & concidental chemotherapy. Cure or marked regression 90→100% (Eur J Radiol 32:76, 1999). NOTE: If cyst spillage secondary to trauma or surgery, need **praziquantel** and then several cycles of **albendazole** to prevent implantation of secondary cysts.	

[1] **CDC** = Available from CDC Drug Service

NOTE: All dosage recommendations are for adults (unless otherwise indicated) and assume normal renal function. See page 101 for abbreviations.

TABLE 12A (8)

INFECTING ORGANISM	SUGGESTED REGIMENS		COMMENTS
	PRIMARY	ALTERNATIVE	
CESTODES (Tapeworms) (continued)			
Echinococcus multilocularis (alveolar cyst disease)	**Albendazole** efficacy not clearly demonstrated, can try in dosages used for hydatid disease. Wide surgical resection only reliable rx; technique evolving (Radiology 198:259, 1996).		
Intestinal tapeworms			
Diphyllobothrium latum (fish), Dipylidium caninum (dog), Taenia saginata (beef), and	**Praziquantel** 5–10 mg/kg po x1 dose for children and adults. **Alternative: Niclosamide** 2 gm po x1.		
Taenia solium (pork), Hymenolepis diminuta (rats) and H. nana (humans)	**Praziquantel** 25 mg/kg po x1 dose for children and adults		
Cerebral (neuro) cysticercosis. Larval stage of T. solium—see Comment. Management refs. Ann Rev Med 51:187, 2000; J Child Neurol 15:207, 2000	No controlled trial has shown benefit of antiparasitic drug over anticonvulsant therapy alone. See Comment	**Albendazole** x8–30 d by weight: >60 kg, 400 mg po bid with meals; <60 kg, 15 mg/kg/d po div bid with meals (max. daily dose 800 mg) or **praziquantel** 50 mg/kg/d po in 3 div. doses x30 d	Dexamethasone ± seizure meds may be needed to control rx-induced inflammation from cyst death. Subarachnoid cysts or giant cysts in fissures: **albendazole** x30+ days (NEJM 345:879, 2001). Examine optic fundi for cysts.
Sparganosis (Spirometra mansonoides) Larval cysts: source—frogs/snakes	Surgical resection or ethanol injection of subcutaneous masses (NEJM 330:1887, 1994).		
ECTOPARASITES Ref: Ln 355:819, 2000			
Pediculus humanus corporis (body lice)	Treat the clothing. Organism lives in, deposits eggs in seams of clothing. Discard (if not possible, treat clothing with 1% malathion powder or 10% DDT) powder.		Body louse leaves clothing only for blood meal. Nits in clothing viable for 1 month. Ref.: Med Lett 38:6, 1997.
P. humanus var. capitis (**head louse**, nits) Ref.: Ln 356:523, 2000	**Permethrin**, 5% prescription strength (ELIMITE) or 1% non-prescription (Nix). Wash hair, apply lotion for 10 min., then rinse off. comb. 2nd treatment 7–10 days after 1st to kill newly hatched lice (all products).	Benefit of residual permethrin on hair reduced by shampoos or vinegar. No residual effect with lindane or pyrethrin products. Nit removal important adjunct. Use nit comb ± enzymatic egg remover (CLEAR is one example).	
Phthirus pubis (crabs)	**Lindane (Kwell)** 1%, less effective (use only if failed other therapy). Seizures can occur from overuse of broad areas or ingestion. For head lice treatment failures, anecdotal reports of success with **ivermectin** 200 µg/kg single dose po, does not kill eggs. Another option (not in neonates/infants): **Malathion 0.5% lotion** (Ovide). Apply for 8–12 hrs. Study shows no need to comb for lice after malathion (Ln 356:540, 2000).	Treat sex partners if body or pubic lice. Cost: Permethrin 60 gm $9.20, lindane 60 ml $6.35–16.40, malathion $31.25; ivermectin $9.97. For failures with 1% permethrin, repeat permethrin + po TMP/SMX 10 mg/kg/d. in 2 div. doses x10 days (Ped 107:E30, 2001).	
Sarcoptes scabiei (**scabies**) (mites)			
Immunocompetent patients	**Primary: Permethrin** 5% cream (ELIMITE). Apply entire skin from chin to toes. Leave on 8–10 hrs. Repeat in 1 week. Safe for children >2 mos. old. **Alternative: Lindane** 1% lotion. Apply as for permethrin OR ivermectin 200 µg/kg po x1 (NEJM 333:26, 1995). Do not use in pregnancy (see Comment)	Trim fingernails. Reapply to hands after handwashing. Pruritus may persist x2 wks after mites gone. Do not use lindane in pregnancy or in young children—absorbed through skin; can use 6–10% precipitated sulfur in petrolatum daily x3 days. Repeated lindane application associated with seizures in children.	
AIDS patients, CD4 <150/mm³ (Norwegian scabies—see Comments)	For Norwegian scabies: Permethrin as above on day 1, then 6% sulfur in petrolatum daily or ivermectin 200 µg/kg po x1 reported effective.	Norwegian scabies in AIDS pts: Extensive, crusted. Can mimic psoriasis. Not pruritic. ELIMITE: 60 gm $18.10, lindane 60 ml $2.60–10.50. Highly contagious—isolate!	

NOTE: All dosage recommendations are for adults (unless otherwise indicated) and assume normal renal function. See page 101 for abbreviations.

TABLE 13B: DOSAGE, PRICE, AND SELECTED ADVERSE EFFECTS OF ANTIPARASITIC DRUGS

NOTE: Drugs available from CDC Drug Service indicated by "CDC." Call (404) 639-3670 (or 2888).

Doses vary with indication. For convenience, drugs divided by type of parasite; some drugs used for multiple types of parasites, e.g., albendazole.
COMMENT: Cost data represent average wholesale prices as listed in 2002 Drug Topics Red Book, Medical Economics.

CLASS, AGENT GENERIC NAME (TRADE NAME)	USUAL ADULT DOSAGE (Cost)	ADVERSE REACTIONS/COMMENTS
Antiprotozoan Drugs		
Intestinal Parasites		
Albendazole (Albenza)	Doses vary with indication, 200–400 mg bid po 200 mg tab $1.32	Teratogenic, Pregnancy Cat. C; give after negative pregnancy test. Abdominal pain, nausea/vomiting, alopecia, ↑ serum transaminase. Rare leukopenia.
Dehydroemetine (CDC)*	1.5 mg/kg/d to max. of 90 mg IM	Local pain, ECG changes, cardiac arrhythmias, precordial pain, paresthesias, weakness, peripheral neuropathy. GI: nausea/vomiting, diarrhea. Avoid strenuous exercise for 4 wks after rx.
Dioxanide furoate (CDC)*	500 mg po tid	GI: flatulence, abdominal distention, nausea/vomiting. Pruritus, urticaria.
Furazolidone (Furoxone)	Peds: 6 mg/kg/d div. qid. Not for infants <1 mo. old. Liquid: 50 mg/15 ml. 473 ml $100	Only liquid antigiardiasis drug in U.S. Disulfiram-like reaction with alcohol. Occasional side-effects: Fever, urticaria, ↓ BP, arthralgia, nausea/vomiting, headache. Hemolysis if G6PD deficient. May turn urine brown.
Iodoquinol (Yodoxin) (650 mg $0.75)	Adults: 650 mg po tid; children: 40 mg/kg/d div. tid. See metronidazole in Table 9A, page 68	Rarely causes nausea, abdominal cramps, rash, acne. Contraindicated if iodine intolerance.
Metronidazole/Ornidazole (Tiberal)/Tinidazole (Fasigyn)	Side-effects similar for all. See metronidazole in Table 9A page 62, 6 9B, page 68	Drug is aminoglycoside similar to neomycin; if absorbed due to concomitant inflammatory bowel disease can result in oto/nephrotoxicity. Doses >3 gm assoc. with nausea, abdominal cramps.
Paromomycin (Humatin) Aminosidine in U.K.	Up to 750 mg qid. 250 mg caps $3.03	
Quinacrine (Atabrine, Mepacrine)	100 mg tid. No longer available in U.S.; 2 pharmacies will prepare as a service: (1) Connecticut 203-785-6818; (2) California 800-247-9767	Contraindicated for pts with history of psoriasis or psychosis. Yellow staining of skin. Dizziness, headache, vomiting, toxic psychosis (1.5%), hemolytic anemia, leucopenia, thrombocytopenia, urticaria, rash, fever, minor disulfiram-like reactions.
Tinidazole (Fasigyn)	For giardiasis: 2 gm po x1 dose	Chemical structure similar to metronidazole but better tolerated. Can obtain from Panorama Pharm. 1-800-247-9767. Avoid concomitant alcohol intake.
Extraintestinal Parasites		
Antimony compounds Stibugluconate sodium (Pentostam, Tricostam) (CDC) Meglumine antimonate (Glucantime, Glucontim)—French tradenames	Solution containing 30–34% pentavalent antimony	Cough/vomiting if IV infusion too fast. Arthralgia 50%, Others: myalgia, bradycardia, cramps/diarrhea, pruritus/rash, renal toxicity, amylase. **NOTE: EKG abnormalities occur. Combination rx with, or sequential rx with, ampho B may trigger fatal arrhythmias (Ln 351:1928, 1998).**
Artesunate	Adults: 4 mg/kg po x3 d., can give IM	Drug fever, abdominal pain, diarrhea, primary heart block. Refs.: CID 33:2009, 2001; Ln 359:1365, 2002; AAC 46:778, 2002
Atovaquone (Mepron) Ref.: AAC 46:1163, 2002	Suspension: 1 tsp (750 mg) po bid 750 mg/5 ml. Cost: 210 ml $709.00	No. pts stopping rx due to side-effects was 9%; rash 22%, GI 20%, headache 16%, insomnia 10%, fever 14%
Atovaquone and proguanil (Malarone) For prophylaxis of P. falciparum; little data on P. vivax	Prophylaxis: 1 tab po (250 mg + 100 mg), qd with food Treatment: 4 tabs po (1000 mg + 400 mg) once daily with food x3 days. Either 250/100 mg or 62.5/25 mg. Peds dosage: footnote 2 page 92. Cost: 250/100 mg tab $4.70	Adverse effects in rx trials: Adults—abd. pain 17%, N/V 12%, headache 10%, dizziness 5%. Rx stopped in 1%. Asymptomatic mild ↑ in ALT/AST. Children—cough, headache, anorexia, vomiting, abd. pain. See drug interactions, Table 21. Safe in G6PD-deficient pts. Can crush tabs for children and give with milk or other liquid nutrients.
Benznidazole (Rochagan, Roche, Brazil)	7.5 mg/kg/d	Photosensitivity in 50% of pts. GI: abdominal pain, nausea/vomiting/ anorexia. CNS: disorientation, insomnia, twitching/seizures, polyneuritis.
Chloroquine phosphate (Aralen)	Dose varies—see Malaria prophylaxis and rx. 500 mg tabs $5.24; IM 250 mg ampule $22.00	Minor: anorexia/nausea/vomiting, headache, dizziness, blurred vision, pruritus in dark-skinned pts. Major: protracted rx in rheumatoid arthritis can lead to retinopathy. Can exacerbate psoriasis. Can block response to rabies vaccine.

* All doses are for adults (unless otherwise indicated) and assume normal renal function. See page 101 for abbreviations.

TABLE 12B (2)

CLASS, AGENT, GENERIC NAME (TRADE NAME)	USUAL ADULT DOSAGE (Cost)	ADVERSE REACTIONS/COMMENTS
Antiprotozoan Drugs/Extraintestinal Parasites *(continued)*		
Dapsone Ref.: *CID 27:191, 1998*	100 mg po 100 mg tabs $0.20	Usually tolerated by pts with rash after TMP/SMX. Adverse effects: nausea/vomiting, rash, oral lesions *(CID 18:630, 1994)*. Methemoglobinemia (usually asymptomatic); if > 10–15%, stop drug. Hemolytic anemia, if G6PD deficient. Sulfone syndrome: fever, rash, hemolytic anemia, atypical lymphocytes, and liver injury *(West J Med 156:303, 1992)*.
Eflornithine (Ornidyl) 3656	Approved in U.S. for trypanosome infections but not marketed. Contact Hoechst Marion Roussel, (800) 552-	Diarrhea in ⅓ pts, vomiting, abdominal pain, anemia/leucopenia in ⅓ pts, seizures, alopecia, jaundice, ↓ hearing
Fumagillin	Eyedrops + po. Call 800-547-1392	
Halofantrine (Halfan)	Adults: 500 mg po q6h x3 doses Children: 8 mg/kg po q6h x3 doses 250 mg tab $3.88	Poor oral bioavailability ↑ with fatty meal. Causes delay in A-V conduction: **do not use if long QT interval or pt taking drugs known to ↑ QT interval (e.g., quinine/quinidine, astemizole, chloroquine, antidepressants, neuroleptic drugs).** Other side-effects: nausea, abdominal pain, diarrhea. Do not use in pregnancy.
Mefloquine (Lariam)	One 250 mg tab/week for malaria prophylaxis; for rx, 1250 mg x1 or 750 mg x1 & then 500 mg 1 in 6–8 hrs. 250 mg tab $10.76. In U.S.: 250 mg tab = 228 mg base; outside U.S., 275 mg tab = 250 mg base	Side-effects in roughly 3%. Minor: headache, irritability, insomnia, weakness, diarrhea. Toxic psychosis, seizures can occur. Teratogenic—do not use in pregnancy. Do not use with quinine, quinidine, or halofantrine. Rare: Prolonged QT interval and toxic epidermal necrolysis *(Ln 349:101, 1997)*. Not used for self-rx due to neuropsychiatric side-effects.
Melarsoprol (CDC) **(Mel B, Arsobal)** (Manufactured in France)	See Trypanosomiasis for adult dose. Peds dose ≥ 0.36 mg/kg IV, then gradual ↑ to 3.6 mg/kg q1–5 days for total of 3 doses	Post-rx encephalopathy (10%) with 50% mortality overall; risk of death 2° to rx 4–8%. Prednisolone 1 mg/kg/d po may ↓ encephalopathy. Other: myocardial damage, albuminuria, abdominal pain, vomiting, peripheral neuropathy. Herxheimer-like reaction, pruritis.
Miltefosine^{NUS} (Zentaris, Impavido)	Visceral leishmaniasis 2.25 mg/kg/d. po Kala-azar: 50 mg po bid x21 d. Cutaneous leishmaniasis 2.25 mg/kg po qd x6 wks	Contact Astra Medica. Ger. **Pregnancy—No:** teratogenic. Side-effects vary: kala-azar pts, vomiting in majority, cutaneous leishmaniasis, vertigo & nausea
Nifurtimox (Lampit) (CDC) Registered in Germany by Bayer	8–10 mg/kg/d po qiv. 4x/day	Side-effects in 40–70% of pts. GI: abdominal pain, nausea/vomiting. CNS: polyneuritis (1/3), disorientation, insomnia, twitching, seizures. Skin rash. Hemolysis with G6PD deficiency
Nitazoxanide (Cryptaz)	0.5–1.0 gm po bid	Investigational. Contact Romark Labs. (813) 282-8544. www.romarklaboratories.com. Ref.: *TRSTM 92:663, 1998.*
Pentamidine (NebuPent)	300 mg via aerosol q month. Also used IM. 300 mg $98.75 + admin. costs	Hypotension, hypocalcemia, hypoglycemia followed by hyperglycemia, pancreatitis. Neutropenia (15%), thrombocytopenia. Nephrotoxicity. Others: nausea/vomiting, ↑ liver tests, rash.
Primaquine phosphate	26.3 mg (= 15 mg base) po	In G6PD def. pts, can cause hemolytic anemia with hemoglobinuria, esp. African, Asian peoples. Methemoglobinemia. Nausea/abdominal pain if pt. fasting.
Pyrimethamine (Daraprim, Malocide) Also combined with sulfadoxine as **Fansidar**	100 mg po, then 25 mg qd 25 mg $0.43. Cost of folinic acid (leucovorin) 5 mg $2.36	Major problem is hematologic: megaloblastic anemia, ↓ WBC, ↓ platelets. Can give 5 mg folinic acid/day to ↓ bone marrow depression and not interfere with antitoxoplasmosis effect. If true pyrimethamine, folinic acid to 10–50 mg/d. Other: Rash. vomiting, diarrhea, xerostomia
Quinacrine^{NUS}	For giardiasis: 100 mg po tid x5 d. Peds dose: 2 mg/kg po tid x5 d. Can Mfr., 390 mg/vl x5 d.	Compounded by Med. Center Pharm., New Haven, CT: (203) 688-8816 or Panorama Compound. (800) 247-9767.
Quinidine gluconate	Loading dose of 10 mg/kg IV over 1–2 hrs., and then constant infusion of 0.02 mg of quinidine gluconate/kg/minute. 80 mg/1 vl $20.53	Adverse reactions of quinidine/quinine similar. (1) IV bolus injection can cause fatal hypotension. (2) hyperinsulinemic hypoglycemia, esp. in pregnancy, (3) ↓ rate of infusion of IV quinidine if QT interval ↑ >25% of baseline, (4) reduce dose by 3 due to ↓ renal clearance and ↓ vol. of distribution

NOTE: All dosage recommendations are for adults (unless otherwise indicated) and assume normal renal/renal function. See page 101 for abbreviations.

TABLE 12B (3)

CLASS, AGENT, GENERIC NAME (TRADE NAME)	USUAL ADULT DOSAGE (Cost)	ADVERSE REACTIONS/COMMENTS
Antiprotozoan Drugs/Extraintestinal Parasites (continued)		
Quinine sulfate (300 mg salt = 250 mg base)	325 and 650 mg tabs. No IV prep. in U.S. Oral rx of chloroquine-resistant falciparum malaria: 650 mg po tid x5d, then tetracycline 250 mg po qid x7 d. 325 mg po x7 d. $0.16	Cinchonism; tinnitus, headache, nausea, abdominal pain, blurred vision. Rarely: blood dyscrasias, drug fever, asthma, hypoglycemia. Transient blindness in <1% of 500 pts (AnIM 136:339, 2002).
Spiramycin² (Rovamycine) (JAC 42:572, 1998)	Up to 3–4 gm/d	GI and allergic reactions have occurred. Not available in U.S.
Sulfadiazine	1.0–1.5 gm po q6h 500 mg $0.34	See Table 9B, page 69, for sulfonamide side-effects
Sulfadoxine and pyrimethamine combination (Fansidar)	Contains 500 mg of sulfadoxine and 25 mg of pyrimethamine One tab $3.57	Very long mean half-life of both drugs: Sulfadoxine 169 hrs, pyrimethamine 111 hrs allows weekly dosage. Fatalities reported due to Stevens-Johnson syndrome and toxic epidermal necrolysis. Renal excretion—use with caution in pts with renal impairment.
DRUGS USED TO TREAT NEMATODES, TREMATODES, AND CESTODES		
Bithionol (CDC)	Adults & children: 30–40 mg/kg (to max. of 2 gm/d) po qod x10–15 doses	Photosensitivity, skin reactions, urticaria, GI upset
Diethylcarbamazine² (Hetrazan) (CDC)	Used to treat filariasis. Licensed (Lederle) but not available in U.S.	Headache, dizziness, nausea, fever. Host may experience inflammatory reaction to death of adult worms: fever, urticaria, asthma, GI upset (Mazzotti reaction).
Ivermectin (Stromectol, Mectizan)	Strongyloidiasis dose: 200 µg/kg x1 dose po Onchocerciasis: 150 µg/kg x1 po Scabies: 200 µg/kg po x1 3 mg tabs $5.45	Mild side-effects: fever, pruritus, rash. In rx of onchocerciasis, can see tender lymphadenopathy, headache, bone/joint pain. Can cause Mazzotti reaction (see above).
Mebendazole (Vermox)	Doses vary with indication. 100 mg tab $4.55	Rarely causes abdominal pain, nausea, diarrhea. Contraindicated in pregnancy and children <2 yrs old.
Oxamniquine (Vansil)ᴺᵁˢ	For S. mansoni. Some experts suggest 40–60 mg/kg over 2–3 days in all of Africa.	Rarely: dizziness, drowsiness, neuropsychiatric symptoms, GI upset EKG/EEG changes. Orange/red urine.
Praziquantel (Biltricide)	Doses vary with parasite; see Table 12A. 600 mg $11.90	Mild: dizziness/drowsiness; N/V, rash, fever. Only contraindication is ocular cysticercosis. Metab.-induced by anticonvulsants and steroids; can negate effect with cimetidine 400 mg po tid.
Pyrantel pamoate (over-the-counter as Reese's Pinworm Medicine)	Oral suspension. Dose for all ages: 11 mg/kg (to max. of 1 gm) x1 dose	Rare GI upset, headache, dizziness, rash
Suramin (Germanin) (CDC)	For early trypanosomiasis. Drug powder mixed to 10% solution with 5 ml water and used within 30 minutes.	Does not cross blood-brain barrier, no effect on CNS infection. Side-effects: vomiting, pruritus, urticaria, fever, paresthesias, albuminuria (discontinue drug if casts appear). Do not use if renal/liver disease present. Deaths from vascular collapse reported.
Thiabendazole (Mintezol)	Take after meals. Dose varies with parasite; see Table 12A. 500 mg $1.25	Nausea/vomiting, headache, dizziness. Rarely: liver damage, ↓ BP, angioneurotic edema, Stevens-Johnson syndrome. May ↓ mental alertness.

Abbreviations: **Clinda** = clindamycin; **CQ** = chloroquine phosphate; **MQ** = mefloquine; **NUS** = not available in the U.S.; **PQ** = primaquine; **Pyri** = pyrimethamine; **QS** = quinine sulfate; **TMP/SMX** = trimethoprim/sulfamethoxazole

¹ Available from FDA, (301) 443-5680
² Available from Wyeth-Ayerst, (610) 971-5509

* All doses for adults with normal renal function unless pediatric dose given.

Average wholesale costs from 2002 Drug Topics Red Book, Medical Economics.

TABLE 13A: METHODS FOR PENICILLIN DESENSITIZATION
[Penicillin Allergy Reviews: CID 35:26, 2002 & MMWR 51(RR-6):28–30, 2002]

Perform in ICU setting. Discontinue all β-adrenergic antagonists. Have IV line, ECG and spirometer (Curr Clin Topics Inf Dis 13:131, 1993). Once desensitized, rx must not lapse or risk of allergic reactions ↑. A history of Stevens-Johnson syndrome, exfoliative dermatitis, erythroderma are nearly absolute contraindications to desensitization (use only as an approach to IgE sensitivity).

Oral Route: If oral prep. available and pt has functional GI tract, oral route is preferred. 1/3 pts will develop transient reaction during desensitization or treatment, usually mild.

Step *	1	2	3	4	5	6	7	8	9	10	11	12	13	14	15	16	17
Drug (mg/ml)	0.5	0.5	0.5	0.5	0.5	0.5	0.5	5.0	5.0	5.0	50	50	50	50	1000	1000	1000
Amount (ml)	0.1	0.2	0.4	0.8	1.6	3.2	6.4	1.2	2.4	4.8	1.0	2.0	4.0	8.0	0.16	0.32	0.64

* Interval between doses: 15 min. After Step 14, observe for 30 minutes, then 1.0 gm IV

Parenteral Route:

Step **	1	2	3	4	5	6	7	8	9	10	11	12	13	14
Drug (mg/ml)	0.1	0.1	0.1	0.1	0.1	1.0	1.0	10	10	10	100	100	100	100
Amount (ml)	0.1	0.2	0.4	0.8	0.16	0.32	0.64	0.12	0.24	0.48	0.1	0.2	0.4	0.8

** Interval between doses: 15 min. After Step 17, observe for 30 minutes, then 1.0 gm IV

[Adapted from Sullivan, TJ, in Allergy: Principles and Practice, Middleton, E., et al, Eds. C.V. Mosby, 1993, p. 1726, with permission]

TABLE 13B: RAPID ORAL TMP/SMX DESENSITIZATION*

Hour	Dose TMP/SMX (mg)
0	0.004/0.02
1	0.04/0.2
2	0.4/2
3	4/20
4	40/200
5	160/800

Comment
Perform in hospital or clinic. Use oral suspension [40mg TMP/200 mg SMX/5 ml (tsp)]. Take 6 oz water after each dose. Corticosteroids, antihistamines NOT used. Refs: CID 20:849, 1995; AIDS 5:311, 1991

All dosage recommendations are for adults

TABLE 14A: ANTIVIRAL THERAPY (Non-HIV)
(See *NEJM* 340:1255, 1999)

VIRUS/DISEASE	DRUG/DOSAGE	SIDE EFFECTS/COMMENTS
Adenovirus Common cause of respiratory tract infections including fatal pneumonia in young adults—esp. severe in immunocompromised children		No proven rx to date, but case reports of possible success with ribavirin (2/5 with severe immunosuppression survived) (*Ped* 110:e9, 2002)
Enterovirus—Meningitis: most common cause of aseptic meningitis. PCR on CSF valuable for early dx (*Scand J Inf Dis* 34:359, 2002). New strain 71 identified in Taiwan in 1998, appears particularly neurotropic & assoc. with ↑ mortality (78/408 children died) (*CID* 34(Suppl 2):S52, 2002)	No rx currently recommended; however, **pleconaril** still under investigation. [For compassionate use (for chronic enteroviral meningoencephalitis in pts with immunodeficiency, neonatal sepsis syndrome, myocarditis, enterovirus infection complicating bone marrow transplant or vaccine-associated paralytic polio), call Viropharma (610) 458-7300); ext. 6297 (Donna Kolbush, RN)]	2/16 with chronic enterovirus meningoencephalitis rx with pleconaril had favorable clinical response & 12/13 had virologic response (*CID* 32:228, 2001). Caused breakthrough bleeding in 3% of women taking oral contraceptives in large cold trial
Hemorrhagic Fever Viral Infections		
Congo-Crimean Hemorrhagic Fever (HF)	**Ribavirin** po 4 gm qd x4 d, then 2.4 gm qd x6 d (see Comment), with complete recovery in Pakistan (*Ln* 346:472, 1995)	For oral drug, contact Virazole, ICN Pharmaceuticals, Costa Mesa, CA, USA
Ebola/Marburg HF (Central Africa)	No data to date on antiviral therapy	An intense inflammatory response within 4 d. after infection may control viral proliferation and result in asymptomatic infection (*Ln* 355:2210, 2000). A vaccine may be near (*Nature* 408:527, 2000)
With pulmonary syndrome: Hantavirus pulmonary syndrome, "sin nombre virus"	No benefit from ribavirin has been demonstrated to date (controlled trial in progress). Refs.: *JID* 173:1297, 1996; *Emerg Inf Dis* 3:95, 1997; *Curr Int Dis* Rep 3.258, 2001.	Acute onset of fever, headache, myalgias, non-productive cough, thrombocytopenia and non-cardiogenic pulmonary edema with respiratory insufficiency following exposure to rodents. Persistent presence of myalgias, nausea, diarrhea, dramatic (↓ shift on blood smear, ↓ platelets, & ↑ PCO_2 predicted Hanta pulmonary syndrome (HPS) (*CID* 34:293, 2002). Serological studies available through CDC (*Ln* 347:739, 1996). Inhaled nitric oxide associated with single case(*PCCM* 17:749, 1996)
With renal syndrome: Lassa, Venezuelan, Korean, HF, Sabia, Argentinian HF, Junin, Machupo	**Ribavirin** IV 2 gm loading dose, then 1 gm q6h x4 days, then 0.5 gm q8h x6 d (See Comment, Congo-Crimean HF)	Toxicity low, hemolysis reported but recovery when treatment stopped. No significant changes in WBC, platelets, hepatic or renal function. Effective in Lassa and in 2 cases of Bolivian HF (*CID* 24:718, 1997). No data on others. Venezuelan HF may look like dengue (*CID* 26:308, 1998)
Dengue and dengue hemorrhagic fever (DHF) Aedes aegypti major vector (*JID* 176:313, 1997)	No proven rx to date. Appropriate fluid replacement with careful hemodynamic monitoring critical (*Ln* 352:971, 1998). Rx of DHF with colloids may be more effective than crystalloids in pts with low pulse pressures (*CID* 32:204, 2001; *J Ped* 140:629, 2002)	Resurgence in Southeast Asia, Central and South America and Caribbean. No vaccine; best prevention is to limit mosquito contact (*AnIM* 128:931, 1998) gives specifics. *BMJ* 324:1563, 2002)
West Nile virus A flavivirus introduced in the U.S. in 1999. NYC), transmitted by mosquitoes, blood transfusions, and transplanted organs, & spread throughout the U.S. by Nov. 2002 (*AnIM* 137:173, 2002; *MMWR* 51:973, 2002)	No proven rx to date. Ribavirin and interferon under study; to enroll pt, see www.nyho.org/posting/nihal.html. High titer IMIG from Israel (ron@omrix.co.il) under study; U.S. IVIG has no WNV antibody	1/150 infected develops severe neurological disease, severity ↑ in older persons. Encephalitis > meningitis & assoc. with muscle weakness & flaccid paralysis. Dx by ↑ IgM in serum & CSF (contact State Health Dept./CDC).
Yellow fever	No data on antiviral rx	Reemergence across Africa and South America (200,000 cases/yr). Vaccination effective and should be used (*JAMA* 276:1157, 1996)
Hepatitis Viral Infections		
Hepatitis A (*Ln* 351:1643, 1998)	No therapy recommended. If within 2 wks of exposure, gamma globulin 0.02 ml/kg IM injection x1 is protective.	For vaccine recommendations, see Table 20 (*MMWR* 48:RR-12, 1999). 40% of pts with chronic Hep C who developed superinfection with Hep A developed fulminant hepatic failure in 1 study (*NEJM* 338:286, 1998).
Hepatitis B		
Acute	No therapy recommended	

TABLE 14A (2)

VIRUS/DISEASE	DRUG/DOSAGE	SIDE EFFECTS/COMMENTS
Hepatitis Viral Infections/Hepatitis B **Chronic** (AnIM 132:326, 2000; NEJM 336:347, 1997; 337:1733, 1997) In general, **consider ↑ in pts with persistent ↑ of aminotransferase; detectable levels of HBsAg, HBeAg and HBV DNA in serum for at least 6 mos; hepatitis (at least 6 mos) & compensated liver disease**	**B** *(continued)* **For HBeAg+, ↑ ALT, HBV DNA+:** Lamivudine 100 mg po (dc 6 mos. after HBe Ag seroconversion) ↑ HBV DNA after 3-6 mos rx suggests emergence of YMDD mutations; add or switch to either Adefovir 10 mg po qd and/or interferon alfa 2a x16 wks **OR** Interferon alfa-2b 5 million units daily or 10 million units tiw sc x 16 weeks (was gold standard in the past) **For anti-HBeAb+, ↑ ALT, HBV DNA+:** Rx with lamivudine achieve virologic & biochemical remission)	**Goal of rx: ↓ liver inflammation, stop progression of cirrhosis, & prevent hepatocellular carcinoma.** Both INF & lamivudine work; response measured by loss of HBe Ag & undetectable DNA (20–30%), return of ALT to normal (41–72%). This usually followed by appearance of HBs antibody, loss of HBs Ag, & appearance of HBe antibody. Sustained viral response (**SVR:** lack of relapse after rx dc) seen in 50–60%. Histological improvement seen in >80%. In chronic Hep B with ↓ persistence of HBV DNA. Both drugs work best when baseline ALT ↑ & ALT ↑ high (*Viral Hep 9:208, 2002*). SVR after LAV rx with ALT 2x normal = only 5%, 2–5x normal 26%, >5x normal 64% (*Hepatol 36:186, 2002*). SVR also ↑ with ↑ duration of LAV rx: 1 year 22%, 3 yrs 40%, 6 yrs +65%, but if ALT >2x normal at initiation of LAV rx: SVR 38%, 65%, & 77% respectively. **Major problems with INF:** ↑ cost & toxicity (myalgias, bone marrow suppression, depression, thyroid abnormalities) (*Clin Enzio 56:780, 2002*); but duration of rx shorter (4 vs 16 wks). Pegylated interferons under study. **LAV remarkably nontoxic, but resistant mutations to LAV predictably emerge over time.** esp. when HBV DNA levels high: 1 yr 15%, 2 yrs 38%, 3 yrs 56%, 4 yrs 67%. While mutants appear to be less virulent than wild type virus, breakthrough may be assoc. with ↑ biochemical (↑ ALT) relapse & occasionally but not always to hepatic decompensation (*J Gastro Hepat 17:765, 2002*). Clinical significance still unclear? Combination rx with LAV + INF will ↓ emergence of YMDD mutants & ↑ effectiveness of rx in INF non-responders (*J Gastro Hepat 100:39?, 2002*). LAV also effective in Asians. while INF less effective in Asians (perhaps due to tolerance to virus associated with infections occurring at birth). Pretreatment with LAV in children (*NEJM 346:1706, 2002*). Future direction of rx of Hep B infection will likely be increased use of combination chemotherapy. **Adefovir** (approved by FDA 1-2002) effective as single agent in ↓ HBV DNA + HBV DNA ↓ 3.6 logs copies/mL from baseline. ALT normalization in 48–72% respectively. Histological improvement in 53–64%; but only 12% seroconversion (HBeAg+) at 48 wks. **Active against lamivudine-resistant mutants in vitro & in vivo in 2 studies** (435 & 461). In both studies, HBV DNA ↓ 3.8 & 3.1 logs at 48 wks. Lamivudine alone in combination with adefovir added nothing. Adefovir-resistant mutations have **not** emerged after 60 mos of rx (*Hepatol 36:464, 2002*). Other new nucleoside analogs look impressive (**tenofovir, entecavir, AMC-265, emtricitabine**). Famciclovir shows activity in vitro, but less effective in vivo (*Scand J Inf Dis 34:505, 2002; J Med Wro 67:334, 2002*).
Prevention Re-transplantation after transplantation for hepatitis B-induced cirrhosis (See Table 15A, page 120 for post-exposure prophylaxis recommendations)	Lamivudine 100 mg po. Start at least 4 wks pre-transplant and continue for at least 12 months post-transplant	Based on 3 uncontrolled studies, data suggest that lamivudine may reduce the rate of HBV reinfection post-transplant. Most pts were clinically stable at 1 yr. Post-transplant recurrence of HBV was lowest with lamivudine in some pts & "YMDD variant" HBV was detected in some pts (*Hpt 30:1302, 1999; Tpt 62:1456, 1996; Ln 348:1212, 1996*). Lamivudine (when combined with HBIG (*Hpt 28:585, 1998*) but has not been used alone in low-risk pts (*NEJM 34:888, 2001*). Optimal dose and duration of HBIG unknown.
Hepatitis C (up to 3% of world infected, 4 million in U.S.) See *NEJM 345:41, 2001; CID 33:1728, 2001; AnIM 136:747, 2002* **Acute:** Most pts asymptomatic (>75%), occasionally non-specific complaints such as fatigue.	PEG INF + ribavirin, occasionally INF alone, but controversial; requires confirmation (*NEJM 346:1091, 2002*)	Data emerging that early rx of acute hepatitis C with INF alfa 2b may reduce progression to chronic Hep C (mean 54 days to start of rx after exposure/infection) had neg. HCV RNA & normal ALT after 24 wks of INF alfa 2b rx (*NEJM 345:1452, 2001*). A review of published trials (206 pts) concluded that SVR following rx of acute Hep C with INF alfa 2b was 32% vs 4% with placebo (p=0.000001) (*Cochrane Database Sys S Rev:CD000369, 2002*).

NOTE: All dosage recommendations are for adults (unless otherwise indicated) and assume normal renal function.

TABLE 14A (3)

VIRUS/DISEASE	DRUG/DOSAGE	SIDE EFFECTS/COMMENTS
Hepatitis Viral Infections/Hepatitis C *(continued)*		

Chronic: see JAMA 284 consensus statement, www.niddk.nih.gov/health/digest/pubs/chrnhepc/chrnhepc.htm. Genotype 1 is most common in U.S. (>90%), & least responsive to rx. Once infected only 15% clear virus, 85% become chronic. Chronic infection: 10–15% progress to cirrhosis (med. time 28–32 yrs), 4% hepatocellular (HCCA) carcinoma. 5–10,000 deaths in U.S./yr. Co-infection with HIV: extremely common.
 	
Consider dx in high-risk pts *(see Prevention, below)* with ↑ ALT ↑ max value. Dx: antibody screen by EIA for HCV antibody, sensitivity & specificity >99%; in at-risk populations & those with liver disease. Qualitative HCV PCR used for confirmation of acute or chronic HCV infection without obvious risk factors or no evidence of liver disease. Immunoblot assay used as confirmatory test for pos. EIA in non-clinical settings or neg. HCV RNA pos. 1–3 wks after initial exposure. EIA later (6–8 wks) & **+HCV PCR pos 1–3 wks** after initial exposure. **Persistent infection (dx by +HCV RNA pos 6 mos** (>6 mos). Progressive liver disease associated with older age, immunosuppressed state (HIV), concurrent Hep B & esp. ↑ alcohol use (>30 gm/d). 50% pos for serum cryoglobulins, but clinical manifestations uncommon.
	Ref.: www.hcv.gov/hepatitis
	Rx indicated for persistent elevations ALT, HCV RNA+, & findings of fibrosis & at least moderate inflammation by liver bx.
	
	When genotype 1, for 48 wks:
	
	Pegylated INF-
	    Wt
	  Alfa 2a (Pegasys) + Ribavirin
	  180 μg sc q wk 600 mg po p.m. <75 kg
	    or and
	  Alfa 2b (PEG-Intron) 600 mg po bid >75g]
	  1.5 μg/kg sc q wk
	
	[Sustained viral response (SVR) = 42–51% for genotype 1 after 48 wks of rx with PEG INF & ribavirin. 50% relapse if rx only for 24 wks or 3 after 24 weeks).]
	
	When genotype 2 or 3 (non-1), alternatives are for 24 wks:
	  Standard INF alfa + Ribavirin as above
	  3 mU sc 3x/wk
	    or
	  PEG INF alfa (either + Ribavirin 400 mg
	  2a or 2b) as above po bid
	  [since SVR SVR similar to PEG INF for genotypes 2&3]
		Obtain baseline CBC and at wks 2, 4 of rx *(see Table 14B, page 111)* & HCV RNA at 24 wks; hemolytic anemia very common with ribavirin.
		Sustained viral response [neg. HCV RNA (<50 IU/ml) at least 24 wks after end of rx] assoc. with resolution in hepatic injury, reduction of fibrosis & **low likelihood of HCV relapse.**
		
		3 large pivotal trials have demonstrated superiority of pegylated interferon + ribavirin over standard interferon-ribavirin combination or PEG INF alone. Rates similar with PEG INF + ribavirin similar to PEG INF alfa-2a & -2b where different doses & 3 where PEG INF + ribavirin similar to PEG INF after 24 wks). Factors that ↑ success: genotypes other than 1, lower baseline viral levels, less fibrosis, lower body wt & surface area *(NEJM Aug 2002).*
		
		Excessive alcohol consumption (>5 oz/d.) **dramatically accelerates hepatic fibrosis** from HCV *(Lancet 349:825, 1997)*. Occult HBV HCV infection might account for lack of response to rx in some pts *(NEJM 341:22, 1999)*. **HIV accelerates HCV disease progression** *(CID 35:562, 2001)*. Rx associated with reduction of hepatocellular carcinoma *(AnIM 131:174, 1999).*
		
		Decisions regarding re-treatment of non-responders or relapses complex. Only about 15–20% of non-responders to with INF-Rib combination will respond to retreatment with PEG INF-Rib. Pts with advanced fibrosis/cirrhosis have ↑ risk of hepatic decompensation & should probably be monitored *(2002 NIH Consensus Conference).*

Duration of rx: **Genotype 1:** check quantitative HCV RNA after 12 wks of rx. If ↓<2 log, continue for total of 48 wks (up to 51% SVR reported). If ↓>2 log ↓: dc rx (unlikely to respond & consider rx failure). **Other genotypes: Rx for total of 24 wks**		Side effects significant: 10–14% receiving PEG INF-Rib: dc rx secondary to side effects flu-like symptoms, hematological & particularly neuropsychiatric abnormalities. **2002 FDA warning:** Intron can cause or aggravate life-threatening, neuropsychiatric, auto-immune, ischemic & infectious disorders—monitor closely). *See drug section, Table 14B.* **Ribavirin is teratogenic and must not be used if pregnancy possible in pt or partner.** Because of toxicity, rx of pts with minimal inflammation by liver bx or low to normal ALT is usually **not** recommended.
Prevention of acute and chronic infection **Risk factors:** (1) contaminated blood via transfusion (1/100,000 per unit in U.S.); (2) injection drug use (highest, prevalence of HCV ↑ 79% with continued injection from needlesticks from hollow-bore needles *(AIMA 287:2406, 2002)*; (4) sexual activity risk low (but ♂ > ♀ > ♀ → ♂); (3) occupational exposure such as HCV+ mothers have 5–6% risk of transmission to child (w HIV, risk is 14%)		*See MMWR 47(RR-19), Oct. 16, 1998.* Although interferon + ribavirin is now approved for rx of chronic hepatitis C *(see Table 14B, page 111)*, no data on use as post-exposure prophylaxis.
Herpesvirus Infections *(see review CID 26:541, 1996)*		
Cytomegalovirus (CMV) **Normal host**	No rx indicated for acute mononucleosis-like infection in healthy and not established for congenital CMV *(see Comment)*	A study of newborns with symptomatic congenital CMV infection suggests 8 and 12 mg/kg/d IV ganciclovir has limited efficacy in suppressing CMV disease.
Immunocompromised host	**Treatment of AIDS patients with highly active antiretroviral therapy (HAART)** without specific CMV therapy and note developed retinitis *(AIDS 17:1203, 1999).*	
Colitis/esophagitis	Ganciclovir as with retinitis except induction period extended for 3–6 wks then maintenance. No agreement on use of maintenance *(AIM 98:109, 1995)*. Foscarnet 90 mg/kg q12h effective in 9/10 (hs CMV-effective in 16/16 hs CMV-negative by PCR).	Responses less predictable than for retinitis *(AIM 98:109, 1995)*. Valganciclovir also likely effective. Switch to oral valganciclovir when po tolerated.

NOTE: All dosage recommendations are for adults (unless otherwise indicated) and assume normal renal function.

TABLE 14A (4)

VIRUS/DISEASE	DRUG/DOSAGE	SIDE EFFECTS/COMMENTS
Herpesvirus Infections/Cytomegalovirus/Immunocompromised host *(continued)*		
CMV of the nervous system: Encephalitis & ventriculitis. Treatment not defined, but disease develops while taking ganciclovir as suppressive therapy. Lumbosacral polyradiculopathy. Mononucleosis multiplex.	Not defined. Consider combination of ganciclovir and foscarnet [if prior CMV rx used. Switch to valganciclovir when possible.]	*(Neurol 29:139, 1991.)* About 50% will respond to antiviral rx *(AnNeurol 29:139, 1991)*.
CMV pneumonia — seen predominantly in transplants (esp. bone marrow), rare in HIV	Ganciclovir 2.5 mg/kg q8h IV x20 days + IVIG 500 mg/kg qod x10 doses, then ganciclovir 5 mg/kg q3–5 x/week for 20 doses + IVIG 500 mg/kg 2x/week x8 more doses *(AnIM 109:777, 1988)*	Due to vasculitis and may not be responsive to antiviral rx. 11/16 pts showed initial improvement with either ganciclovir or foscarnet but disease eventually progressed despite maintenance *(CID 23:76, 1996)*. In BMT recipients, serial measure of pp65 antigen was useful in establishing early dx of CMV pneumonia and good results of CMV was initiated within 6 days of antigen positivity *(Bone Marrow Transplant 26:413, 2000)*. For preventive therapy, see *Table 15, page 122.*
Retinitis (most common in AIDS) 19/20 pts (63%) with inactive CMV retinitis who responded to HAART (↑ of CD4 cells/ml develop ped immune recovery vitreitis. Vision ↓ & floaters with posterior segment inflammation—vitreitis, papillitis & macular edema. In an average of 43 days from start of HAART, 19 of 30 developed inflammatory complications *(AIDS 14:1163, 2000)*. See Guidelines of International Panel *(ArIM 158: 957, 1998)*	**Induction therapy, primary:** **Valganciclovir** 900 mg po bid with food x 21 days [equal to IV GCV with advantage of oral over IV administration *(NEJM 346:1119, 2002)*] OR **Ganciclovir** (GCV) 5 mg/kg IV q12h (adjust for renal function) x14–21 days OR **Foscarnet** (FOS) 90 mg/kg q12h (adjust for renal function) IV at constant rate (requires infusion pump) over minimum of 1 hr x14–21 days OR Combination of intraocular ganciclovir (GCV) implant (delivers 1–2 μg/hr x6–7 mos.) + (either concomitant IV GCV or oral valganciclovir 900 mg qd with food) **Induction therapy, alternative:** **Cidofovir** 5 mg/kg IV q week x2 wks then 5 mg/kg IV q2 weeks with probenecid (2 gm po 3 hrs before cidofovir dose, 1 gm 2 hrs immediately after dose, and 1 gm 8 hrs after dose) and 1 liter of normal saline IV 1 hr before cidofovir infusion *(AIDSHR 17:339, 1998; Blood 97:388, 2001)* OR **Fomivirsen** 330 mg by direct intravitreal injection q2wk x2, then q month in combination with valganciclovir as above For pts who fail monotherapy with GCV or FOS, consider combination rx with both: (1) GCV 5 mg/kg q12h or q24h IV and FOS 90 mg/kg qd IV OR (2) FOS 90 mg/kg q12h up to total of 125 mg/kg qd *(CID 34:1337, 2000)*. **Suppression** (maintenance therapy): See *CID 28:334, 1999*. **Primary:** **Valganciclovir** 900 mg po qd or GCV 5 mg/kg IV qd or 6 mg/kg IV qd 5 days/week or OR **FOS** 90–120 mg/kg qd IV with hydration and dose adjusted for renal function (NOTE: oral and IV hydration found equally effective; 1700 ml/day about 298 from 4th CRV, 1997) OR Combination of GCV intraocular implant q6 mos. + **valganciclovir** 900 mg po qd **Alternative:** **Cidofovir** 5 mg/kg IV q2 wks + probenecid and hydration (as above under induction rx)	Comprehensive reviews of most important clinical issues: *J AIDS & HR 14(Suppl. 1), 1997* and *Arch Ophthal 114:863, 1996.* Corticosteroid rx ↓ inflammatory reaction of immune recovery vitreitis without reactivation of CMV retinitis *(5th CRV, Abst 757)*. Differential dx: HIV retinopathy, herpes simplex retinitis *(Arch Ophthal 114:834, 1996)*, varicella-zoster retinitis (rare, hard to diagnose) *(CID 24:620, 1997; NEJM 337:83, 1997)*. Similarly, intraocular injections of fomivirsen will not prevent contralateral eye or systemic/visceral disease *(NEJM 337:83, 1997)*. Risk ↓ with systemic rx *(CID 24:620, 1997; NEJM 337:83, 1997)*. Similarly, intraocular injections of fomivirsen will not prevent contralateral eye or systemic/visceral disease. IVIG 500 mg/kg q2wk x6–7 mos.) **Corticosteroid rx** ↓ inflammatory reaction of immune recovery vitreitis without reactivation of CMV retinitis *(5th CRV, Abst 757)*. Ocular use of GCV ocular implant alone as approx. 50% risk of CMV retinitis other eye at 6 mos. and 31% risk visceral disease *(Arch Ophthal 12: 153, 1994)*. Risk ↓ with systemic rx *(CID 24:620, 1997; NEJM 337:83, 1997)*. Response rates similar to other therapies (med. time to progression 267–403 days) although retinal inflammation & detachment were common side effects. Because of unique mode of action, fomivirsen may have a role if isolates become resistant to other therapies. **Corticosteroid rx** ↓ inflammatory reaction of immune recovery vitreitis. Watch for retinal detachments; 50–60% within 1 yr of dx of retinitis. Equal efficacy of IV GCV and FOS. FOS rx takes more time to administer due to saline hydration. GCV avoids nephrotoxicity of FOS; FOS avoids bone marrow suppression of GCV. Reports indicate success of combination rx with GCV at ½ to dose 5 mg/kg/d q24h & FOS up to 125 mg/kg/d for GCV-resistant isolates in solid organ transplants *(CID 34:1337, 2002)*. Others used higher doses *(Transplant 62:576, 1996)*. Hypomagnesemia is major problem. Probenecid emergence of resistant CMV, 27% pts treated developed resistant CMV isolates resistant to GCV *(JID 177:770, 1998)*, hence may be reason for clinical failure. DC rx a great advantage since IV catheter complications are common. 12 person-yr with mortality rate of 5.8% *(AIDS 12:2321, 1999)*.
EBV—Mononucleosis *(NEJM 343:481, 2000; JAMA 281:454, 1999)*	**No treatment.** Corticosteroids for tonsillar obstruction of airway or Acyclovir and prednisolone inhibited oropharyngeal EBV replication but did not affect duration of symptoms *(JID 174:324, 1996)*.	EBV replication but did not affect duration of CNS complications.

NOTE: All dosage recommendations are for adults (unless otherwise indicated) and assume normal renal function.

TABLE 14A (5)

VIRUS/DISEASE	DRUG/DOSAGE	SIDE EFFECTS/COMMENTS
Herpesvirus Infections (continued)		
HHV-6 a probable cause of roseola (exanthem subitum) & other febrile diseases of childhood; 100% of adults have antibodies. Fever & rash documented in some pts but association with pneumonitis & prolonged bone marrow suppression plant pts but association with pneumonitis & prolonged bone marrow suppression. HHV-6 isolated from CSF (*J Ped* 138:921, 2001); HHV-6,6,-7 DNA both found in CSF in cases of without rx (*J Ped* 138:921, 2001); HHV-6 & -7 DNA both found in CSF in cases of encephalitis. Reactivation with immunosuppression (*Blood* 93:1658, 1999).	**No rx** or prophylaxis currently uncertain. Dx depends on separating latent virus from active infection. The rapid shell vial assay, serum PCR assay or immunohistochemical stain for viral proteins may be of value (*AnM* 124:1065, 1996). Rx with ganciclovir and foscarnet did lower CSF HHV-6 DNA levels in BMT pts (*BMT* 25:787, 2000).	
HHV-7—a ubiquitous virus that probably accounts for 10% of roseola. Role in disease has not been clearly elucidated (some cases of exanthem subitum and other febrile illnesses of childhood).	**No antiviral treatment** currently recommended.	Role of rx or prophylaxis currently uncertain. Dx depends on separating latent virus from active infection. The rapid shell vial assay, serum PCR assay or immunohistochemical stain for viral proteins may be of value (*AnM* 124:1065, 1996). Rx with ganciclovir and foscarnet did lower CSF HHV-6 DNA levels in BMT pts (*BMT* 25:787, 2000).
HHV-8 probable agent of Kaposi's sarcoma and body cavity lymphoma—may cause interstitial pneumonia and saliva (*JID* 177:213, 1998).		Localized lesions: radiotherapy, laser surgery or intralesional chemotherapy. Systemic: chemotherapy. Anecdotal report of remission in 5 pts given foscarnet 80 mg/kg/d. (*Scand J Inf Dis* 26:749, 1994). Also, less KS in pts given foscarnet for CMV and associated with ↓ KS in retrospective analysis (*Sci* 267:1078, 1995). HHV-8 implicated in Castleman's disease (*CID* 28:678, 1999).
Herpes simplex virus (HSV Types 1 & 2) (See in: 357:1513, 2001)		
Bell's palsy (May also be caused by H. zoster, Lyme disease, HHV-6) (*CID* 30:529, 2000)	Either **no rx** for **herpesvirus** or [Acyclovir (400 mg po 5x/d for 10 days)] with or without **prednisone** po (30 mg bid po 1 mg/kg daily given bid x5 d, then taper to 5 mg for 5 days after total of 10 days)]	HSV-1 genomes were detected in 11/14 pts in facial nerves by PCR (*AnIM* 124:27, 1996). In one study, 99 pts with symptoms <3 days had better recovery and less neural degeneration when rx with acyclovir + prednisone compared to prednisone alone (*Ann Oto/Rhino/Laryngol* 105:371, 1996), but another study was inconclusive. More data needed to support this recommendation (*Cochrane Database Syst Rev* 2:CD001869, 2001). If caused by VZV (Ramsay Hunt syndrome), acyclovir may be of value (*PIDJ* 21:615, 2002).
Encephalitis See excellent reviews: *CID* 23:219, 1996; 25:89, 1997; *CID* 35:254, 2002	**Acyclovir** 10 mg/kg (IV infuse over 1 hr) q8h x14–21 days	HSV-1 is most common cause of sporadic encephalitis. Survival and recovery from neurological sequelae are related to mental status at time of initiation of rx. Early dx and rx imperative! PCR analysis of CSF for HSV-1 DNA is 100% specific and 75–98% sensitive but 3 cts, 1–3 days after onset of symptoms had neg. HSV-1 DNA. All 3 turned pos. 4–7 days later (*CID* 34:1154, 2002). CSF IgG M was positive in 7/27 (27%) children. Observe: Up to 20 mg/kg q8h in relapse. Relapse after successful rx reported in 1/27 (4%) pts (*CID* 30:185, 2000).
Genital, immunocompetent		
Primary (initial episode) See comments (*JAMA* 289:(Suppl 1):1, 54, 1999 & 7, 1999 & 7; *AnIM* 137:20, 2002 or CDC 2002 Guidelines)	**Acyclovir** (Zovirax or generic) 400 mg po bid x7–10 days (FDA-approved dosage is 200 mg 5x/d po x10 days). OR [NB: $90/course, G $50/course]; **Valacyclovir** (Valtrex) 1000 mg po bid x7–10 days [$96/course] **Famciclovir** (Famvir) 250 mg po tid x7–10 days (not FDA-approved for this indication) [$50–190/course]	An ester of acyclovir, which is well absorbed, bioavailability 3–5x greater than acyclovir. Found to be equal to acyclovir (*Sex Trans Dis* 24:481, 1997). Metabolized to penciclovir, which is active component. Side effects and activity similar to acyclovir. Found to be equal to acyclovir (200 mg 5x/d) tid (*IDCP* 6:512, 1997).
Episodic recurrences	**Acyclovir** 400 mg po tid x5 days or **Famciclovir** 125 mg po bid x5 days or **valacyclovir** 500 mg po bid x5 days	All effective with few differences. Choice can be made on basis of cost & convenience (*AnIM* 156:3:358, 1996; *JAMA* 276:44, 1996; *Genitourin Med* 73:110, 1997). Trend is to ↓ duration of rx. (*CID* 26, 2002)
Chronic suppression (*JAMA* 280:928, 1998; *JID* 178:603, 1998; *MMWR* 51(RR-6):1, 2002). Decision to rx arbitrary, but rx significantly improves quality of life over 1 yr (*Sex Trans Infect* 75:398, 1999).	**Suppressive rx reduces the frequency of genital herpes recurrences (i.e., >6 recurrences/yr) & many report no recurrences** **Acyclovir** 400 mg po bid **Famciclovir** 250 mg po bid ($2327), or **valacyclovir** 1 gm po qd or 500 mg po qd (costs $1867), or ($2231), May use 1000 ($1055). May use 1000	Suppresses subclinical HSV-2 shedding between episodes of active disease and ↓ symptomatic recurrences (*JCI* 96:1092, 2001; *JAMA* 280:887, 1998). Drug resistance unlikely to develop with use (*J Clin Virol* 21:261, 2001). Since in a large natural hx study 2/3 of pts demonstrated ↓ in recurrences between yrs 1 & 5 (approx. median 6 to 3 episodes/yr), daily suppressive rx should be reassessed periodically after ~5 yrs episodic rx may be practical (*NEJM* 131:14, 1999).
Gingivostomatitis, primary (children)	**Acyclovir** 15 mg/kg po 5x/d x7 d	Efficacy demonstrated in randomized double-blind placebo-controlled trial (*BMJ* 315:1800, 1992).
Kerato-conjunctivitis and recurrent epithelial keratitis	**Trifluridine** (Viroptic), 1 drop 1% solution q2h (max. 9 drops/d) for max. of 21 days (see *Table 1, page 9*)	In controlled trials, response % > idoxuridine. Topical suppressive rx with acyclovir (400 mg bid) reduced recurrences of ocular HSV from 32% to 19% over 12-month period (*NEJM* 339:300, 1998).

NOTE: All dosage recommendations are for adults (unless otherwise indicated) and assume normal renal function.

TABLE 14A (6)

VIRUS/DISEASE	DRUG/DOSAGE	SIDE EFFECTS/COMMENTS
Herpesvirus Infections/Herpes simplex virus (HSV Types 1 & 2) *(continued)*		
Mucocutaneous		
Oral labial, "fever blisters"	Rx usually not indicated; however, some use **penciclovir 1%** cream applied q2h while awake for 4 d. (see Comment) or oral **acyclovir** 2 gm po given twice 12 hrs apart (4-duration of "cold sore" episodes by 1 day if started within 2 hrs of onset of symptoms *(15th Conf on Antiviral Research 2002, Abst. 653)* Cost approx. $25)	Penciclovir given topically ↓ duration of pain (3.4 vs 4.1 days) *(J Derm Treat 13:67, 2002; JAMA 277:1374, 1997)*. Resistance has not developed *(JAC 46:2423, 2000)*. In immunocompromised pts, severe blisters associated with other infections (e.g., pneumococcal sepsis) may benefit from acyclovir 400 mg po x5 days (reduces viral shedding and ↓ healing time). Oral famciclovir 500 mg 3x/d. for 5 d. when started 48 hrs after experimental herpes labialis, ↓ healing time from 6 to 4 days mean (p < 0.01) *(JID 179:303, 1999)*. Topical fluoronucleosides (0.6% Lidex gel) q6h x5 in combination with famciclovir 1 tab po qd when compared to famciclovir alone *(JID 181:1906, 2000)*.
Herpes Whitlow	See Table 1, page 18	
Immunocompromised (includes pts with AIDS) and critically ill pts in ICU setting	**Acyclovir** 5 mg/kg IV (infused over 1 hr) q8h x7 d. or 400 mg (4 [250 mg/M²] or 400 mg po 5x/d x14–21 d. (see Comment if suspect acyclovir-resistant).	Acyclovir-resistant HSV occurs, esp. in large ulcers. Most will respond to **IV foscarnet**, but recur after drug discontinued (median 6 weeks) *(NEJM 325:551, 1991)*. Suppressive rx with famciclovir (500 mg po bid) reduced viral shedding and clinical recurrences (total days with lesions 18% vs 9%) in HIV-infected pts *(AnIM 128:21, 1998)*, 38% similar to findings with acyclovir & valacyclovir 500 mg po bid [at 6 mos. 60% of valacyclovir were recurrence-free vs 38% of placebo-rx *(JID 177:892, 1997)*. Cidofovir (topical) has been used with moderate success *(NEJM 337:509, 1997)*.
	Famciclovir 500 mg po bid x7 d (approved for AIDS pts.)	
Perinatal (genital) in pregnancy at delivery	**Acyclovir** 12 mg/kg IV q8h or **ganciclovir** 5 mg/kg IV q12h until lesion heals. Some use **acyclovir** 800 mg po bid for prolonged duration. (Prompt Rx may limit infection to ↓ site.)	25% HSV reactivated during last month of pregnancy. Infant exposure to primary lesion 50% risk, if recurrent lesion 4%. 50% mortality in infected neonates. If visible genital lesion, deliver by **C-section**, regardless of duration of membrane rupture. If no lesions or symptoms, vaginal delivery. Routine HSV cultures no longer recommend and **acyclovir** useful in dose of 10 mg/kg (20 mg/kg if premature) q8h x10–21 days IV *(PID 14:827, 1995; NEJM 337:509, 1997)*.
Herpes simiae—Monkey bite (Herpes B virus)		*(JID 20:421, 1995*. Fatal human cases of hemorrhagic encephalitis have been reported following bites, scratches, or eye inoculation of saliva from monkeys. Incubation period of 2–14 days. headache, myalgias and diffuse adenopathy.)
Herpes Varicella-Zoster Virus (VZV)		
Varicella		
Normal host (chickenpox)		
Child (2–12 years)	**Rx not recommended** by American Academy of Pediatrics. Oral acyclovir for healthy persons at ↑ risk for moderate to severe varicella, i.e., > 12 yrs of age, chronic cutaneous or pulmonary diseases, chronic salicylate rx (↑ risk of Reye syndrome). Use **acyclovir 20 mg/kg** po qid x5 days (start within 24 hrs of rash).	Modest response to acyclovir. Slowed development and ↓ number of new lesions. Analgesic requirements decreased *(J Ped 116:633, 1990; NEJM 325:1539, 1991)*. Oral dose of acyclovir in children should not exceed 80 mg/kg/d or 3200 mg/d.
Adolescents, young adults	**Acyclovir** 800 mg po 5x/d x5–7 days (start within 24 hrs of rash) or **valacyclovir** 1000 mg po 3x/d. x5 d. *(not FDA-approved for this indication)*. Famciclovir 500 mg po 3x/d. also probably effective but not FDA-approved for this indication and data lacking *(AnIM 130:922, 1999)*.	↓ duration of fever, time to healing, and symptoms *(AnIM 117:358, 1992)*.
Pneumonia or chickenpox in 3rd trimester of pregnancy	**Acyclovir** 800 mg po 5x/d or 10 mg/kg IV q8h x5 days. Risks and benefits to fetus and mother still unknown. Many experts recommend rx, especially in 3rd trimester. Some would add VZIG (varicella-zoster immune globulin).	Varicella pneumonia severe in pregnancy (41% mortality, Ob Gyn 25:734, 1965) and acyclovir ↓ incidence and severity *(JID 185:422, 2002)*. If varicella-susceptible mother exposed and respiratory symptoms develop within 10 days after exposure, start acyclovir *(CCTID 13:123, 1993)*. Acyclovir is pregnancy category B; no evidence of ↑ birth defects *(MMWR 42:806, 1993)*.
Immunocompromised host	**Acyclovir** 10–12 mg/kg IV (infused over 1 hr) q8h x7 days (500 mg/M²)	Acyclovir (given to 31 immunocompromised children) was used successfully in 1 pt with severe hemorrhagic varicella *(NEJM 336:732, 1997)*. Mortality high (43%) in AIDS pts *(Int J Inf Dis 6:6, 2002)*.

NOTE: All dosage recommendations are for adults (unless otherwise indicated) and assume normal renal function.

TABLE 14A (7)

VIRUS/DISEASE	DRUG/DOSAGE	SIDE EFFECTS/COMMENTS
Herpesvirus Infections/Herpes Varicella-Zoster Virus (VZV)/Varicella	**Varicella-Zoster Virus (VZV)/Varicella** (continued)	
Prevention (See NEJM 347:26, 2000)	**CDC Recommendations for Prevention:** Since <5% of cases of varicella but >50% of varicella-related deaths occur in adults >20 yrs of age, the CDC recommends a more aggressive approach in this age group. **1st, varicella-zoster immune globulin (VZIG)** (125 U/10 kg (22 lbs) body weight IM up to a max. of 625 U; minimum dose is 125 U) is recommended for post-exposure prophylaxis in susceptible persons at greater risk for complications (immunocompromised such as HIV, malignancies, pregnancy, and newborn) as soon as possible after exposure (48 hrs optimal; up to 96 hrs post-exposure). **2nd,** persons with negative or uncertain hx of varicella (10–30% will be Ab-neg.) and vaccinate those who are Ab-neg. **3rd,** susceptible children should receive vaccination. Recommended routinely before age 12–18 mos. but OK at any age (MMWR 4:10, 19 May 1997). Varicella is the leading cause of vaccine-preventable deaths in children in the U.S. (MMWR 47:365, 1998).
Herpes zoster (shingles) *(See JID 197:S228, 2008)* **Normal host** Effective rx most evident in pts >50 yrs. *(For rx of post-herpetic neuralgia, see Ln 353:1636, 1999.)* 25-fold ↓ in zoster after immunization (MMWR 48:R-6, 1999)	**[NOTE: Trials showing benefit of rx: only in pts treated within 3 days of onset of rash]** **Valacyclovir** (Valtrex) 1000 mg po q8h x7 days. Adjust dose for renal failure. *or* **Famciclovir** (Famvir) 500 mg po q8h x7 days. Adjust for renal failure (see Table 17). *or* **Acyclovir** 800 mg po 5x/d x7–10 days. **Prednisone** po 30 mg bid days 1–7, 15 mg bid days 8–14 and 7.5 mg bid days 15–21 also recommended by some authorities in pts >50 yrs of age (NEJM 335:32, 1996)] and especially when pt has large number of lesions (>21) and/or severe pain at presentation (JID 178:9, 1998)	**Valacyclovir** ↓ post-herpetic neuralgia more rapidly than acyclovir in pts >50 yrs. Or median duration of zoster-associated pain was 38 days with valacyclovir and 51 days on acyclovir (AAC 39:1546, 1995). Toxicity of both drugs similar (Arch Fam Med 9:863, 2000). Time to healing more rapid. Reduced post-herpetic neuralgia (PHN) vs placebo in pts >50 yrs of age. Famciclovir similar to acyclovir in reduction of acute pain and PHN (Int. J Antimicrob Agents 4:241, 1994; AnIM 77:23-89, 1995). A meta-analysis of 4 placebo-controlled trials (691 pts) demonstrated that acyclovir accelerated by approx. 2-fold pain resolution by all measures employed and reduced post-herpetic neuralgia at 3 & 6 mos (JID 22:341, 1996). Prednisone added to acyclovir improved quality of life measurements (↓ acute pain, sleep, and return to normal activity) (AnIM 125:376, 1996). In post-herpetic neuralgia, antidepressant (amitriptyline, desipramine), ↓ pain (Arch Neurol 35:550, 1994; J Fam Practice 51:121, 2002).
immunocompromised host Not severe Severe: >1 dermatome, trigeminal nerve or disseminated	**Acyclovir** 800 mg po 5x/d x7 days (famciclovir and valacyclovir not FDA-approved for this indication). **Acyclovir** 10–12 mg/kg (500 mg/m²) IV (infusion over 1 hr) q8h x7–14 days. In older pts, ↓ to 7.5 mg/kg if nephrotoxicity and adjust dose for renal function. Rx for 14 days (AnIM 115:19, 1991)	If progression, switch to IV. If immune, consider switch to po. Acyclovir-resistant VZV occurs in HIV+ pts previously treated with acyclovir. Rx must be begun within 72 hrs. Acyclovir-resistant VZV successful in 4/5 pts but 2 relapsed in 7 and 14 days.
Influenza (A & B) (MMWR 49:18, 2000; NEJM 343:1778, 2000; CID 31:1166, 2000; CID 35:729, 2002) Suspect or proven acute disease Rapid diagnostic tests are now available (J Clin Virol 25:15, 2002)	**If fever & cough; known community influenza activity; and 1st 48 hrs of illness, consider:** **For influenza A & B** **Oseltamivir** 75 mg po bid x5 d. (also approved for rx of children age 1–12 yrs, dose 2 mg/kg up to a total of 75 mg bid x5 d.) *or* **Zanamivir** 2 inhalations (2x5 mg) bid x5 d. **For influenza A only:** **Rimantadine** 100 mg po bid x5 d. **Amantadine** or rimantadine—Age 1–9 yrs, 5 mg/kg/d to max. of 75 mg po bid; 10–65 yrs, 100 mg po bid; >65 yrs, 100 mg qd (adjust for ↓ renal function) for 3–5 d. or 1–2 d after the disappearance of symptoms	Pts with COPD or asthma, **potential risk of bronchospasm with zanamivir.** If using inhaled bronchodilator, use before dose of zanamivir. Amantadine & rimantadine equally effective, but rimantadine ↓ side effects (Cochrane Database Sys Rev CD 001169, 2002). Both zanamivir & oseltamivir are neuraminidase inhibitors, effective against influenza A & B and are equally effective as amantadine & rimantadine against influenza A, all reduce duration of symptoms by approx. 50% (1–2 d.) if given within 30–36 hrs after onset of symptoms (AnIM 137:225, 2002; AJM 82:11, 1987). Prevention of influenza A: give vaccine followed by rimantadine or amantadine (dosages as above) for duration of influenza A activity in community (Consider oseltamivir in non-responsive populations as immunization recommendations). Immunization contraindicated in those with hypersensitivity to hen's eggs. Both amantadine and rimantadine are about 70–90% effective against influenza A. Both oseltamivir and zanamivir are reported effective as prophylaxis in clinical trials (JAMA 282:31 & 75, 1999; NEJM 341:1336 & 1387, 1999; JAMA 285:748, 2001).
Prevention. See MMWR 50:RR-4, 2001 Annual vaccination is recommended (preferably Oct.–Nov.) for the following who are at ↑ risk for complications from influenza: >65 yrs of age, residents of nursing homes and other facilities that house persons with chronic medical conditions, those with chronic pulmonary or cardiac conditions, chronic metabolic diseases (diabetes, renal failure, etc.), immunosuppression, children on chronic ASA, women in 2nd or 3rd trimester of persons who can transmit virus to above (HCWs, etc.)	**Prevention of influenza A & B:** give vaccine and if ≥13 yrs age, consider **oseltamivir** 75 mg po qd for duration of peak influenza activity in community (Consider in non-responsive populations as immunization recommendations).	

NOTE: All dosage recommendations are for adults (unless otherwise indicated) and assume normal renal function.

TABLE 14A (8)

VIRUS/DISEASE	DRUG/DOSAGE	SIDE EFFECTS/COMMENTS
Measles	No therapy or **vitamin A** 200,000 IU po x2 days	Vitamin A ↓ severity of measles in one study (NEJM 323:160, 1990), not in others.
	No rx. or **ribavirin** IV (i) 20–35 mg/kg/d x7 days	↓ severity of illness in adults (CID 20:454, 1994).
Papillomavirus		
Anogenital Warts Condyloma acuminatum	See CID 27:796, 1998, for consensus statement: **Podofilox** (Condylox) 2x daily application with cotton swabs for 3 days followed by 4 days without rx; repeat cycle 4–6x as necessary) **OR** (25% **podophyllin** in tincture of benzoin	Podofilox: Local reactions—pain, burning, inflammation 50%. No systemic effects. Efficacy in penile warts 74% vs placebo 8%. Recurrences 60%. (NEJM 328:263, 1993.)
Children		
Adults	(Podophyllin) apply once weekly for up to 6 wks. wash after 1–4 hrs.) If no regression after 4 weekly applications, use alternate rx.	55.6% Warts recur in 1/3 with either agent within 1st month after rx.
[NOTE: Results of Pap smear should be available prior to rx. **avoid rx in pregnant women**]	**interferon alfa-2b** (intron A), **alfa-n3** (Alferon N) 1 million units (0.1 ml) into lesion 3x/week x3 weeks	Painful; dilute to 10 million units/1 ml. Other concentrations are hypertonic (CID 28:SS37, 1999). Use when other rx. fails, esp. in AIDS.
NOTE: Recurrences common after all treatments	Cryodestruction or electrosurgery	
	imiquimod (5% cream). Apply 3x/week prior to sleep; remove 6–10 hrs later when awake. Continue until cleared or max. of 16 wks.	Apply 3x/wk overnight for up to 16 wks or until warts completely cured, produced clearance rates of 52% vs 14% for controls (AAC 42:789, 1998). Cost of 1–4 wks rx: $108–432. Imiquimod local reactions—mild: erythema 60%, erosion 30% (AJM 102(5A):34, 1997).
Parvo B19 Virus (Erythrovirus B19)		
Uncomplicated or self-limited acute arthritis. May be chronic in children.	No treatment recommended	Bone marrow shows selective erythrocyte maturation arrest with giant pronormoblasts. IgM antibody available for diagnosis. Specialty Labs, Santa Monica, CA. Parvo B19 also associated with respiratory distress syndrome (CID 28:1343, 1999).
Acute profound anemia in utero, in hemolytic anemia, in HIV	**IVIG** 0.4 gm/kg IV qd x5 d in immune def. states with severe anemia has been reported successful.	IVIG contains anti-parvo B19 antibody. In pts with pre-existing hemolytic anemia, parvo B19-induced bone marrow arrest can result in sudden severe anemia. See An J Hematol 61:16, 1999 for new suggestions on management.
Papovavirus/Polyoma Virus		
Progressive multifocal leuco-encephalopathy (PML)(JC virus) Usually in pts with advanced HIV disease & organ transplant (CID 35:1081, 2002)	See SANFORD GUIDE to HIV/AIDS THERAPY. **HAART** ↑ survival (545 d. vs 60 d., p < 0.001) and either improved (50%) or stabilized (25%) neurological deficits in 12 pts (AIDS 12:2467, 1999). Others less optimistic (CID 28:1152, 1999).	Cytarabine of no value in controlled trial (NEJM 338:1345, 1998). Camptothecin, a human topoisomerase I inhibitor, was administered to a single pt with slowing of progression (Lin 349:1366, 1997).
Respiratory Syncytial Virus		
Major cause of morbidity in neonates/infants (JID 180:41, 1999.) T recognition in adults, 2–9% of cols in pts with advanced HIV with pneumonia requiring hospitalization are due to RSV (JID 179:25, 1999).	**RSV immune globulin intravenous** (RSV-IVIG) 100 mg/kg IV once monthly Nov. through April (for northern hemisphere) (1st year of life for premature infants) **OR**	Ribavirin was reported to ↓ fever and other symptoms and signs. However, in a retrospective case controlled study of children on mechanical ventilators for severe RSV & in a prospective placebo-controlled trial of otherwise normal children, ribavirin had **no beneficial effect** (J Pediatr 126:422, 1996; AJRCCM 160:829, 1999). Still recommended by some authorities in immunocompromised patients. See Ln 354:847, 1999 for updated review.
Prevention		
(1) Children <24 mos. old with bronchopulmonary dysplasia (BPD) requiring supplemental O₂	**Palivizumab** 15 mg/kg IM q month Nov.–April as above (Scand J Inf Dis 33:323, 2001)	Palivizumab reduced hospitalization rates for RSV in 1500 premature infants & children with chronic lung disease from 10.6% to 4.8% (Pediatrics 102:531, 1998). Cost: $3300–5000/yr
(2) Perhaps premature infants (<26 wks gestation) and <6 mos. old at start of RSV season		
Rhinovirus (Colds) (NEJM 346:1300, 2002)	No antiviral rx indicated. Symptomatic. • **ipratropium** bromide nasal (2 sprays/nostril tid) • **Clemastine** 1.34 mg, 1–2 tab po bid-tid (OTC)	Sx relief: ipratropium nasal spray ↓ rhinorrhea and sneezing vs placebo (Ann IM 125:89, 1996). Clemastine (an antihistamine) ↓ sneezing, rhinorrhea but was associated with dry nose, mouth and throat in 6–19% (CID 31:1202, 2000). intranasal cidofovir (dosage uncertain), contact CDC: 770-488-7100
Contact vaccinia (JAMA 288:1901, 2002)	**Smallpox vaccine** (within 4 days of exposure) + cidofovir (dosage uncertain). From vaccination: Progressive vaccinia—vaccinia immune globulin may provide benefit & reduce duration and severity of symptoms in 2 clinical trials (CID 33:1865, 2001).	Vaccinia immune globulin, contact CDC: 770-488-7100

NOTE: All dosage recommendations are for adults (unless otherwise indicated) and assume normal renal function.

TABLE 14B: ANTIVIRAL DRUGS (Other Than Retroviral)

DRUG NAME(S) GENERIC (TRADE)	DOSAGE/ROUTE/COST*	COMMENTS/ADVERSE EFFECTS
CMV (See SANFORD GUIDE To HIV/AIDS THERAPY)		
Cidofovir (Vistide)	5 mg/kg IV q week x2, then q2 weeks. (375 mg $846) Properly timed IV prehydration with normal saline and administration of probenecid (see pkg insert for details). Renal function (serum creatinine and urine protein) must be monitored prior to each dose (see pkg insert for details).	**Adverse effects: Nephrotoxicity;** dose-dependent proximal tubular injury (Fanconi-like syndrome); proteinuria, glycosuria, bicarbonaturia, phosphaturia, polyuria (nephrogenic diabetic insipidus now reported, *Ln 350:413, 1997*). ↑ creatinine. Concomitant saline prehydration, probenecid, prolonged, extended dosing intervals allowed use. 25% of pts dc IV cidofovir due to nephrotoxicity. Other toxicities: nausea 48%, fever 43%, alopecia 16%, myalgia 16%, proteinuria 16%, neutropenia 29%. No effect on hematocrit, platelets, LFTs. **Comment**: Recommended dosage, frequency or infusion rate of cidofovir must not be exceeded. Dose must be reduced or discontinued if changes in renal function occur during rx. For ↑ of 0.3-0.4 mg/dl in serum creatinine, cidofovir dose must be ↓ from 5 to 3 mg/kg; discontinue cidofovir if ↑ of 0.5 mg/dl above baseline or 3+ proteinuria develops (for 2+ proteinuria, observe pts carefully and consider discontinuation).
Fomivirsen (Vitravene)	330 µg by direct intravitreal injection q2 wks x2, then q month (330 µg $1,000)	This is an antisense drug approved for local treatment of CMV retinitis in AIDS pts who are intolerant of, have a contraindication to or were unresponsive to other treatments for CMV. It inhibits production of proteins responsible for regulation of viral gene expression essential for virulence. **Adverse effects:** ocular inflammation (uveitis), iritis and vitreitis, ↑ intraocular pressure, abnormal vision, anterior chamber inflammation. Do not give if rx'd IV or intravitreal cidofovir (Vistide) within last 2-4 wks; may exaggerate ocular inflammation (*Priority Pharmacy 3, #8, Oct. 30, 1998*).
Foscarnet (Foscavir)	90 mg/kg q12h IV (induction) 90 mg/kg qd (maintenance) Dosage adjust. with renal dysfunction (see Table 17) (6 gm $76)	**Adverse effects: Major clinical toxicity is renal impairment (1/3 of patients)**—↑ creatinine, proteinuria, nephrogenic diabetes insipidus. ↓ K+, ↓ Ca++, ↓ Mg++. [↓ toxicity ↑ with other nephrotoxic drugs (amphotericin B, aminoglycosides or pentamidine (especially severe ↓ Ca++))]. Adequate hydration may ↓ toxicity. Other: headache, mild (100%), fatigue (100%), nausea (80%), fever (25%). CNS: seizures. Hemato.: ↓ WBC, ↓ Hgb. Hepatic: liver function tests. ↑. Neuropathy. Penile ulcers.
Ganciclovir (Cytovene)	IV: 5 mg/kg q12h x14 days (induction) 5 mg/kg IV qd or 6 mg/kg 5x/wk (maintenance) Dosage adjust. with renal dysfunction (see Table 17) (500 mg IV $37). Oral: 1.0 gm tid with food (fatty meal) (250 mg cap $6.10)	**Adverse effects:** Absolute neutrophil count dropped below 500/mm³ in 15%, thrombocytopenia 21%, anemia 6%. Fever 48%. GI 50%, nausea, vomiting, diarrhea, abdominal pain 19%, rash 10%. Retinal detachment 11% (relationship to ganciclovir?). Infusion: headache, psychiatric disturbances. ANC <500 common, neutropenia may respond to granulocyte colony-stimulating factor (G-CSF or GM-CSF). Severe myelosuppression when used with concomitant administration of zidovudine or azathioprine. 32% discontinued rx, principally for neutropenia. Hematologic less frequent than with IV. Granulocytopenia 18%, anemia 12%, thrombocytopenia 6%. GI: skin same as with IV. Retinal detachment 8%.
Ganciclovir (Vitrasert)	Intraocular implant (~$5000/device + cost of surgery)	**Adverse effects:** ↑ late retinal detachment (7/30 eyes). Does not prevent CMV retinitis in good eye or visceral dissemination. **Comment**: Replacement every 6 months recommended.
Valganciclovir (Valcyte)	900 mg PO bid x 21 d (induction) followed by 900 mg po qd. Take with food (450 mg cap $29 - $1,755 for 60 caps)	A prodrug of ganciclovir with better bioavailability. 60% with food. **Adverse effects:** Similar to ganciclovir.
Herpesvirus (non-CMV)		
Acyclovir (Zovirax or generic)	Doses see Table 14A po: 400 mg tab NB $2.72, G $0.70 IV 500 mg NB $65, G $4.75 Suspension 200 mg/5 ml 473 ml $121 Ointment 5% 15 gm $62.41	**po:** Generally well-tolerated with occ. diarrhea, vertigo, arthralgia. Less frequent rash, fatigue, insomnia, fever, menstrual abnormalities, acne, sore throat, muscle cramps, lymphadenopathy. **IV:** Phlebitis, caustic with local vesicular lesions with IV infiltration. CNS (1%): lethargy, tremors, confusion, hallucinations, delirium, seizures, coma. Nephrotoxicity—crystalluria with renal insufficiency after rapid IV (1%): ↑ creatinine, hematuria, ↑ BUN. Crystals in renal tubules → obstructive uropathy. Adequate pre-hydration may prevent such nephrotoxicity. Hepatic: ↑ ALT, AST. Uncommon: neutropenia (*CID 20; 1557, 1995*), rash, diaphoresis, hypotension, headache, nausea.
Famciclovir (Famvir)	250 mg cap $3.66 500 mg cap $7.36	Metabolized to penciclovir (like acyclovir; included headache, nausea, diarrhea, and dizziness but incidence did not differ from acyclovir). **Adverse effects:** Similar to acyclovir. (*AAC 39; 1546, 1996*). May be taken without regard to meals. Dose should be reduced if CrCl <60 ml/min (see package insert & Table 14, page 106 & Table 17, page 130).
Penciclovir (Denavir)	Topical 1% cream 1.5 gm $24	Apply to area of recurrence of herpes labialis with start of sx, then q2h while awake x4 d. Well tolerated.
Trifluridine (Viroptic)	1% solution q2h (max. 9 drops/d) for max. of 21 d. (7.5 ml 1% solution $99)	Mild burning (5%), palpebral edema (3%), punctate keratopathy, stromal edema.

* See page 116 for footnotes and abbreviations

TABLE 14B (2)

DRUG NAME(S) GENERIC (TRADE)	DOSAGE/ROUTE/COST*	COMMENTS/ADVERSE EFFECTS
Herpesvirus (non-CMV) *(continued)*		
Valacyclovir (Valtrex)	500 mg cap $3.88	An ester pro-drug of acyclovir that is well-absorbed, bioavailability 3–5x greater than acyclovir. **Adverse effects** similar to acyclovir. Thrombotic thrombocytopenic purpura/hemolytic uremic syndrome reported in pts with advanced HIV disease and transplant recipients participating in clinical trials at doses of 8 gm/day.
Hepatitis		
Adefovir dipivoxil (Hepsera) *Each tab contains ___ mg*	10 mg po qd (with normal CrCl) 20–49 CrCl: 10 mg q48h 10–19 CrCl: 10 mg q72h Hemodialysis: 10 mg q7 days following dialysis	Adefovir dipivoxil is a diester prodrug of the active moiety adefovir. It is an acyclic nucleotide analog with activity against hepatitis B (HBV) at 0.2–2.5 mM (IC₅₀). Peak plasma concentration after 10 mg po was 18.4 ± 6.26 ng/ml. 1–4 hrs after dose. Terminal elimination t½ was 7.48 ± 1.65 hrs. Primarily renal excretion—adjust dose. No drug interactions. Generally remarkably low side effects. Nephrotoxicity was found with higher doses in HIV with 60 & 120 mg/d & early studies in Hep B with 30 mg/d. Not yet reported in hepatitis B pts; nonetheless, esp. with pre-existing renal impairment, monitor for risks for renal impairment. Pregnancy Category C. Hepatitis may exacerbate when rx dc. 6–25% of pts developed ALT ↑ 10x normal within 12 wks, usually respond to retreatment or are self-limited, but hepatic decompensation has occurred.
Interferon alfa (s) available as alfa-2a (Roferon-A), alfa-2b (Intron-A)	3 million units (Roferon $37, Intron $43; Intergen 9 µg $39)	**Adverse effects:** Flu-like syndrome is common, esp. during 1st week of rx: fever 98%, fatigue 89%, myalgia 73%, headache 71%, GI: anorexia 46%, diarrhea 29%, CNS: dizziness 21%. Rash 18%, later profound fatigue & psychiatric effects (depression, anxiety, emotional lability and agitation), alopecia. ↑ TSH, autoimmune thyroid disorders in pts with history. Acute reversible hearing loss and/or tinnitus in up to 1/3 (*Ln* 343:1134, 1994). Side-effects ↑ with ↑ doses and dose reduction necessary in up to 46% receiving critical rx for HBV.
PEG interferon alfa-2b (PEG-Intron)	0.5–1.5 µg/kg sc q wk (120 µg) ($340)	Attachment of INF to polyethylene glycol (PEG) prolongs half-life and allows weekly dosing. Better efficacy data with similar adverse effects profile compared to regular formulation.
Pegylated-40k interferon alfa-2a (Pegasys)	180 µg sc q wk x48 wks (180 µg) ($355)	
Lamivudine (3TC) (Epivir-HBV)	100 mg po qd x1 yr for hepatitis B.	**Adverse effects:** See *Table 14D, page 117*. NOTE: 100 mg po qd x1 yr for hepatitis B.
Ribavirin+Interferon alfa-2b combination pack (Rebetron)	Ribavirin tab contains 2 wk supply of INF and 42, 70, or 84 caps of 200 mg ribavirin. **Dose:** INF 3 million U sc tw AND ribavirin 400 mg po a.m. + 600 mg po p.m. (<75 kg) or 600 mg po bid (>75 kg) x 48 wks. Rebetron (1000 mg/d ribavirin dose pack). ($307/24 wk course)	Ribavirin/interferon alfa see above. Hemolytic anemia common (mean reduction in Hgb 3 gm/dl) but usually responds to ↓ ribavirin dosage (see package insert). **Severe psychiatric effects, esp. depression, most common reason for discontinuation of therapy** in (25–36%) of pts on biologic. Significant hypothyroidism, alopecia 6%. & pulmonary disease reported (*Mayo Clin Proc 74:367, 1999*). **Since ribavirin is teratogenic, drug must not be used during pregnancy** (and for 6 months after). Also should not be used in pts with endstage renal failure, severe heart disease, or hemoglobinopathies.

	Interferon	Ribavirin
Dose changes		
Hgb: <10	→ to 200 mcg a.m, 400 mg q.p.m.	
<8.5	DC	DC
WBC: <1500	No change	
<1000	DC	
Abs. PMNs <750	No change	
<500	DC	
Platelets: <50,000	No change	
<25,000	DC	

	Interferon	
Hgb: <10	→ to 1.5 mIU sc 3x/wk	
<8.5	DC	
WBC: <1500	→ to 1.5 mIU sc 3x/wk	
<1000	DC	
Abs. PMNs <750	→ to 1.5 mIU sc 3x/wk	
<500	DC	
Platelets: <50,000	No change	
<25,000	DC	

| **Ribavirin (Rebetol)** | For use only with an interferon for hepatitis C & was unbundled from the combination Rebetron (see above), mostly for use with the new PEG interferons (alfa-2a & 2b). Available in 200 mg capsules. Dose: <75 kg BW 2 caps in a.m. & 3 caps p.m. >75 kg BW 3 caps in a.m. & 3 caps in p.m. Cost: 200 mg $9.60 | Response to rx in some complex renal disease: *A/M 106:347, 1999*. Side-effects as above. Hemolytic anemia (drop 1–2 wks of rx) with hemoglobin ↑ of 3–4 gm. Should not be used with CrCl <50 ml/min & cautiously with cardiac disease. |

NOTE: *All dosage recommendations are for adults (unless otherwise indicated) and assume normal renal function.*
* From 2002 Red Book, Medical Economics Data and Hospital Formulary Pricing Guide. Price is average wholesale price (AWP). **NB** = name brand, **G** = generic, **DC** = discontinue

TABLE 14B (3)

DRUG NAME(S) GENERIC (TRADE)	DOSAGE/ROUTE/COST*	COMMENTS/ADVERSE EFFECTS
Influenza A		
Amantadine (Symmetrel) or Rimantadine (Flumadine)	Amantadine and rimantadine doses are the same (rimantadine approved only for prophylaxis in children, not treatment). Amantadine 100 mg po bid; >65 y.o., 100 mg po qd. G: cap $0.20, 100 mg/10 ml soln. $1.50. Rimantadine 100 mg tab/syrup $2	**Side-effects/toxicity:** CNS (nervousness, anxiety, difficulty concentrating, and lightheadedness). Symptoms occurred in 6% on amantadine vs 14% on rimantadine. They usually ↓ after 1st week and disappear when drug dc. GI (nausea, anorexia). Some serious side-effects—delirium, hallucinations, and seizures—are associated with high plasma drug levels resulting from renal insufficiency, esp. in older pts, those with prior seizure disorders, or psychiatric disorders. In pts with impaired renal function, dosage of both drugs should be reduced (amantadine: creatinine clearance <50 ml/min, rimantadine: CrCl <10 ml/min); see package inserts and Table 17, pages 130 & 131. Both drugs teratogenic in animals and contraindicated during pregnancy (Med Lett 39:72, 1997).
Influenza A and B—For both drugs, initiate within 48 hrs of symptom onset		
Zanamivir (Relenza) For pts ≥12 yrs of age	2 inhalations (2 x 5 mg) bid x5 d. Powder is inhaled using specially designed breath-activated device. Each medication-containing blister contains 5 mg of zanamivir. $48/course	Active by inhalation against neuraminidase of both influenza A and B and inhibits release of virus from epithelial cells of respiratory tract. Approx. 4–17% of inhaled dose absorbed into plasma. Excreted by kidney but with low absorption, dose reduction not necessary in renal impairment. Minimal side-effects: <3% cough, sinusitis, diarrhea, nausea and vomiting. **Reports of respiratory adverse events in pts with or without hx airway disease; should be avoided in pts with respiratory disease.**
Oseltamivir (Tamiflu)	75 mg po bid for treatment [pediatric suspension (12 mg/ml) approved for treatment, not prevention, in children age 1–12 at dose of 2 mg/kg (up to 75 mg total) bid x5 d]. For prevention: 75 mg po qd for duration of peak of flu epidemic. $65/5 day course	Well absorbed (80% bioavailable) from GI tract as ethyl ester of active compound GS 4071. T½ 6–10 hrs; excreted unchanged by kidney. Adverse effects in 15% include nausea, vomiting, headache. Nausea ↓ with food. Also available as 12 mg/ml oral suspension.
Respiratory Syncytial Virus (RSV) and other		
Palivizumab (Synagis) (See Med Lett 41:1, 1999) Used only for prevention of RSV infection in high-risk children (Ped 102:1211, 1998)	15 mg/kg IM q month 100 mg vial (for 1 injection) $1369	A monoclonal antibody directed against the F glycoprotein on surface of virus; side-effects are nominal; occ. ↑ ALT (JID 176:1215, 1997).
Ribavirin (Virazole)	1.1 gm/day (6 gm vial for inhalation $1320)	**Ribavirin side-effects:** Anemia, rash, conjunctivitis: Read package insert. Avoid procedures that lead to drug precipitation in ventilator tubing with subsequent dysfunction. Significant deterioration in animals. **Contraindicated in pregnant women and partners.** Pregnant health care workers should avoid direct care of pts receiving aerosolized ribavirin.
RSV-IV immunoglobulin (IG) (RespiGam)	100 mg/kg IV q month (50 ml $816)	RespiGam side-effects rare but include fatal anaphylaxis, pruritus, rash, wheezing, fever, joint pain.
Warts (See JAMA CID 28:S37, 1999)		
Interferon alfa-2b or alfa-n3	Apply 1 million units into lesion	Interferon alfa-2b or alfa-n3: 1 million units/0.5 ml, interferon alfa-n3 5 mIU/1 ml. Cost: $10.
Podofilox (Condylox)	3.5 ml for topical application, $110	**Side-effects:** Local reactions—pain, burning, inflammation in 50%. No systemic effects.
Imiquimod (Aldara)	Cream applied 3x/week to maximum of 16 wks. 250 mg packets $12	Mild erythema, erosions, itching and burning

NOTE: All dosage recommendations are for adults (unless otherwise indicated) and assume normal renal function.

* From 2002 Red Book, Medical Economics Data and Hospital Formulary Pricing Guide. Price is average wholesale price (AWP). **NB** = name brand, **G** = generic, **DC** = discontinue

TABLE 14C: ANTIRETROVIRAL THERAPY IN ADULTS 2002

2002 has continued to bring enormous changes to the care of the HIV-infected individual. With increased experience in clinical practice, a reduction in cost and a better understanding of the meaning of quantitative measures of viral RNA (see *Table 2 of the SANFORD GUIDE TO HIV/AIDS THERAPY*) and increased experience of utilizing **Highly Active Antiretroviral Therapy (HAART)**, clinicians have gained valuable lessons in managing this increasingly complex disease. The current practice is moving towards later (but before CD4 counts get below 200/mm³) initiation of HAART, more liberal use of resistance testing, more attention to adherence (with construction of less frequent (dosing schedules) and more time spent on managing toxicities. See www.hivatis.org; AnIM 137:381, 2002.

The following concepts guide therapy:

- **Goal of rx: To adequately inhibit viral replication allowing re-establishment and persistence of an effective immune response against pathogenic organisms.**

- **The lower the vRNA levels can be driven the longer the therapeutic effect will last!**

- **Achieving the maximum therapeutic response is most successful in patients not previously treated (antiretroviral naive).**

- **Keep trough drug concentrations > inhibitory concentration of the virus.** This has led to the use of 2 PIs; one chosen for ↑ activity (indinavir, nelfinavir and saquinavir) and the other to ↑ $T_{1/2}$ (ritonavir) by inhibiting metabolism of the 1ˢᵗ drug (P450 inhibition) and allowing bid (and maybe qd) dosing. Thus dual PIs are emerging as drugs of choice in combination with NRTIs as described below.

- **Adequate response to antiviral therapy. Continue current regimen.**
  - 0.5–0.75 log₁₀ ↓ in plasma HIV RNA by 4 weeks but generally effective rx reduces VL by >1 log (90% or 10-fold ↓) within 2 weeks
  - Undetectable levels by 4–6 months
  - In certain individuals undetectable viral loads may not be achieved, esp. when initial viral load is high (>100,000 copies/ml)
  - A sustained rx in CD4 counts: counts typically ↑ ≥50 cells/ml at 4 to 8 weeks after rx initiated or changed followed by 50 to 100 cells/ml per year thereafter

- **Virologic/Clinical failure to antiretroviral therapy: Change current regimen**
  - <0.5–0.75 log₁₀ reduction in plasma HIV RNA by 4 weeks
  - <1 log₁₀ reduction in plasma HIV RNA by 8 weeks
  - Failure to suppress plasma HIV RNA to undetectable levels within 4–6 months of initiating therapy
  - Repeated detection of significant level of virus in plasma after initial suppression to undetectable levels, suggesting the development of resistance
  - Persistent decline in CD4 counts, as measured on at least 2 separate occasions
  - Clinical deterioration

- **Disconnect syndrome: Continue current regimen if tolerance good until CD4 cells ↓ or if good alternative options available, some experts would change regimen (data not available to make definitive recommendation)**
  - ↑ of plasma HIV RNA by 3-fold or to detectable level but HIV RNA remains 0.5 log (3-fold ↓) below original setpoint (pretreatment level)
  - CD4 count is unchanged or increasing
  - No sign of clinical progression
  - Some experts recommend changing regimens if options are available
  - If alternative option not available, continue present rx and follow CD4 cell count

- **When changing rx because of clinical or virological failure, all 3 drugs (2 RTIs and the PI or NNRTI) should be changed** if possible, because the emergence of resistant viruses is likely (similar to the management of tuberculosis). **Genotype and phenotype testing should be considered.**

- **If failure is the result of drug toxicity (bone marrow suppression, neuropathy or pancreatitis) without virological relapse, one can change the offending drug alone (ZDV, ddI or ddC).**

* See page 116 for footnotes and abbreviations

TABLE 14C (2)

1. When should antiretroviral treatment be started?

The most important factor in answering this question is to find out if the patient is ready to comply with the difficult regimens.

- **Acute retroviral (HIV) syndrome:** Most authorities would treat immediately with HAART as suggested below, in an attempt to rapidly control viral proliferation, establish a lower viral set-point and preserve the immunologic defenses (virus-specific cytotoxic T-cells and CD4 helper cells) against HIV *(AIDS 14:2643, 2000; J Exp Med 193:169, 2001)*. Addition of cyclosporine A to HAART ↑ CD4 cells in one study *(JCI 109:681, 2002)*.
- **Therapy is recommended in symptomatic patients.**
- **In asymptomatic pts, 2002 guidelines recommend using CD4 count to guide time of initiation of rx:** *(Int'l AIDS Soc USA Panel, 2002; WHO treatment guidelines issued 4/22/2002: www.who.int)*.
- **If possible, rx when CD4 count between 200 and 350/mm³.**
   - If CD4 <200, less predictable rise in CD4, ↓ chance of complete immune reconstitution (esp. naïve cells), less effective viral suppression, more rapid progression to AIDS & ↓ survival
   - If >350, no apparent benefit in survival and unnecessary drug toxicity.
   - Since many pts today initially present with very low (0–<200) CD4 cells, rx should still be offered since at least partial immune recovery can be expected with associated survival benefit.
- Using viral load level as an independent indicator for initiating rx is **not** supported by available data, however, pts with **>50,000–100,000 HIV RNA copies/ml should be frequently monitored** because rx of pts with CD4 count even with VL >55,000 copies/ml even with CD4 counts between 350 & 500/mm³ *(See www.hivatis.org)*. Previous guidelines recommended initiating antiretroviral rx when CD4 counts between 350 & 500/mm³ *(See www.hivatis.org)*.

2. Available drugs: categories, names, and dosages *(Summary in Med Letter 43:103, 2001; Mayo Clin Proc 74:1284, 1999; Deeks & Volberding in MEDICAL MANAGEMENT OF AIDS, Sande & Volberding, Eds., 6th Ed., 1999)*

DRUG NAME(S)	DOSE/FREQUENCY	DOSAGE FORM(S)/COST
Nucleoside Analog Reverse Transcriptase Inhibitors (NRTI)		
Abacavir (Ziagen)	300 mg po bid No dietary restrictions	300 mg tab ($408/month) Oral solution 20 mg/ml
Didanosine (ddI, Videx)	>60 kg: 400 mg po qd <60 kg: 250 mg po qd On empty stomach	125, 200, 250, 400 mg delayed release enteric-coated cap ($285/month) 25, 50, 100, 150, 200 mg chewable tab 100, 167, 250 mg powder **Reduce dose to 200 mg qd if with tenofovir**
Lamivudine (3TC, Epivir)	150 mg bid or 300 mg po qd No dietary restrictions	150, 300 mg tab ($316/month) Oral solution 10 mg/ml ($81/8 oz)
Stavudine (d4T, Zerit)	>60 kg: 40 mg po bid <60 kg: 30 mg po bid No dietary restrictions	15, 20, 30, 40 mg cap ($318/month) Oral solution 1 mg/ml ($59/200 ml)
	NOTE: Extended release formulation available soon—stavudine XR, 100 mg qd	
Zalcitabine (ddC, Hivid)	0.75 mg bid No dietary restrictions	0.375, 0.75 mg tab ($246/month)
Zidovudine (ZDV, AZT, Retrovir)	300 mg po bid No dietary restrictions	100, 300 mg tab ($355/month) 10 mg/ml injectable ($18/20 ml vial) Oral solution 50 mg/5 ml ($56/30 ml) 10 mg/ml IV solution
ZDV/3TC (Combivir)	One combination tablet po bid No dietary restrictions	300 mg ZDV/150 mg 3TC ($658/month)
ZDV/3TC/Abacavir (Trizivir)	One combination tablet po bid No dietary restrictions	300 mg ZDV/150 mg 3TC/300 mg abacavir ($1,005/month)
Nucleotide Analog Reverse Transcriptase Inhibitor (NtRTI)		
Tenofovir (Viread)	300 mg po qd With food	300 mg tab ($408/month)

NOTE: All dosage recommendations are for adults *(unless otherwise indicated) and assume normal renal function.*

* From 2002 Red Book, Medical Economics Data and Hospital Formulary Pricing Guide. Price is average wholesale price (AWP). **NB** = name brand, **G** = generic, **DC** = discontinue

DRUG NAME(S)	DOSE/FREQUENCY	DOSAGE FORM(S)/COST
Non-Nucleoside Reverse Transcriptase Inhibitors (NNRTI)		
Delavirdine (Rescriptor)	400 mg po bid No dietary restrictions	100, 200 mg tab ($304/month)
Efavirenz (Sustiva)	600 mg po qd hs No dietary restrictions	600 mg tab; 50, 100, & 200 mg cap ($432/month)
Nevirapine (Viramune)	200 mg po qd x14 days, then 200 mg po bid No dietary restrictions	200 mg tab ($336/month) 50 mg/5 ml oral suspension (pediatric)
Protease Inhibitors (PI)		
Amprenavir (Agenerase)	1200 mg po bid No dietary restrictions When combined with efavirenz, consider adding ritonavir 200 mg po bid	50, 150 mg cap ($706/month) Oral solution 15 mg/ml Oral solution contains large amount of propylene glycol, which is contraindicated in pts <4 yrs of age, pregnancy, pts with hepatic or renal failure, and pts on disulfiram or metronidazole
Indinavir (Crixivan)	800 mg po q8h On empty stomach or with low-fat meals Most commonly used with ritonavir (see *SANFORD GUIDE TO HIV/AIDS THERAPY for details*) If indinavir is combined with efavirenz or nevirapine, consider ↑ the dose to 1000 mg po tid unless ritonavir is used, then no dosage adjustment necessary	100, 200, 333, 400 mg cap ($522/month)
Lopinavir/Ritonavir (Kaletra)	400 mg/100 mg po bid With food When combined with efavirenz or nevirapine, ↑ the dose to 533.6 to 533.3 mg lopinavir/133.3 mg ritonavir (4 capsules) po bid	133.3 mg lopinavir/33.3 mg ritonavir cap ($703/month) Once dispensed, drug can be stored at room temperature for 2 months Oral solution 80/20 mg/ml
Nelfinavir (Viracept)	1250 mg po bid With food	250 mg tab ($756/month) Oral powder 50 mg/gm ($61/144 gm)
Ritonavir (Norvir)	600 mg po bid Starting regimen: 300 mg po bid on day 1; 400 mg po bid on days 2 & 3; 500 mg po bid on days 4 & 5; then 600 mg po bid thereafter. With food Ritonavir is currently used to boost other PIs (dosage 100 mg or 400 mg po bid)	100 mg cap ($571/month) Once dispensed, drug can be stored at room temperature for 1 month Oral solution 80 mg/ml
Saquinavir (Fortovase, softgel capsules) (Invirase, hard capsules)	Fortovase, softgel capsules preferred dosage form because of better bioavailability: Fortovase 1200 mg po tid With food Invirase, hard capsules not usually recommended as single PI because of erratic absorption and ↓ bioavailability, but useful in combination with ritonavir: (Invirase 1600 mg po + ritonavir 100 mg po, both bid) or (Invirase 400 mg po + ritonavir 400 mg po, both bid), with food. Avoid combining saquinavir with efavirenz or nevirapine unless ritonavir is used, then no dosage adjustment is recommended	Fortovase 200 mg softgel cap ($722/month) Once dispensed, drug can be stored at room temperature for 3 months (taken with ritonavir) Invirase 200 mg hard cap ($647/month) (espn. with ritonavir)

Most recommend initiating 3- or 4-drug combinations: Combine 2 NRTIs with either a PI (or double PI) or a NNRTI. Addition of the PI (indinavir) improved results of both clinical & virologic parameters in antiretroviral naive & experienced pts (*NEJM 337:725 & 734, 1997*). Significant drug-drug interactions occur with PIs (*see Table 21B, page 141*). Drug tolerance and the ability of the patient to balance food intake and convenience (quality of life issues) are major considerations.

NOTE: All dosage recommendations are for adults (unless otherwise indicated) and assume normal renal function.
* From 2002 Red Book, Medical Economics Data and Hospital Formulary Pricing Guide. Price is average wholesale price (AWP). **NB** = name brand, **G** = generic, **DC** = discontinue

TABLE 14C (4)

3. Summary of Suggested Initial Treatment of HIV Infection (see text for details) (www.hivatis.org; AnIM 137;381, 2002)
A. Antiretroviral drug regimens are comprised of one choice from columns A and B. Drugs are listed in alphabetical, not priority order.

PREFERRED		ALTERNATIVE	
Column A (PI, 2 PIs, or NNRTI)	Column B (2 NRTIs)	Column A (NRTI, PI, 2 PIs, NNRTI)	Column B (2 NRTIs)
Efavirenz	Didanosine + lamivudine	Abacavir	Didanosine + lamivudine
Indinavir + ritonavir	Stavudine + didanosine	Amprenavir ± ritonavir	Stavudine + didanosine
Lopinavir/ritonavir (Kaletra)	Stavudine + lamivudine	Delavirdine	Stavudine + lamivudine
Nelfinavir	Zidovudine + didanosine	Nelfinavir ± (saquinavir)	Zidovudine + didanosine
Ritonavir + saquinavir	Zidovudine + lamivudine	Nevirapine[1]	Zidovudine + lamivudine
		Ritonavir	
		Saquinavir SGC[1]	

Abbreviations: **NRTI** = nucleoside reverse transcriptase inhibitor; **NNRTI** = non-nucleoside reverse transcriptase inhibitor; **PI** = protease inhibitor; **ZDV** = **zidovudine**; **3TC** = lamivudine; **d4T** = stavudine; **ddI** = didanosine; **SGC** = softgel capsules
[1] Substitute nevirapine for efavirenz in pregnant women or when contraception cannot be assured.

B. Examples of common regimens used in 2002 as initial therapy:
Efavirenz 600 mg + didanosine (ddI) 400 mg + lamivudine 300 mg, all po qd
OR
Lopinavir/ritonavir 400/100 mg (Kaletra) + zidovudine/lamivudine 300/100 mg (Combivir), all po bid
OR
Nelfinavir 1250 mg po bid + (Combivir 1 tab po bid or stavudine 40 mg po bid + ddI 400 mg po qd)

4. Monitoring of patients
Patients on HAART:
  • Check viral load and CD4 count 4 weeks after initiation of treatment
  • Then every month until goal viral load achieved (usually viral load <50 copies/ml)
  • Then every 3-4 months
  • Consider more frequent monitoring if CD4 count drops, clinical symptoms appear, or progress
Patients not on treatment:
  • Check viral load and CD4 count every 3-4 months

5. What is appropriate when antiretroviral regimen fails? (as defined above)
Failure of rx may be due to many different reasons and it is important to attempt to identify the cause.
A. **Non-adherence:** One may initially reinstitute original regimen, especially if patient stopped all drugs at once (it has been shown that even after a year on rx when drugs are stopped simultaneously, the viral isolates will still be sensitive to all 3 drugs and patients will again respond to reinitiation of original rx).
B. **The patient took the drug erratically or the drug was incompletely absorbed and broke through with a rise in vRNA:** The virus may well be resistant to all drugs and a change in rx is warranted. It is recommended that all drugs be changed (possible, as outlined below (JID 177;1521, 1998)
C. **Drug malabsorption or drug-drug interactions that ↓ effective plasma drug concentrations:** In several studies, plasma indinavir concentrations correlated with therapeutic effect: mean trough concentrations were 0.133 mg/L in responders and 0.023 mg/L in non-responders. In addition, levels above the IC50 (concentration of drug required to inhibit 90% of viruses in vitro) were present 90% of the dosing interval for responders but only 58% for those who failed (ICAAC Absts. A-15, A-19, & IDSA Abst. I-173, 1997). Use of plasma drug levels in instances when the cause of failure is not apparent may be of value.
D. **Mutations that confer resistance:** Genotyping and phenotypic tests for resistance to antiretroviral drugs are commercially available and are recommended for clinical decision-making (see Table 2 of the SANFORD GUIDE TO HIV/AIDS THERAPY).

[1] Use of saquinavir hard-gel capsule is not recommended, except in combination with ritonavir
NOTE: All dosage recommendations are for adults (unless otherwise indicated) and assume normal renal function.
* From 2002 Red Book, Medical Economics Data and Hospital Formulary Pricing Guide. Price is average wholesale price (AWP). **NB** = name brand, **G** = generic, **DC** = discontinue

TABLE 14C (5)
POSSIBLE THERAPEUTIC OPTIONS FOR PATIENTS WHO FAIL THEIR INITIAL ANTI-HIV DRUG REGIMEN

CLINICAL CIRCUMSTANCE:	SOME OPTIONS:	NOT RECOMMENDED:
Failure of initial therapy	1. As for treatment-naive, but switch to a different PI and a different combination of NRTIs, consider ritonavir enhanced PI to replace single PI. 2. Double PI rx (ritonavir + saquinavir–SGC ±NRTI) 3. Efavirenz + a different combination of NRTIs 4. Double PI + 2 different NRTIs 5. Lopinavir/ritonavir (Kaletra) + 2 different NRTIs 6. Add tenofovir to new regimen (results encouraging in 2 Phase 3 studies)	Change of only 1 or 2 drugs of 3-drug regimen

TABLE 14D: ANTIRETROVIRAL DRUGS AND ADVERSE EFFECTS (*I.n. 358:1322, 2001*)

DRUG NAME(S): GENERIC (TRADE)	ADVERSE EFFECTS
Nucleoside Reverse Transcriptase Inhibitors (NRTI)	All NRTIs have potential for causing **mitochondrial toxicity** (*Curr Opin ID 13:13, 2000*) All NRTIs have been associated with **lactic acidosis** with severe steatosis and hepatomegaly (rare) (*see Table 10 of the Sanford Guide to HIV/AIDS Therapy*) NRTIs have also been associated with **lipodystrophy** (*AIDS 14:F25, 14:37, 2000; AIDS 14:F25, 2000; AIDS 13:1659, 1999*)
Abacavir (Ziagen)	**Most common:** Headache 16%, nausea/vomiting 16%, diarrhea 12%, loss of appetite/anorexia 11%, malaise **Most significant: Hypersensitivity** reaction in 5% with malaise, fever, GI upset, rash, lethargy, & respiratory symptoms most commonly reported; myalgia, arthralgia, edema, paresthesia less commonly reported. **Rechallenge contraindicated; may be life-threatening.**
Didanosine (ddI) (Videx)	**Most common:** Diarrhea 28%, nausea 6%, headache 7%, fever 12%, hyperuricemia 2% **Most significant: Pancreatitis 1–9%.** Cases of fatal and nonfatal pancreatitis have occurred in pts receiving ddI, especially when used in combination with d4T or d4T + hydroxyurea. Peripheral neuropathy in 20%, 12% required dose reduction; **see drug-drug interaction with tenofovir (*Table 21*)**
Lamivudine (3TC) (Epivir)	Well tolerated. Headache 35%, nausea 33%, diarrhea 18%, abdominal pain 9%, insomnia 11%. Pancreatitis rare in common in pediatrics (15%).
Stavudine (d4T) (Zerit)	**Most common:** Diarrhea, nausea, vomiting, headache **Most significant: Peripheral neuropathy** 15–20%. Pancreatitis 1%. Appears to produce lactic acidosis more commonly than other NRTIs. Fatal lactic acidosis/steatosis in pregnant women receiving d4T + ddI
Zalcitabine (ddC) (Hivid)	**Most common:** Oral ulcers 13%, rash 8% **Most significant:** Pancreatitis <1%, **peripheral neuropathy 22–35%.** Severe continuous pain, slowly reversible when ddC is discontinued, ↑ risk with diabetes mellitus.
Zidovudine (ZDV, AZT) (Retrovir)	**Most common:** Nausea 50%, anorexia 20%, vomiting 17%, **headache 62%,** malaise 53%, pigmentation of nails, asthenia, insomnia, myalgias **Most significant: Anemia** (<8 gm 1%), granulocytopenia (<750 1.8%). Macrocytosis expected with all dosage regimens. Anemia may respond to epoetin alfa if endogenous serum erythropoietin levels are <500 mU/ml.
Nucleotide Reverse Transcriptase Inhibitor (NRTI) Tenofovir (Viread)	**Most common:** Nausea 11%, diarrhea 9%, vomiting 5%, flatulence 4% (generally well tolerated); **drug interaction with didanosine** **Most significant:** Lactic acidosis with hepatic steatosis. Affinity of tenofovir for polymerase gamma is lower than NRTI.
Non-Nucleoside Reverse Transcriptase Inhibitors (NNRTI) Delavirdine (Rescriptor)	**Most common:** Nausea, diarrhea, vomiting, headache **Most significant: Skin rash** has occurred in 18%; can continue or restart drug in most cases. Stevens-Johnson syndrome and erythema multiforme have been reported rarely. ↑ in liver enzymes rarely. DC in <5% of patients.

NOTE: All dosage recommendations are for adults (unless otherwise indicated) and assume normal renal function. **NB** = name brand, **G** = generic, **DC** = discontinue

* From 2002 Red Book, Medical Economics Data and Hospital Formulary Pricing Guide. Price is average wholesale price (AWP).

TABLE 14D (2)

DRUG NAME(S): GENERIC (TRADE)	ADVERSE EFFECTS
Efavirenz (Sustiva)	**Most common: CNS side-effects 52%;** symptoms include dizziness, insomnia, somnolence, impaired concentration, and abnormal dreams; symptoms are worse after 1st or 2nd dose and improve over 2-4 weeks; discontinuation rate 1.7%. Rash 26%; improves with oral antihistamines; discontinuation rate 1.7%. Can cause false-positive urine test results for cannabinoid with CEDIA DAU multi-level THC assay. **Most significant:** Elevation in liver function tests. **Teratogenicity reported in animals; not recommended in pregnant women** (see Table 6)
Nevirapine (Viramune)	**Most common: Rash 37%;** occurs during 1st 6 wks of therapy. Women experience 7-fold ↑ in risk of severe rash (CID 32:124, 2001). 50% resolve within 2 wks of dc drug and 80% by 1 month. 6.7% discontinuation rate. Severe life-threatening skin reactions reported: Stevens-Johnson syndrome, toxic epidermal necrolysis, and hypersensitivity reaction or drug rash with eosinophilia and systemic symptoms (DRESS) (AHM 161:2501, 2001). For severe rashes, dc drug immediately and do not restart. In a clinical trial, the use of prednisone ↑ the risk of rash. **Most significant: Life-threatening hepatotoxicity reported.** 2/3 during the first 12 wks of rx. Overall 1% develop hepatitis. Pts with pre-existing ↑ in ALT or AST and/or history of chronic Hep B or C most susceptible. Monitor pts monthly (clinical and LFTs), esp. during the first 12 wks of rx. If clinical hepatotoxicity occurs, dc drug and never rechallenge.
Protease inhibitors (PI)	Spontaneous bleeding episodes have been reported in HIV+ pts with hemophilia being treated with PI. All PIs may be associated with hyperglycemia and/or hyperlipidemia. 2 published studies reported 6-7% of pts given PIs developed symptomatic diabetes mellitus. 16% had impaired glucose tolerance (Ln 353:2093, 1999; An Pharmacother 34:580, 2000). **Lipodystrophy common with all PIs.** Central obesity, gynecomastia, and buffalo hump fatty distributions [median time after initiation of PI rx 2 wks] (CID 27:65 & 68, 1998). Pts with lipodystrophy were more likely to have ↓ glucose tolerance, diabetes, ↑ triglycerides, ↓ HDL cholesterol than pts without lipodystrophy (CID 32:130, 2001; CID 34:248, 2002). Pts taking PI may be at increased risk for developing osteopenias and osteoporosis.
Amprenavir (Agenerase)	**Most common:** Nausea 38-73%, vomiting 19-20%, diarrhea 33-56%, paresthesias 26-30% **Most significant:** Skin rash 28%. Most maculopapular of mild-moderate intensity. Severe or life-threatening rash, including Stevens-Johnson syndrome in 1% of pts. Skin rash onset 7-73 days, median 10 days
Indinavir (Crixivan)	**Most common:** ↑ in indirect bilirubin 10-15% (≥2.5 mg/dl), due to a drug-induced Gilbert's syndrome (of no clinical significance). Severe hepatitis reported in 3 cases (JJ 349:924, 1997). Nausea 12%, vomiting 4%, diarrhea 5%, Paronychia of big toe reported (CID 32:140, 2001) **Most significant: Kidney stones.** Due to indinavir crystals in collecting system (2-3% on 2.4 gm/d but higher in ↑hot climates" (AIDS 12:296, 1997). 12/174 (6.9%) developed nephrolithiasis within 4 months of starting indinavir; 5/6 who continued rx had a 2nd episode (ICAAC Abst. 183, 1997). Prevent (minimize) by good hydration (at least 48 oz. water/day) (AAC 42:332, 1998)
Nelfinavir (Viracept)	**Most common:** Mild to moderate **diarrhea** 14-52%. Oat bran tabs, calcium, or oral anti-diarrheal agents (e.g., loperamide, diphenoxylate/atropine sulfate) can be used to manage diarrhea.
Ritonavir (Norvir)	**Most common:** GI: bitter aftertaste ↓ by taking with chocolate milk. Ensure, or Advera, nausea 23%, ↓ by initial dose escalation (titration) regimen; vomiting 13%, diarrhea 15%. Circumoral paresthesias 5-6%. ↑ dose > 100 mg bid assoc. with ↑ GI side-effects &.↑ in lipid abnormalities. **Most significant:** Hepatic failure (AHM 129:670, 1998). Many important drug-drug interactions—inhibits P450 CYP3A system (see Table 21).
Saquinavir (Invirase: hard cap) (Fortovase: softgel cap)	**Most common:** GI: **diarrhea** 16-20%, abdominal discomfort 9-13%, nausea 11-18%. Headache 5-9%.
Lopinavir/Ritonavir (Kaletra)	**Most common:** GI: **diarrhea** 14-24%, nausea 2-16%, lipid abnormalities in up to 30% **Most significant:** Pancreatitis

NOTE: All dosage recommendations are for adults (unless otherwise indicated) and assume normal renal function.
* From 2002 Red Book, Medical Economics Data and Hospital Formulary Pricing Guide. Price is average wholesale price (AWP). **NB** = name brand, **G** = generic, **DC** = discontinue

TABLE 15A
PREVENTION OF INFECTION WITH CHEMOTHERAPY

CLASS OF ETIOLOGIC AGENT/DISEASE/CONDITION	PROPHYLAXIS: AGENT/DOSE/ROUTE/DURATION	COMMENTS
Group B streptococcal disease (GBS), neonatal: Vaginal colonization with GBS assoc. with ↑ neonatal sepsis & maternal peripartum and postpartum infectious complications (*IJID 179:1410, 1999; Ln 353:51, 1999).*		
Pregnant women—intrapartum antimicrobial prophylaxis—The use of standard orders and forms by most US hospitals by 1999 correlates with a ↓ in neonatal GBS infection (*MMWR 49:936, 2000; J Perinatol 21:9, 2001).* Approaches to management [CDC Guidelines, *MMWR 51:(RR-11):1, 2002*]: **1. Prenatal screening cultures**—Rx during labor if culture pos. from vagina & rectum, by swab, at 35–37 wks gestation. Use transport media (Amies); survive at room temp. up to 96 hr. **2. Risk factor approach**—Rx if any of the following is present: (a) previously delivered infant with invasive GBS infection; (b) GBS bacteriuria during this pregnancy; (c) delivery at <37 wks gestation; (d) duration of ruptured membranes ≥18 hrs; (e) intrapartum temp. ≥100.4°F (≥38.0°C)	**Rx mother during labor:** ampicillin 2 gm IV (load) then 2.5 MU IV q4h until delivery or **pen G** 5 MU IV (load) then 2.5 MU IV q4h until delivery. Alternate rx: **Ampicillin** 2 gm IV (load) then give 1 gm IV q4h until delivery. **Pen-allergic: Pts not at high risk for anaphylaxis: Cefazolin** 2 gm IV initial dose, then 1 gm IV q8h until delivery. **Pts at high risk for anaphylaxis:** GBS susceptible to clinda & erythro: **Clindamycin** 900 mg IV q8h until delivery or **erythromycin** 500 mg IV q6h until delivery.	If culture positive or risk factors dictate prophylaxis (but not if pre-labor, planned C-section without ruptured membranes).
Neonate delivered from mother who received prophylaxis	Careful observation of signs & symptoms (*see MMWR 45:RR-7, 1996 for specifics); 95%* of infants will show clinical signs of infection during the 1st 24 hrs whether mother received intrapartum antibiotics or not (*Pediatrics 106:244, 2000).*	
Preterm, premature rupture of the membranes in Group B strep-negative women (*JAMA 278:989, 1997*)	(IV **ampicillin** 2 gm q6h + IV **erythromycin** 250 mg q8h) for 48 hrs followed by po **amoxicillin** 250 mg q8h + po **erythromycin** base 333 mg q8h x5 d. Effective in ↓ infant morbidity.	Antibiotic rx reduced infant respiratory distress syndrome (50.6% to 40.8%, p = 0.03), necro-tizing enterocolitis (5.8% to 2.3%, p = 0.03) and prolonged pregnancy (2.9 to 6.1 days, p < 0.001) vs placebo. In 1 large study (4809 pts), erythromycin improved neonatal outcomes vs placebo (11.2% vs 14.4% poor outcomes, p=0.02 for single births) but not co-AM/CL or both drugs in combination (both assoc. with ↑ necrotizing enterocolitis) (*Ln 357:979, 2001).*
Influenza (*see Table 14, page 108*)		
Meningitis prevention: Hemophilus and Neisseria meningitidis—See Table 1, pages 5, 6		
Neutropenic patients, afebrile, e.g., post-chemotherapy *See CID 25:551, 1997; CID 27:235, 1998*	IDSA guidelines for afebrile neutropenic pts: **Routine prophylaxis should be avoided** even though TMP/SMX 2 double strength tablets po bid or **FQ** (**norfloxacin** 400 mg po bid, **ofloxacin** 400 mg po bid, or **ciprofloxacin** 500 mg po bid) have been shown to reduce febrile episodes. No reduction in mortality and ↑ resistance prompt this recommendation.	**TMP/SMX** (>30 studies) reduces infection rates (vs placebo) with fewer adverse effects (*JID 161:381, 1990).* In a meta-analysis of 19 randomized studies, **quinolone** use reduced Gm-neg. bacteremia (OR = 0.09) but not Gm+ bacteremia (OR = 1.05). Addition of penicillin, vancomycin, macrolide or rifampin reduced Gm+ bacteremia (OR = 0.46) but had no impact on fever-related morbidity (OR = 0.83) or infection-related mortality (OR = 0.74) (*CID 23:795, 1996; AnIM 125:183, 1996*). Ampho 0.2 gm/kg/day, oral fluconazole and itraconazole shown to reduce fungal infections but use remains controversial (*CID 28:331, 1999; CID 28:250, 1999; BMT 8:853, 2000*).

TABLE 15A (2)

Management of Exposure to Blood, Vaginal/Penile Secretions With Risk of Transmission of Hepatitis B/C and/or HIV (Needlestick Injury) *(Adapted from CDC recommendations: MMWR 47:R-7, 1998; also see JAMA 281:931, 1999; Emerg Inf Dis 7:254, 2001; MMWR 50:RR-11, 2001).* For free consultation for clinicians treating occupational exposures, call CDC PEPLine 1-888-HIV-4911 or website, http://www.cdc.gov/ncidod/

General steps in management:
1. Wash clean wounds/flush mucous membranes immediately (use of caustic agents or squeezing the wound is discouraged; data lacking regarding antiseptics).
2. Assess risk by doing the following: (a) Characterize exposure; (b) Determine/evaluate source of exposure by medical history, risk behavior, & testing for hepatitis B/C, HIV; (c) Evaluate and test exposed individual for hepatitis B/C & HIV

Hepatitis B Exposure

Exposed Person	Exposure Source		
	HBs Ag+	**HBs Ag−**	**Status Unknown**
Unvaccinated	Give HBIG 5 ml IM & initiate HB vaccine	Initiate HB vaccine	Initiate HB vaccine and if possible, do HBs Ag on source person
Vaccinated (antibody status unknown)	Do anti-HBs on exposed person If titer ≥10 MIU/ml, no rx If titer <10 MIU/ml, HBIG + 1 dose HB vaccine	No rx necessary	Do anti-HBs on exposed person If titer ≥10 MIU/ml, no rx If titer <10 MIU/ml, give 1 dose HB vaccine + HBIG

Hepatitis C Exposure

Determine antibody to hepatitis C for both exposed person and, if possible, exposure source. If source +, follow-up HCV testing advised. **No recommended prophylaxis**, immune serum globulin not effective. *See Table 14.*

HIV: Occupational exposure management *(for sexual exposure to HIV, see below)*
- The decision to initiate post-exposure prophylaxis (PEP) for HIV is a clinical judgment that should be made in concert with the exposed healthcare worker (HCW). It is based on:
  1. Likelihood of the source patient having HIV infection: ↑ with history of high-risk activity—injection drug use, sexual activity with known HIV+ person, unprotected sex with multiple partners (either hetero- or homosexual), receipt of blood products 1978–1985. ↑ with clinical signs suggestive of advanced HIV (unexplained weight loss, night sweats, seborrheic dermatitis, etc.). Remember, the vast majority of persons are **not** infected with HIV (1/200 women infected in larger U.S. cities) and likelihood of infection **extremely rare** if not in above risk groups.
  2. Type of exposure (approx. 1 in 300–400 needlesticks from infected source will transmit HIV).
  3. Limited data regarding efficacy of PEP (PEP with ZDV alone reduced transmission by 90% in 1 retrospective case-controlled study—*NEJM 337:1485, 1997*).
  4. Significant adverse effects of PEP drugs.

- If source is **known positive for HIV or likely to be infected** and **status of exposure warrants PEP**, antiretroviral drugs should be started **immediately** (at least within 72 hrs). If ELISA for HIV is negative, drugs can be stopped. The HCW should be re-tested at **3–4 weeks, 3 & 6 months** whether **PEP is used or not** (the vast majority of seroconversions will occur by 3 months; delayed conversions after 6 months are exceedingly rare). Tests for HIV RNA should not be used for dx of HIV infection because of false-positives (esp. at low titers) & these tests are only approved for established HIV infection [a possible exception is if pt develops signs of acute HIV (mononucleosis-like) syndrome within the 1st 4–6 wks of exposure when antibody tests might still be negative.]
- PEP for HIV is usually given for **4 weeks** and monitoring of adverse effects recommended: baseline **complete blood count, renal and hepatic panel** to be repeated at **2 weeks** at 2 weeks of HCW on PEP demonstrate mild side-effects (nausea, diarrhea, myalgias, headache, etc.) but in up to ⅓ severe enough to discontinue PEP(*Antivir Ther 3:195, 2000*). Consultation with infectious diseases/ HIV specialist valuable when questions regarding PEP arise.

TABLE 15A (3)

3 Steps to HIV Post-Exposure Prophylaxis (PEP) After Occupational Exposure: *(MMWR 50:RR-11, 2001)*

Step 1: Determine the exposure code (EC)

Is source material blood, bloody fluid, semen/vaginal fluid or other normally sterile fluid or tissue?

- Yes → What type of exposure occurred?
- No → No PEP

What type of exposure occurred?

- Mucous membrane or skin integrity compromised (e.g., dermatitis, open wound)
  - Volume
    - Small: Few drops → No PEP / EC1
    - Large: Major splash and/or long duration → EC2

- Intact skin → No PEP

- Percutaneous exposure → Severity
  - Less severe: Solid needle, scratch → EC2
  - More severe: Large-bore hollow needle, deep puncture, visible blood, needle used in vein of source (risk 1:300/400) → EC3

Step 2: Determine the HIV Status Code (HIV SC)

What is the HIV status of the exposure source?

- HIV negative → No PEP

- HIV positive
  - Low titer exposure: asymptomatic & high CD4 count → HIV SC 1
  - High titer exposure: advanced AIDS, prim. HIV high viral load or low CD4 count → HIV SC 2

- Status unknown → HIV SC unknown

- Source unknown → HIV SC unknown

Step 3: Determine Post-Exposure Prophylaxis (PEP) Recommendation

EC	HIV SC	PEP
1	1	May not be warranted
1	2	Consider basic regimen[†]
2	1	Recommend basic regimen[†]
2	2	Recommend expanded regimen[†]
3	1 or 2	Recommend expanded regimen[†]
2 or 3	Unknown	If exposure setting suggests risks of HIV exposure & EC in 2 or 3, consider basic regimen.

Post-Exposure Prophylaxis (after high-risk sex or parenteral drug exposure) *(JID 183:707, 2001) (Adapted from MMWR 47:RR-17, 1998; also see Int J STD AIDS 11:424, 2000; NEJM 336:1097, 1997).* Since the probability of transmission of HIV via sexual contact may approach that of a needlestick, it is reasonable to consider PEP in persons who have had a sexual encounter with an HIV+ person. Currently there are no data on effectiveness of PEP in this setting. The same assessment as suggested above for occupational exposure might be followed in an attempt to determine relative risk. It has been **estimated that transmission of HIV following an episode of receptive penile-anal sexual exposure is 0.1–0.3%, for receptive vaginal exposure 0.1–0.2%,** and unknown for receptive oral intercourse (although less risky than other exposures).
PEP should not be used for low-risk exposure (potentially involving body fluids on intact skin) or for persons who seek care too late for anticipated effect (>72 hrs after exposure). **Consideration might be given for PEP when risk is high, PEP can be initiated promptly, and adherence is likely.** It is prudent to weigh per-act probability of transmission with reported exposure against uncertain toxicities, potential toxicities, and cost (approx. $600–1000/course).
Management and drug selection as above. Patient should also be screened for other sexually transmitted diseases.

[1] Treat for 4 weeks. Monitor for drug side-effects q2 weeks

Basic regimen: ZDV + 3TC, DDI + d4T, or d4T + 3TC
Expanded regimen: Basic regimen + one of the following: indinavir, nelfinavir, abacavir, or efavirenz. [Do not use nevirapine; 22 HCWs receiving drug for PEP had serious adverse events including 3 with hepatic necrosis *(MMWR 49:1153, 2001)*].

[†] If possible, use two antiretroviral drugs that the source pt is not currently taking or for which resistance is unlikely.

TABLE 15A (4)

CLASS OF ETIOLOGIC AGENT/DISEASE/CONDITION	PROPHYLAXIS: AGENT/DOSE/ROUTE/DURATION	COMMENTS
HIV transmission from mother to neonate (vertical transmission)	**Standard for developed countries with prenatal care: Zidovudine** (ZDV) 300 mg & lamivudine (3TC) 150 mg po bid, then 2 mg/kg IV loading dose then 1 mg/kg/hr during labor & then 2 mg/kg po q6h beginning 8-12 hrs after birth for 6 weeks. (Cost: $200/mother-baby pair) If mother already receiving antiretroviral rx, consult with HIV/ID specialist. **For infants born to HIV-infected mother who received no antiretroviral rx during labor or before delivery:** 2 mg/kg po q6h to baby beginning 6-12 hrs after birth for 6 wks. **Suggested regimen for less-developed countries: Nevirapine** 200 mg po to mother at onset of labor & a single 2 mg/kg dose to baby within 72 hrs of birth (not FDA-approved indication). (Cost: $4.00/mother-baby pair)	This is ACTG 076 trial which reduced infection in neonates to **8.3% vs 25.5%** in placebo. None of the mothers breast-fed (NEJM 331:1173, 1994). Standard course for mother (starting at 28th wk of gestation) superior to short course (starting at 35th wk). Shorter course to infant (3 d) similar to standard 6 wks if mother rx at 28th wk (NEJM 343:982, 2000). Observational study of 900 births showed ZDV rx to infant reduced transmission from 30% to 10% (NEJM 339:1409, 1998). Nevirapine rx reduced HIV transmission to neonate to **8.2% at birth, 11.9% by 6-8 wks & 13.1% by 14-16 wks** as compared to ZDV rx given at onset of labor & to baby bid for 1 wk: birth 10.4%, 6-8 wks 21.3%, **14-16 wks 25.1%, 98% of mothers breast-fed.** No evidence for drug-associated fetal abnormalities, but follow-up short (Ln 354:795, 1999)
Lyme Disease (see Table 1, page 39)		
Otitis media (see Table 1, page 7)	**Penicillin V** Children——Age <5 yrs 125 mg po bid, >5 yrs 250 mg po bid. Adults 250 mg po bid. (Alternatives: **Amoxicillin, TMP/SMX**) NOTE: Repeat pneumococcal vaccine every 6 years	
Post-splenectomy bacteremia. Likely agents: Pneumococci, meningococci, H. influenzae type b (also at ↑ risk of fatal malaria, severe babesiosis) (immunization important, see Comments)		Daily antimicrobial prophylaxis effective with sickle-cell disease, but should be considered for asplenic children <5 yrs. Also recommended in children and adolescents for 3 yrs post splenectomy. **Adjunct measures for all ages: meningococcal A & C, pneumococcal & Hib vaccines before elective splenectomy.** Some authorities prescribe AM/CL for self-administration with onset of any fever for all ages. Compliance with recommendations poor (J Clin Path 54:214, 2001)
Rheumatic fever, acute (see Table 1, page 41)		
Sexual Exposure		
Sexual assault victim (likely agents and risks, see NEJM 322:713, 1990	(**Ceftriaxone** 125 mg IM) + (**doxycycline** 100 mg po x7 d) + (**metronidazole** 2 gm po single dose) (NEJM 332: 234, 1995)	Perform bimanual pelvic exam. Examine wet mount for motile sperm, T. vaginalis. Culture for gonococci, chlamydia (if available), syphilis & HIV antibody test. Pregnancy test. Follow-up exam at 2 wks. Repeat STS & serology for HIV at 12 weeks (MMWR 42:78-14, 1993)
Sexual contacts, likely agents: N. gonorrhoeae, C. trachomatis	(**Ceftriaxone** 125 mg IM) + (**doxycycline** 100 mg po bid, or **azithromycin** 1 gm po), each as single dose)	Be sure to check for syphilis since all regimens may not eradicate incubating syphilis (JID 174:689, 1996)
Sickle cell disease. Likely agent: S. pneumoniae (see post-splenectomy, above)	3 mos—5 yrs: **Amoxicillin** 125 mg po bid >5 yrs: **Penicillin V** 250 mg po bid	Rx for exposure within 3 months. Make effort to dx syphilis Start prophylaxis before age 4 mos (Am Acad Ped Red Book 1994, p. 375). Children with SCD should receive vaccines: DTP, OPV, MMR, Hep B, Hib, pneumococcus, influenza ± meningococcal. Treat febrile episodes with ceftriaxone (50 mg/kg IV) (NEJM 329:472,1993)
Transplantation (also see Table 1C, page 47)		
Bone marrow	Regimens continue to evolve. Current 'standard' regimens include drugs active vs bacteria, fungi, pneumocystis, herpes simplex and CMV. Many use **TMP/SMX** 1 single-strength tab po qid for 4-12 mos. post-transplant. Special concern for CMV infection (see Comment)	Details of specific drugs and timing of administration vary from one transplant center to another. Representative regimen presented in AnlM 123:205, 1995. Similar regimen for solid organ transplants.
Solid organ transplants: liver, kidney, heart, lung (See CID 33:S26, 2001 & 32:596, 2001)		Range of opportunistic infections and variability in prophylaxis protocols is greater than in bone marrow recipients. For extent of infections, see NEJM 338:1741, 1998. For "optimal" CMV prophylaxis, see Transplantation 61:1279, 1996. Hard to define best regimens, as unethical to use placebo control. Ganciclovir better than acyclovir in prevention of CMV (Ln 346:69, 1995). Valacyclovir also effective (NEJM 340:1462, 1999).
Varicella-Zoster (see Table 14, page 108)		
Wegener's granulomatosis	**TMP/SMX** 800/160 tab po bid	Reduced relapses of pts in remission [18% (TMP/SMX) vs 40% (placebo)] over 24 months (NEJM 335:16, 1996)

TABLE 15B: SURGICAL ANTIBIOTIC PROPHYLAXIS (*MMWR* 48(15):316, 1999; *EID* 7:220, 2001)

Surgical Procedures: To be optimally effective, antibiotics must be started in the interval: 2 hrs before time of surgical incision (*NEJM* 326:281, 1992). For most procedures the number of doses needed for optimal coverage has not been defined. Current practice is to give a single dose (*Ln* 344:1547, 1994; *Med Lett* 43:92, 2001) although FDA-approved product labeling is often for 2 or more doses. If surgical procedure lasts >3 hrs, intraoperative doses should be given at approx. 3-hr intervals. (Note: The dose/route/durations listed below are for the most part those approved in FDA product labeling; these at times will differ from single-dose regimens, and the dosage & route are the same.)

TYPE OF SURGERY	PROPHYLAXIS	COMMENTS
Cardiovascular Surgery Antibiotic prophylaxis in cardiovascular surgery has been proven beneficial only in the following procedures: • Reconstruction of abdominal aorta • Procedures on the leg that involve a groin incision • Any vascular procedure that inserts prosthesis/foreign body • Lower extremity amputation for ischemia • Cardiac surgery • Perhaps permanent pacemakers (see *Comment*)	**Cefazolin** 1 gm IV as a single dose or q8h x1–2 d. or **cefuroxime** 1.5 gm IV as a single dose or q12h for total of 6 doses. **Dosage as with C-** section, above, except **cefazolin 1 gm** IV, repeat at 12–24 hrs (AAC 40:70, 1996) Consider **intranasal mupirocin** evening before, day of surgery add bid x5 days, post-op in pts with pos. nasal culture for S. aureus.	Single injection just before surgery probably as effective as multiple doses (*Eur J Cardiothor Surg* 9:840, 2000). Not recommended for cardiac catheterization. For prosthetic heart valves, customary to give a single dose (but only if coverage either after removal of retrosternal drainage catheters or just a 2nd dose after coming off bypass). Vancomycin may be preferable in hospitals with ↑ frequency of MRSA but no coverage for Gm-neg. bacilli, therefore would add cefazolin for groin incisions. A meta-analysis of 7 placebo-controlled randomized studies of antimicrobial prophylaxis for implantation of permanent pacemakers, sig. ↓ in incidence of infection (*Circ* 97:1796, 1998). Intranasal mupirocin ↓ sternal wound infections from S. aureus in 1850 pts; used historical controls (*Ann Thoracic Surg* 71:1572, 2001).
Gastric, Biliary and Colonic Surgery		
Gastroduodenal/Biliary Gastroduodenal, includes percutaneous endoscopic gastrostomy (high-risk only; see *Comments*) Biliary, includes laparoscopic cholecystectomy (high-risk only; see *Comments*)	**Cefazolin or cefoxitin or cefotetan or ceftizoxime or cefuroxime** 1.5 gm IV as a single dose (some give additional doses q12h x2–3 d.)	Gastroduodenal: High-risk is marked obesity, obstruction, ↓ gastric acid or ↓ GI motility. Biliary: Cephalosporins not active vs enterococci yet clinically effective as prophylaxis in biliary surgery. With cholangitis, treat as infection, not prophylaxis (*Cl-Cl*, 3.1 gm q4–6h IV or *PIP/T* 2.3.375 gm q6h or 4.5 gm q8h IV) or AM/SB 3.0 gm q4–6h IV. Biliary high-risk: age >70, acute cholecystitis, non-functioning gallbladder, obstructive jaundice or common duct stones. NOTE: Meta-analysis supports use in percutaneous endoscopic gastrostomy (*Am J Gastro* 93:2155, 1998).
Endoscopic retrograde cholangiopancreatography	No rx without obstruction. If obstruction: **Ciprofloxacin** 500 mg–1 gm po 2 hr prior to procedure	Most studies show that **achieving adequate drainage** will prevent postprocedural cholangitis or sepsis and no further benefit from prophylaxis. With inadequate drainage antibiotics may be of value. American Society for GI Endoscopy recommends use for known or suspected biliary obstruction (*CID* 23:380, 1996).
	Ceftizoxime 1.5 gm IV 1 hr prior to procedure or **Piperacillin** 4 gm IV 1 hr prior to procedure	Oral CIP as effective as cephalosporins in 2 studies & less expensive (*CID* 23:380, 1996).
Colorectal, Includes appendectomy Elective surgery	**Neomycin + erythromycin** po (see *Comment for dose*) **Cefazolin** 1–2 gm IV + **metronidazole** 0.5 gm IV (single dose) or **cefoxitin or cefotetan** 1–2 gm IV	Elective colorectal prep: Pre-op day: (1) 10 am 4 L polyethylene glycol electrolyte solution (GoLYTELY) po over 2 hr. (2) Clear liquid diet only. (3) 1 pm, 2 pm and 10 pm, neomycin 1 gm + erythro base 1 gm po. (4) NPO after midnight. There are alternative regimens which have been less well studied. GoLYTELY 1–6 pm, then neomycin 2 gm po + metronidazole 2 gm po at 7 am and 11 pm. Oral regimen as effective as parenteral. For emergency colorectal surgery, use parenteral.
Emergency surgery	**Cefoxitin** 2 gm IV then 1 gm IV q8h x 25 d. (base on clinical signs) or (**clindamycin** 600 mg IV q8h x 25 d.)	(*CID* 15:Suppl. 1:S313, 1992).
Ruptured viscus: See *Peritonitis, Table 1, p. 31*		
Head and Neck Surgery (*Ann Otol Rhinol Laryngol* 101:Suppl:16, 1992) (Prophylaxis in head & neck surgery is efficacious only for procedures involving oral/pharyngeal mucosa (i.e. laryngeal or pharyngeal tumor) but even with prophylaxis, wound infection rate high (41% in 1 center) (*Head Neck* 23:447, 2001). Uncontaminated head & neck surgery does not require prophylaxis.	**Cefazolin** 2 gm IV, then 1.0 gm IV q8h x 25 d. **Clindamycin** 600–900 mg IV (single dose) + **gentamicin** 1.5 mg/kg IV q8h) x 25 d.	
Neurosurgical Procedures [Prophylaxis not effective in ↓ infection rate with intracranial pressure monitors in retrospective analysis of 215 pts (*J Neurol Neurosurg Psych* 69:381, 2000). Clean (e.g. craniotomy) Clean contaminated (cross sinuses, or nasopharynx) CSF shunt surgery: controversial (Meta-analysis *CID* 17:98, 1993)	**Cefazolin** 1 gm IV, 1 dose. Alternative: **vanco** 1 gm IV x1. **Clindamycin** 900 mg IV (single dose) **Vancomycin** 10 mg into cerebral ventricles + **gentamicin** 3 mg into cerebral ventricles (*Ln* 344:1547, 1994)	Referenced: *Lancet* 344:1547, 1994; *Neurosurgery* 35:422, 1994. British trial: cefuroxime 1.5 gm IV + (cefuroxime 1.5 gm IV + metronidazole 0.5 gm) IV. Alternative: TMP/SMX (160 mg) + SMX (800 mg) IV pre-op and metronidazole 0.5 gm x3 doses. Efficacy when infection rate >15%. Alternative: TMP (160 mg) + SMX (800 mg) IV pre-op and metronidazole 0.5 gm x3 doses.

TABLE 15B (2)

TYPE OF SURGERY	PROPHYLAXIS	COMMENTS
Obstetric/Gynecologic Surgery		
Vaginal or abdominal hysterectomy	**Cefazolin** 1–2 gm or cefotixin 1–2 gm or **cefotetan** 1–2 gm or **cefoxitan** 1.5 gm all IV 30 min. before surgery. See Comment NOTE.	1 study found cefotetan superior to cefazolin (CID 20:677, 1995). For prolonged procedures, doses can be repeated q4–8h for duration of procedure. NOTE: Also approved is trovafloxacin 200 mg IV/po 1 to 2 hrs pre-op.
Cesarean section for premature rupture of membranes or active labor	**Cefazolin** x1, administer IV as soon as umbilical cord clamped.	Not effective in elective C-section in a large suggested double-blind randomized trial (BJOG 106:143, 2001). However, meta-analysis of 7 trials suggested benefit (Am J Ob Gyn 184:656, 2001).
Abortion	1st trimester: high-risk only (see Comments) aqueous penicillin G 1 million units IV or **doxycycline** 300 mg po. 2nd trimester: **cefazolin** 1 gm IV	High-risk: Pts with previous pelvic inflammatory disease, gonorrhea or multiple sexual partners (Drugs 41:19, 1991).
Orthopedic Surgery (Generally pts with prosthetic joints do not require prophylaxis for dental procedures. Individual considerations prevail (J Am Dental Assn 128:1004, 1997). See Table 1, pages 21, 22		
Hip arthroplasty, spinal fusion	Same as cardiac.	Customarily stopped after "Hemovac" removed.
Total joint replacement (other than hip)	**Cefazolin** 1–2 gm IV pre-op (± 2nd dose) or **vancomycin** 1 gm IV on call to OR	Post-op: some would give no further rx (Med Lett 39:98, 1997)
Open reduction of closed fracture with internal fixation	**Ceftriaxone** 2 gm IV or IM x1 dose	8.3% vs 3.6% (for placebo) reduction found in Dutch trauma trial (Lancet 347:1133, 1996).
Peritoneal Dialysis Catheter Placement	**Vancomycin** single 1000 mg dose 12 hrs prior to procedure	Effectively reduced peritonitis during 14 days post-placement in 221 pts: vanco 1%, cefazolin 7%, placebo 12% (p=0.02) (Am J Kidney Dis 36:1014, 2000).
Urologic Surgery/Procedures		
Antimicrobials not recommended in pts with sterile urine. Pts with pre-operative bacteriuria should be treated.	Recommended antibiotic to pts with pre-operative bacteriuria: **Cefazolin** 1 gm IV q8h x1–3 doses perioperatively, followed by oral antibiotics (**nitrofurantoin** or **TMP/SMX**) until catheter is removed or for 10 d.	
Transrectal prostate biopsy	**Ciprofloxacin** 500 mg po 12 hrs prior to biopsy and repeated 12 hrs after biopsy (levo, norflox should work)	CIP reduced bacteremia from 37% (in gentamicin-rx group) to 7% (Urology 38:84, 1991; and review in JAC 39:115, 1997).
Others		
Breast surgery, herniorrhaphy	**P: Ceph 1,2**, dosage as C-section above	
Traumatic (non-bite) wound	Either **cefazolin** 1 gm IV q8h or **ceftriaxone** 2 gm IV q24h x 25 d (base on clinical signs)	

TABLE 15C: ANTIMICROBIAL PROPHYLAXIS FOR THE PREVENTION OF BACTERIAL ENDOCARDITIS IN PATIENTS WITH UNDERLYING CARDIAC CONDITIONS

[These are the recommendations of the American Heart Association (JAMA 277:1794, 1997). However, a population-based prospective case-controlled study brings into serious question whether dental procedures predispose to endocarditis and whether antibiotic prophylaxis is of any value (see AnIM 129:761, 1998; Br Dent J 189:610, 2000)]

ENDOCARDITIS PROPHYLAXIS RECOMMENDED	ENDOCARDITIS PROPHYLAXIS NOT RECOMMENDED
Cardiac conditions associated with endocarditis	Negligible-risk (same as general population)
High-risk conditions:[1]	Atrial septal defect or repaired ASD/VSD, or PDA (beyond 6 months)
Prosthetic valves—both bioprosthetic and homograft	Previous CABG, mitral prolapse without MI
Previous bacterial endocarditis	Physiologic, functional, or innocent heart murmurs
Complex cyanotic congenital heart disease (CHD), e.g., single ventricle, transposition, tetralogy of Fallot	Previous Kawasaki or rheumatic fever without valve dysfunction
Surgically constructed systemic pulmonic shunts or conduits	Cardiac pacemakers (all) and implanted defibrillators
Moderate-risk conditions:	
Most other CHD, hypertrophic cardiac myopathy, mitral prolapse with regurgitation	

[1] Gentamicin (12.5 mg/gm of acrylic bone cement) is released for at least 3 weeks. Usefulness not proven.

[2] Some now recommend that prophylaxis prior to dental procedures should **only** be used for **extractions** and **gingival surgery** (including implant replacement) and **only** for patients with **prosthetic cardiac valves** or **previous endocarditis** (AnIM 129:829, 1998). If any of these 4 conditions exist = prophylactic antibiotics according to American Heart Association are recommended.

TABLE 15B (3)

ENDOCARDITIS PROPHYLAXIS RECOMMENDED	ENDOCARDITIS PROPHYLAXIS NOT RECOMMENDED

Dental and other procedures where prophylaxis is considered for patients with moderate- or high-risk cardiac conditions[1]
Dental: extractions, periodontal procedures[1]
  Implants, root canal, subgingival antibiotic fibers/strips
  Initial orthodontic bands (not brackets), intraligamentary local anesthetic
  Cleaning of teeth or implants where bleeding anticipated
Respiratory: T&A, surgery on respiratory mucosa, rigid bronchoscopy
GI: Sclerotherapy of esophageal varices; dilation of esophageal stricture; ERCP with biliary obstruction
  Biliary tract surgery on/through intestinal mucosa
GU: Prostate surgery, cystoscopy, urethral dilation
	Dental: Filling cavities with local anesthetic
	  Placement of rubber dams, suture removal, orthodontic removal
	  Orthodontic adjustments, dental x-rays
	  Shedding of primary teeth
	Respiratory: Endotracheal intubation, flexible bronchoscopy[2], tympanostomy tube
	  Transesophageal cardiac: ECHO[2], EGD[2] without biopsy
	GI: Vaginal hysterectomy[2], vaginal delivery[2], C-section
	GU: Uninfected: Foley catheter, uterine D&C, therapeutic abortion, tubal ligation, insert/remove IUD
	Other: Cardiac cath, balloon angioplasty, implanted pacemaker, defibrillators, coronary stents
	  Skin biopsy, circumcision

Abbreviations: CHD = cyanotic heart disease, **T&A** = tonsillectomy/adenoidectomy, **ERCP** = endoscopic retrograde cholangiography, **ASD/VSD** = atrial septal defect/ventricular septal defect, **PDA** = patent ductus arteriosus, **EGD** = esophagogastroduodenoscopy, **D&C** = dilation and curettage

PROPHYLACTIC REGIMENS FOR DENTAL, ORAL, RESPIRATORY TRACT, OR ESOPHAGEAL PROCEDURES

SITUATION	AGENT	REGIMEN[2]
Standard general prophylaxis	Amoxicillin	Adults 2 gm, children 50 mg/kg orally 1 hr before procedure
Unable to take oral medications	Ampicillin	Adults 2 gm IM or IV, children 50 mg/kg IM or IV within 30 min. before procedure
Allergic to penicillin	Clindamycin, OR	Adults 600 mg, children 20 mg/kg orally 1 hr before procedure
	(Cephalexin[3], or cefadroxil[3])[4], OR	Adults 2 gm, children 50 mg/kg orally 1 hr before procedure
	Azithromycin or clarithromycin	Adults 500 mg, children 15 mg/kg orally 1 hr before procedure
Allergic to penicillin and unable to take oral medications	Clindamycin, OR	Adults 600 mg, chidren 20 mg/kg IV within 30 min. before procedure
	Cefazolin[4]	Adults 1 gm, children 25 mg/kg IM or IV within 30 min. before procedure

PROPHYLACTIC REGIMENS FOR GENITOURINARY/GASTROINTESTINAL (EXCLUDING ESOPHAGEAL) PROCEDURES[5]

SITUATION	AGENT[2]	REGIMEN[5]
High-risk patients	Ampicillin + gentamicin	**Adults: ampicillin** 2 gm IM or IV + **gentamicin** 1.5 mg/kg (not to exceed 120 mg) within 30 min. of starting the procedure; 6 hr later, **ampicillin** 1 gm IM/IV or **amoxicillin** 1 gm orally **Children: ampicillin** 50 mg/kg IM or IV (not to exceed 2.0 gm) + **gentamicin** 1.5 mg/kg IM or IV within 30 min. of starting the procedure; 6 hrs later, **ampicillin** 25 mg/kg IM/IV or **amoxicillin** 25 mg/kg orally
High-risk patients allergic to ampicillin/amoxicillin	Vancomycin + gentamicin	**Adults: vancomycin** 1 gm IV over 1–2 hrs + **gentamicin** 1.5 mg/kg IV/IM; complete injection/infusion within 30 min. of starting the procedure. **Children: vancomycin** 20 mg/kg IV over 1–2 hrs + **gentamicin** 1.5 mg/kg IV/IM (not to exceed 120 mg); complete injection/infusion within 30 min. of starting the procedure
Moderate-risk patients	Amoxicillin or ampicillin	**Adults: amoxicillin** 2 gm orally 1 hr before procedure, or **ampicillin** 2 gm IM/IV within 30 min. of starting the procedure **Children: amoxicillin** 50 mg/kg orally 1 hr before procedure, or **ampicillin** 50 mg/kg IM/IV within 30 min. of starting the procedure
Moderate-risk patients allergic to ampicillin/ amoxicillin	Vancomycin	**Adults: vancomycin** 1 gm IV over 1–2 hrs; complete infusion within 30 min. of starting the procedure **Children: vancomycin** 20 mg/kg IV over 1–2 hrs; complete infusion within 30 min. of starting the procedure

[1] Some now recommend that prophylaxis prior to dental procedures should **only** be used for **extractions** and **gingival surgery** (including implant replacement) and **only** for patients with **prosthetic cardiac valves** or **previous endocarditis** (AHA 129:829, 1998). If any of these 4 conditions exist = prophylactic antibiotics according to American Heart Association are recommended.

[2] Prophylaxis optional for high-risk patients

[3] Total children's dose should not exceed adult dose

[4] Cephalosporins should not be used in individuals with immediate-type hypersensitivity reaction (urticaria, angioedema, or anaphylaxis) to penicillins.

[5] No second dose of vancomycin or gentamicin is recommended.

TABLE 16: PEDIATRIC DOSAGES OF SELECTED ANTIBACTERIAL AGENTS
[Adapted from: (1) Nelson's Pocket Book of Pediatric Antimicrobial Therapy, 2002-2003, 15th Ed., J. Bradley & J. Nelson, eds., Lippincott Williams and Wilkins, (2) 1997 Red Book, 24th Ed., American Academy of Pediatrics, pages 607-636, and (3) Mayo Clin. Proc. 75:86, 2000]

DRUG		DOSES IN MG/KG/D OR MG/KG AT FREQUENCY INDICATED[1]			
		BODY WEIGHT <2000 gm		BODY WEIGHT >2000 gm	>28 DAYS OLD
		0–7 days old	8–28 days old	0–7 days old	8–28 days old	

DRUG		0–7 days old (<2000)	8–28 days old (<2000)	0–7 days old (>2000)	8–28 days old (>2000)	>28 DAYS OLD
Aminoglycosides, IV or IM (check levels; some dose by gestational age + wks of life; see Nelson's Pocket Book, page 19)						
Amikacin		7.5 q18–24h	7.5 q12h	10 q12h	10 q12h	10 q8h
Gent/tobra		2.5 q18–24h	2.5 q12h	2.5 q12h	2.5 q12h	2.5 q8h
Aztreonam, IV		30 q12h	30 q8h	30 q8h	30 q6h	30 q6h
Cephalosporins						
Cefaclor						20–40 div tid
Cefadroxil						30 div bid (max 2 g/d)
Cefazolin		20 q12h	20 q12h	20 q12h	20 q8h	20 q8h
Cefdinir						7 q12h or 14 qd
Cefepime						150 div q8h
Cefixime						8 as qd or div bid
Cefotaxime		50 q12h	50 q8h	50 q12h	50 q8h	50 q6h (75 q6h for meningitis)
Cefoxitin			20 q12h			80–160 div q6h
Cefpodoxime						10 div (max 400 mg/d)
Cefprozil						15–30 div bid (max 1 g/d)
Ceftazidime		50 q12h	50 q8h	50 q12h	50 q8h	50 q8h
Ceftibuten						4.5 bid
Ceftizoxime						33–66 q8h
Ceftriaxone		50 qd	50 qd	50 qd	75 qd	50–75 qd (meningitis 100)
Cefuroxime	IV	50 q12h	50 q8h	50 q8h	50 q8h	50 q8h (80 q8h for meningitis)
	po					10–15 div (max 1 g/d)
Cephalexin						25–50 div 4x/d (max 4 g/d)
Loracarbef						15–30 div bid (max 0.8 g/d)
Chloramphen.	IV	25 q24h	25 q24h	25 q24h	15 q12h	12.5–25 q6h (max 2–4 g/d)
Clindamycin	IV	5 q12h	5 q8h	5 q8h	5 q6h	7.5 q6h
	po					5–6 q8h
Ciprofloxacin	po[2]					20–30 div bid (max 1.5 g/d)
Imipenem[3]	IV			25 q12h	25 q8h	15–25 q6h (max 2 g/d)
Macrolides						
Erythro	IV & po	10 q12h	10 q8h	10 q12h	13 q8h	10 q6h
Azithro	po					10–12 day 1, then 5/d[4]
Clarithro	po					7.5 q12h (max. 1 g/d)
Meropenem	IV	20 q12h	20 q8h	20 q12h	20 q8h	60–120 div q8h (120 for meningitis)
Metro	IV & po	7.5 q24h	7.5 q12h	7.5 q12h	15 q12h	7.5 q8h
Penicillins						
Ampicillin		50 q12h	50 q8h	50 q8h	50 q6h	50 q6h
Amp-sulbactam						100–300 div q6h
Amoxicillin	po					25–50 div bid
Amox-Clav	po	30 div bid	30 div bid	30 div bid	30 div bid	45 or 90 (AM/CL-HD) div bid over 12 wks
Cloxacillin						50–100 div 4x/d
Dicloxacillin						12–25 div 4x/d
Mezlocillin		75 q12h	75 q8h	75 q12h	75 q8h	75 q6h
Nafcillin,oxacillin	IV	25 q12h	25 q8h	25 q8h	37 q6h	37 q6h (to max. 8–12 gm/d)
Piperacillin, PIP/tazo	IV	75 mg/kg q12h	75 mg/kg q12h	75 mg/kg q12h	75 mg/kg q8h	100–300 div q4–6h
Ticarcillin, T.clav	IV	75 q12h	75 q8h	75 q8h	75 q6h	75 q6h
Penicillin G, U/kg	IV	50,000 q12h	75,000 q8h	50,000 q8h	50,000 q6h	50,000 U/kg/d
Penicillin V						25–50 mg/kg/d div 3–4x/d
Rifampin	po			10, single dose	20, single dose	20, single dose (max. 600 mg)
Sulfisoxazole	po				120–150	120–150 mg/kg/d div q4–6h
TMP/SMX po,IV; UTI: 8–12 TMP component div bid; Pneumocystis: 20 TMP component div 4x/d						
Tetracycline po (age 8 or older)						25–50 div 4x/d
Doxycycline po,IV (age 8 or older)						2–4 div bid
Vancomycin	IV	12.5 q12h	15 q12h	18 q12h	22 q12h	40–60 div q6h

Abbreviations: **Chloramphen** = chloramphenicol; **Clav** = clavulanate; **div** = divided; **Gent/tobra** = gentamicin/tobramycin; **Metro** = metronidazole; **Tazo** = tazobactam; **TMP** = trimethoprim; **TMP/SMX** = trimethoprim/sulfamethoxazole; **UTI** = urinary tract infection

[1] May need higher doses in patients with meningitis.
[2] With exception of cystic fibrosis, not approved for use under age 18.
[3] Not recommended in children with CNS infections due to risk of seizures.
[4] Dose for otitis; for pharyngitis, 12 mg/kg x5 d.

TABLE 17A: DOSAGE OF ANTIMICROBIAL DRUGS IN ADULT PATIENTS WITH RENAL IMPAIRMENT

Adapted from Drug Prescribing in Renal Failure, 4th Ed., Aronoff et al (Eds.), American College of Physicians, 1999 and Berns et al, Renal Aspects of Antimicrobial Therapy for HIV Infection. In: P. Kimmel &
J. Berns, Eds., HIV Infection and the Kidney, Churchill-Livingstone, 1995, pp. 195–236.

UNLESS STATED, ADJUSTED DOSES ARE % OF DOSE FOR NORMAL RENAL FUNCTION.
Drug adjustments are based on the patient's estimated endogenous creatinine clearance, which can be calculated as:

Ideal body weight for men: 50.0 kg + 2.3 kg per inch over 5 feet
Ideal body weight for women: 45.5 kg + 2.3 kg per inch over 5 feet

$$\frac{(140-age)(ideal\ body\ weight\ in\ kg)}{(72)(serum\ creatinine,\ mg/dL)}\ \ for\ men\ (x\ 0.85\ for\ women)$$

NOTE: For the following drugs, there is no need for adjustment of dosage in patients with renal impairment: abacavir, amphotericin B, amprenavir, azithromycin, caspofungin, ceftriaxone, chloramphenicol, ciprofloxacin-ER, clindamycin, delavirdine, dirithromycin, doxycycline, efavirenz, lopinavir, minocycline, nafcillin, nevirapine, pyrimethamine, rifabutin, rifapentine, trovafloxacin, voriconazole po (not IV form)

ANTIMICROBIAL	HALF-LIFE (NORMAL/ESRD) hr	DOSE FOR NORMAL RENAL FUNCTION[1]	METHOD* (see footnote)	ADJUSTMENT FOR RENAL FAILURE Estimated creatinine clearance (CrCl), ml/min			SUPPLEMENT FOR HEMODIALYSIS, CAPD[‡] (see footnote)	COMMENTS AND DOSAGE FOR CAVH
				>50-90	10-50	<10		
ANTIBACTERIAL ANTIBIOTICS								
Aminoglycoside Antibiotics:		Traditional multiple daily doses—adjustment for renal disease						High-flux hemodialysis membranes lead to unpredictable aminoglycoside clearance, measure post-dialysis drug levels for efficacy and toxicity. With CAPD, pharmacokinetics highly variable—check serum levels. Usual method for CAPD: 2 liters of dialysis fluid (dialysate), 3–4 liters/day (give 8x20 mg lost/L = 160 mg of amikacin supplement IV per day) [Adjust dosing weight for obesity; ideal body weight + 0.4 (actual body weight – ideal body weight)] (CID 25:112, 1997).
Amikacin	1.4–4.2/17–150	7.5 mg/kg q12h	D&I	60-90% q12h	30-70% q12-18h **Same dose for CAVH‡**	20-30% q24-48h	HEMO: Extra ½ of normal renal function dose AD‡ CAPD: 15–20 mg lost/L dialysate/day‡ (see Comment)	
Gentamicin, Tobramycin	2-3/20–60	1.7 mg/kg q8h	D&I	60-90% q8-12h	30-70% q12h **Same dose for CAVH‡**	20-30% q24-48h	HEMO: Extra ½ of normal renal function dose AD‡ CAPD: 3–4 mg lost/L dialysate/day	
Netilmicin[NUS]	2-3/35–72	2.0 mg/kg q8h	D&I	50-90% q8-12h	20-60% q12h **Same dose for CAVH‡**	10-20% q24-48h	HEMO: Extra ½ of normal renal function dose AD‡ CAPD: 3–4 mg lost/L dialysate/day	
Streptomycin	2-3/30–80	15 mg/kg (max. of 1.0 gm) q24h	I	50% q24h	q24-72h **Same dose for CAVH‡**	q72-96h	HEMO: Extra ½ of normal renal function dose AD‡ CAPD: 20–40 mg lost/L dialysate/day	
Once-daily aminoglycoside therapy: adjustment in renal insufficiency (NEJM 336:1303, 1997) usually results in CrCl of approx. 30 ml/min.							**See Table 9C for OD dosing/normal renal function**	
Creatinine Clearance (ml/min.)				40-60	20-30	<10		
				Dose q24h (mg/kg)	Dose q24h (mg/kg)	Dose q48h (mg/kg)		
Gentamicin/Tobramycin		5.1		3.5	4	3		
Amikacin/Kanamycin/streptomycin		15		7.5	7.5	4		
Isepamicin[NUS]		8		8	8	8 q48h		
Netilmicin[NUS]		6.5		4	2.5	2.0		
Carbapenem Antibiotics								
Ertapenem	4/>4	1.0 gm q24h	D	1.0 gm q24h	0.5 gm q24h (CrCl <30)	0.5 gm q24h	HEMO: Dose as for CrCl <10; if dosed <6 hrs prior to HD, give 150 mg supplement AD	↑ potential for seizures if recommended doses exceeded in pts with CrCl <20 ml/min. See pkg insert, esp. for pts <70 kg
Imipenem (see Comment)	1/4	0.5 gm q6h	D&I	250-500 mg q6-8h	250 mg q8-12h **Same dose for CAVH**	125-250 mg q12h	HEMO: Dose AD CAPD: Dose for CrCl <10	
Meropenem	1/6-8	1.0 gm q8h	D&I	1.0 gm q8h	1.0 gm q12h **Same dose for CAVH**	0.5 gm q24h	HEMO: Dose AD CAPD: Dose for CrCl <10	

‡ **CAVH** = continuous arteriovenous hemofiltration (NEJM 336:1303, 1997) usually results in CrCl of approx. 30 ml/min. **AD** = after dialysis. "Dose AD" refers only to timing of dose with NO extra drug. **Supplement** is to replace drug lost via dialysis; extra drug lost beyond continuation of regimen used for CrCl <10 ml/min.
See page 131 for other footnotes and abbreviations.

127

TABLE 17A (2)

ANTIMICROBIAL	HALF-LIFE (NORMAL/ESRD) hr	DOSE FOR NORMAL RENAL FUNCTION†	METHOD* (see footnote)	ADJUSTMENT FOR RENAL FAILURE Estimated creatinine clearance (CrCl), ml/min			SUPPLEMENT FOR HEMODIALYSIS, CAPD† (see footnote)	COMMENTS AND DOSAGE FOR CAVH
				>50-90	10-50	<10		
Cephalosporin Antibiotics: DATA ON SELECTED PARENTERAL CEPHALOSPORINS								
Cefazolin	1.9/40-70	1.0-2.0 gm q8h		q8h	q12h	q24-48h	HEMO: Extra 0.5-1 gm AD CAPD: 0.5 gm q12h	
					Same dose for CAVH			
Cefepime	2.2/18	2.0 gm q8h (max. dose)	D&I	2 gm q8-12h	2 gm q12-24h	1 gm q24h	HEMO: Extra 1 gm AD CAPD: 1-2 gm q48h	CAVH not recommended
Cefotaxime, Ceftizoxime	1.7/15-35	2.0 gm q8h	I	q8-12h	q12-24h	q24h	HEMO: Extra 1 gm AD CAPD: 0.5-1 gm qd	Active metabolite of cefotaxime in ESRD. ↓ dose further for hepatic & renal failure.
Cefotetan	3.5/13-25	1-2 gm q12h	D	100%	50%	25%	HEMO: Extra 1 gm AD CAPD: 1 gm qd	CAVH: 750 mg q12h
Cefoxitin	0.8/13-23	2.0 gm q8h	I	q8h	q8-12h	q24-48h	HEMO: Extra 1 gm AD CAPD: 1 gm qd	May falsely increase serum creatinine by interference with assay.
					Same dose for CAVH			
Ceftazidime	1.2/13-25	2 gm q8h	I	q8-12h	q24-48h	q48h	HEMO: Extra 1 gm AD CAPD: 0.5 gm qd	Volume of distribution increases with infection.
					Same dose for CAVH			
Cefuroxime sodium	1.2/17	0.75-1.5 gm q8h	I	q8h	q8-12h	q8-12h	HEMO: Dose AD† CAPD: Dose for CrCl <10	For CAVH: 1.5 gm, then 750 mg IV q24h
Fluoroquinolone Antibiotics								
Ciprofloxacin	4/6-9	500-750 mg po (or 400 mg IV) q12h	D	100%	50-75%	50%	HEMO: 250 mg po or 200 mg IV q12h CAPD: 250 mg po or 200 mg IV q8h	CAVH: 200 mg IV q12h
Gatifloxacin	7-14/36	400 mg po/IV q24h	D	100%	400 mg q24h	200 mg q24h	HEMO: 200 mg q24h AD CAPD: 200 mg q24h	CAVH: As for CrCl 10-50
Levofloxacin	4-8/76	500 mg po/IV q24h	D†	100%	500 mg x1, then 250 mg q24-48h	500 mg x1, then 250 mg q48h	HEMO/CAPD: Dose for CrCl <10	CAVH: As for CrCl 10-50
Ofloxacin	7.0/28-37	400 mg po/IV q12h	D&I	100%	200-400 mg q12h	200 mg q24h	HEMO: 100-200 mg q24h CAPD: Dose for CrCl <10	CAVH: 300 mg/d
Macrolide Antibiotics								
Clarithromycin	5-7/22	0.5-1.0 gm q12h	D	100%	75%	50-75%	HEMO: Dose AD CAPD: None	ESRD dosing recommendations based on extrapolation
Erythromycin	1.4/5-6	250-500 mg q6h	I	100%	100%	50-75%	HEMO/CAPD/CAVH: None	Ototoxicity with high doses in ESRD. Vol. of distribution increases in ESRD
Miscellaneous Antibacterial Antibiotics								
Linezolid	6.4/7.1	600 mg po/IV q12h	None	600 mg q12h	600 mg q12h	600 mg q12h AD	HEMO: As for CrCl <10 CAPD: No data	CAVH: No data. Accumulation of 2 metabolites—risk unknown.
Metronidazole	6-14/7-21	7.5 mg/kg q6h	D	100%	100%	50%	HEMO: Dose AD CAPD: Dose for CrCl <10	Hemo clears metronidazole and its metabolites (AAC 29:235, 1986)
					Same dose for CAVH			
Nitrofurantoin	0.5/1	50-100 mg q6h	D	100%	Avoid	Avoid	Not applicable CAPD:	
					Same dose for CAVH			
Sulfamethoxazole	10/20-50	1.0 gm q8h	D	q12h	q18h	q24h	HEMO: Extra 1 gm AD CAPD: Dose for CrCl <10	
					Same dose for CAVH			
Teicoplanin[NUS]	45/62-230	6 mg/kg/day	I	q24h	q48h	q72h	HEMO: Dose for CrCl <10 CAPD: Dose for CrCl <10	
Telithromycin	10/15	800 mg qd	I	800 mg qd	400 mg qd (<30 ml/min)	400 mg qd	HEMO: 800 mg AD CAPD: No data	

† Regardless of CrCl, 1st dose is 500 mg, and then adjust dose and interval

‡ CAVH = continuous arteriovenous hemofiltration (NEJM 336:1303, 1997) usually results in CrCl of approx. 30 ml/min; AD = after dialysis. **"Dose AD"** refers only to timing of dose with **NO extra drug.**

See page 131 for other footnotes and abbreviations. **Supplement is to replace drug lost via dialysis; extra drug beyond continuation of regimen used for CrCl <10 ml/min.**

TABLE 17A (3)

ANTIMICROBIAL	HALF-LIFE (NORMAL/ESRD) hr	DOSE FOR NORMAL RENAL FUNCTION‡	METHOD* (see footnote)	ADJUSTMENT FOR RENAL FAILURE Estimated creatinine clearance (CrCl), ml/min >50-90	10-50	<10	SUPPLEMENT FOR HEMODIALYSIS, CAPD† (see footnote)	COMMENTS AND DOSAGE FOR CAVH
Miscellaneous Antibacterial Antibiotics (continued)								
Trimethoprim	11/20-49	100-200 mg q12h	I	q12h	q18h	q24h	HEMO: Dose AD CAPD: q24h	CAVH: q18h
Vancomycin[1]	6/200-250	1 gm q12h	I	q12h	q18h	1 gm q4-7 d.	HEMO/CAPD:Dose for CrCl <10	CAVH: 500 mg q24-48h. New hemodialysis membranes ↑ clear. of vanco; check levels
Penicillins								
Ampicillin	1.0/7-20	250-500 mg q8h		q8h	q8-12h	q12-24h	HEMO: Dose AD‡ CAPD: 250 mg q12h	IV amoxicillin not available in the U.S.
Amoxicillin	1.0/7-20	250 mg-2 gm q8h		q8h	q6-12h	q12-24h		
Amoxicillin/ Clavulanate	1.3 AM/1.0 5.0/20-60 (CL)	500/125 mg q8h (see Comments)	D&I	500/125 mg q8h	250-500 mg AM component q12h	250-500 mg AM component q24h	HEMO: As for CrCl <10; extra dose after dialysis CAPD: Dose for CrCl <10	If CrCl <30/ml, do not use 875/125 or 1000/62.5 AM/CL products
Ampicillin (AM) Sulbactam(SB)	1.0 (AM)/1.0 (SB) 9.0 (AM)/10.0 (SB)	2 gm AM + 1.0 gm SB q6h	I	q6h	q8-12h	q24h	HEMO: Dose AD CAPD: 2 gm AM/1 gm SB q24h	CAVH: 1.5 AM/0.75 SB q12h
Aztreonam	2.0/6-8	2 gm q8h	D	100%	50-75%	25%	HEMO: Extra 0.5 gm AD CAPD: Dose for CrCl <10	Technically is a β-lactam antibiotic.
Mezlocillin	1.1/2.6-5.4	1.5-4.0 gm q4-6h	I	q4-6h	q6-8h	q8h	HEMO/CAPD/CAVH: None	1.9 mEq sodium/gm. Reduce dose further for liver and kidney disease.
Penicillin G	0.5/6-20	0.5-4 million U q4h	D	100%	75%	20-50%	HEMO: Dose for CrCl <10 CAPD: Dose for CrCl <10	1.7 mEq potassium/mU. ↑ potential for seizures. 6 mU/d upper limit dose in ESRD.
Piperacillin	1.0/3.3-5.1	3-4 gm q4-6h	I	q4-6h	q6-8h	q8h	HEMO: Dose AD CAPD: Dose for CrCl <10	1.9 mEq sodium/gm
Pip (P)/Tazo(T)	1.0 P/1.0 T 3.0 P/4.0 T	3.375 gm q6h	D&I	3.375 gm q6h	2.25 gm q6h	2.25 gm q8h	HEMO: Dose for CrCl <10 + 0.75 gm AD CAPD: Dose for CrCl <10	
Ticarcillin	1.2/13	3 gm q4h	D&I	1-2 gm q4h	1-2 gm q8h	1-2 gm q12h	HEMO: Extra 3.0 gm AD CAPD: Dose for CrCl <10	5.2 mEq sodium/gm
Ticarcillin/ Clavulanate	1.0 (TC)/13 (CL) 13 (TC)/4.0 (CL)	3.1 gm q4h	D&I	3.1 gm q4-6h	2.0 gm q4-8h	2.0 gm q12h	HEMO: Extra 3.1 gm AD CAPD: 3.1 gm q12h	
Tetracycline Antibiotics								
Tetracycline	6-10/57-108	250-500 mg qid	I	q8-12h	q12-24h	q24h	HEMO/CAPD/CAVH: None	Avoid in ESRD
ANTIFUNGAL ANTIBIOTICS								
Amphotericin B & amphotericin B lipid complex	24/unchanged	Non-lipid: 0.4-1.0 mg/kg/d ABCD:2 3-6 mg/kg/d ABLC:3 5 mg/kg/d LAB:3 3-5 mg/kg/d		q24h	q24h	q24-48h	HEMO: None CAPD: Dose for CrCl <10	For ampho B, toxicity lessened by saline loading; risk amplified by concomitant cyclosporine A, aminoglycosides, or pentamidine
Fluconazole	37/100	200-400 mg q24h	D	200-400 mg	100-200 mg	100-200 mg	HEMO: 100% of recommended dose AD CAPD: Dose for CrCl <10	
Flucytosine	3-6/75-200	37.5 mg/kg q6h	I	q12h	q12-24h	q24h	HEMO: Dose for CrCl <10 CAPD: 0.5-1.0 gm q24h	Goal is peak serum level >25 µg/ml and <100 µg/ml

1 Vancomycin serum levels may be overestimated in renal failure if measured by either fluorescence polarization immunoassay or radioimmunoassay; vanco breakdown products interfere. EMIT method OK.
2 ABCD = ampho B cholesteryl complex; ABLC = ampho B lipid complex; LAB = liposomal ampho B
‡ **CAVH** = continuous arteriovenous hemofiltration (NEJM 336:1303, 1997) usually requires, in CrCl range (approx. 30 ml/min), dose of drug given in CrCl 10-50 ml/min range.
See page 131 for other footnotes and abbreviations.

TABLE 17A (4)

ANTIMICROBIAL	HALF-LIFE (NORMAL/ESRD) hr	DOSE FOR NORMAL RENAL FUNCTION	METHOD* (see footnote)	ADJUSTMENT FOR RENAL FAILURE Estimated creatinine clearance (CrCl), ml/min			SUPPLEMENT FOR HEMODIALYSIS, CAPD‡ (see footnote)	COMMENTS AND DOSAGE FOR CAVH
				>50-90	10-50	<10		
ANTIFUNGAL ANTIBIOTICS (continued)								
Itraconazole, po soln	35/–	100-200 mg q12h	–	100%	100%	100%	HEMO/CAPD/CAVH: No adjustment with oral solution	
Itraconazole, IV	35/–	200 mg IV q12h	–	200 mg IV bid	Do not use IV itra if CrCl <30 due to accumulation of carrier- cyclodextrin			
Terbinafine	36-200?	250 mg po/day	–	q24h	Use has not been studied. Recommend avoidance of drug.			
Voriconazole, IV	Non-linear kinetics	6 mg/kg IV q12h x2, then 4 mg/kg q12h	–	No change	If CrCl <50 ml/min., accum. of IV vehicle (cyclodextrin). Switch to po or DC			
ANTIPARASITIC ANTIBIOTICS								
Pentamidine	29/118	4 mg/kg/d	I	q24h	q24h	q24-36h	HEMO/CAPD/CAVH: None	
Quinine	5-16/5-16	650 mg q8h	I	650 mg q8h Same dose for CAVH	650 mg q8-12h Same dose for CAVH	650 mg q24h	HEMO: Dose AD‡ CAPD: Dose for CrCl <10	Marked tissue accumulation
ANTITUBERCULOUS ANTIBIOTICS (Excellent review: Nephron 64:169, 1993)								
Ethambutol	4/7-15	15-25 mg/kg q24h	I	q24h Same dose for CAVH	q24-36h	q48h	HEMO: Dose AD‡ CAPD: Dose for CrCl <10	25 mg/kg 4-6 hr prior to dialysis for usual 3x/wk dialysis. Streptomycin recommended in lieu of ethambutol in renal failure.
Ethionamide	2.1/?	250-500 mg q12h	D	100%	100%	50%	HEMO/CAPD/CAVH: None	
Isoniazid	0.7-4/8-17	5 mg/kg (max. 300 mg)	D	100%	100%	100%	HEMO/CAPD/CAVH: Dose for CrCl <10	
Pyrazinamide	9/26	25 mg/kg q24h (max. dose 2.5 gm qd)	D	25 mg/kg q24h	12-25 mg/kg q24h		HEMO: 25-35 mg/kg after each dialysis CAPD: None CAVH: No data	
Rifampin	1.5-5/1.8-11	600 mg/d	D	600 mg q24h	300-600 mg q24h	300-600 mg q24h	HEMO/CAPD: Dose for CrCl <10	Biologically active metabolite
ANTIVIRAL AGENTS								
Acyclovir, IV	2.5/20	5-12.4 mg/kg q8h	D&I	5-12.4 mg/kg q8h	5-12.4 mg/kg q12-24h	2.5 mg/kg q24h	HEMO: Dose AD‡ CAPD: Dose for CrCl <10	Rapid IV infusion can cause renal failure. CAVH: 3.5 mg/kg/d
Adefovir	12/500	10 mg po qd	I	10 mg qd	10 mg q48-72h	10 mg q7 days	HEMO: Dose AD‡ CAPD: q/d AD	
Amantadine	12/500	100 mg po bid	I	100 mg bid	q48-72h	q7	HEMO/CAPD/CAVH: None	
Cidofovir: Complicated dosing—see package insert								
Induction	2.5/unknown	5 mg/kg 1x/wk for 2 wks	–	5 mg/kg 1x/wk	0.5-2 mg/kg 1x/wk	0.5 mg/kg 1x/wk	No data	Major toxicity is renal. No efficacy, safety, or pharmacokinetic data in pts with moderate/severe renal disease.
Maintenance	2.5/unknown	5 mg/kg q2wks	–	5 mg/kg q2wks	0.5-2 mg/kg q2wks	0.5 mg/kg q2wks	No data	
Didanosine tablets	0.6-1.6/4.5	125-200 mg q12h buffered tabs	D	200 mg q12h	200 mg q24h	<60 kg: 150 mg q24h >60 kg: 100 mg q24h	HEMO: Dose AD‡ CAPD/CAVH: Dose for CrCl <10	Based on incomplete data. Data are estimates.
		400 mg qd enteric-coated tabs	D	400 mg qd	125-200 mg q12-24h	Do not use EC tabs	HEMO/CAPD: Dose for CrCl <10	If <60 kg & CrCl <10 ml/min, do not use EC tabs
Famciclovir	2.3-3.0/10-22	500 mg q8h	D&I	500 mg q8h	500 mg q12-24h	250 mg q24h	HEMO: Dose AD‡ CAPD: No data	CAVH: Dose for CrCl <10-50

† Ref. for NRTIs and NNRTIs: the NNRTIs.

‡ **CAVH** = continuous arteriovenous hemofiltration. *Kidney International* 60:821, 2001 ... usually results in CrCl of approx. 30 ml/min., **AD** = after dialysis. **"Dose AD"** refers only to timing of dose with NO extra drug; extra drug lost via dialysis; **Supplement is to replace drug lost via dialysis; extra drug beyond continuation of regimen used for CrCl <10 ml/min.**
See page 131 for other footnotes and abbreviations.

TABLE 17A (5)

ANTIMICROBIAL	HALF-LIFE (NORMAL/ESRD) hr	DOSE FOR NORMAL RENAL FUNCTION†	METHOD* (see footnote)	ADJUSTMENT FOR RENAL FAILURE Estimated creatinine clearance (CrCl), ml/min			SUPPLEMENT FOR HEMODIALYSIS, CAPD‡ (see footnote)	COMMENTS AND DOSAGE FOR CAVH
				>50-90	10-50	<10		

ANTIVIRAL AGENTS (continued)

Foscarnet (CMV) dosage adjustment based on est. CrCl (ml/min) div. by pt's kg — Half-life (Normal/ESRD): Normal half-life (T½) 3 hrs with terminal T½ of 18-88 hrs. T½ very long with ESRD.

Dose for normal renal function: Induction: 60 mg/kg q8h×2-3 wks; Maintenance 90-120 mg/kg/d IV.

Adjustment — CrCl as ml/min/kg body weight—ONLY FOR FOSCARNET:

	>1.4	>1.0-1.4	>0.8-1.0	>0.6-0.8	>0.5-0.6	>0.4-0.5	<0.4
Induction (60 mg/kg)	60 q8h	45 q8h	50 q12h	40 q12h	60 q24h	50 q24h	Do not use
Maintenance (90-120 mg/kg IV)	120 q24h	90 q24h	65 q24h	105 q48h	80 q48h	65 q48h	Do not use

Comments: See package insert for further details

ANTIMICROBIAL	HALF-LIFE (NORMAL/ESRD) hr	DOSE FOR NORMAL RENAL FUNCTION†	METHOD*	>50-90	10-50	<10	SUPPLEMENT FOR HEMODIALYSIS, CAPD‡	COMMENTS AND DOSAGE FOR CAVH
Ganciclovir	2.9/30	IV: Induction 5 mg/kg q12h IV; Maintenance 5 mg/kg q24h IV; po: 1.0 gm tid po	D&I	5 mg/kg q12h; 2.5-5.0 mg/kg q24h; 0.5-1.0 gm tid	2.5-5.0 mg/kg q24h; 0.6-1.25 mg/kg q24h; 0.5-1.0 gm q24h	1.25-2.5 mg/kg 3x/week; 0.625 mg/kg 3x/week; 0.5 gm 3x/week	HEMO: Dose AD†; CAPD: Dose for CrCl <10. HEMO: 0.6 mg/kg AD; CAPD: Dose for CrCl <10. HEMO: 0.5 gm AD; CAPD: Dose for CrCl <10	
Indinavir/nelfinavir/nevirapine		No data on influence of renal insufficiency. Less than 20% excreted unchanged in urine. Probably no dose reduction					HEMO/CAPD/CAVH: No data	
Lamivudine	5-7/15-35	150 mg bid po	D&I	150 mg bid	150 mg qd	25-50 mg qd	HEMO: Dose AD†; CAPD/CAVH: No data	
Oseltamivir	1-3/no data	75 mg bid po	D	75 mg bid	75 mg qd	No data	No data	
Ribavirin		Use with caution in patients with creatinine clearance <10 ml/min.						
Rimantadine	13-65/Prolonged	100 mg bid po	D&I	100 mg bid	100 mg qd-bid	100 mg qd	HEMO/CAPD: No data	Use with caution, little data
Ritonavir & Saquinavir, SGC ‡	1-1.4/5.8			Negligible renal clearance. At present, no patient data.			HEMO/CAPD: No data recommended	
Stavudine, po †		30-40 mg q12h	D&I	100%	50% q12-24h		HEMO: Dose as for CrCl <10 AD†; CAPD: No data	CAVH: Dose for CrCl 10-50
Tenofovir		300 mg q24h	D	300 mg q24h	DO NOT USE IF CrCl <60 ml/min		HEMO: No data	CAVH: No data. Dose for CrCl 10-50
Valacyclovir †	2.5-3.3/14	1.0 gm q8h	D&I	1.0 gm q8h	1.0 gm q12-24h	0.5 gm q24h	HEMO: Dose AD†; CAPD: Dose for CrCl <10	CAVH: Dose for CrCl 10-50
Zalcitabine †	2.0/>8	0.75 mg q8h	D&I	0.75 mg q8h	0.75 mg q12h	0.75 mg q24h	HEMO: Dose AD†; CAPD: No data	CAVH: Dose for CrCl 10-50
Zidovudine †	1.1-1.4/1.4-3	200 mg q8h or 300 mg q12h	D&I	200 mg q8h or 300 mg q12h	200 mg q8h or 300 mg q12h	100 mg q8h; if hemo, AD	HEMO: Dose for CrCl <10; CAPD: Dose for CrCl <10	CAVH: 100 mg q8h

‡ CAVH = continuous arteriovenous hemofiltration (NEJM 336:1303, 1997); AD = after dialysis.
§ Supplement is to replace drug lost via dialysis; extra drug beyond continuation of regimen used for CrCl <10 ml/min. "Dose AD" refers only to timing of dose with NO other drug.
¶ Not recommended for life-threatening infections. D = dosage reduction; I = interval extension; ** Per cent refers to % change from dose for normal renal function.
Abbreviations: HEMO = hemodialysis; **CAPD** = chronic ambulatory peritoneal dialysis; **ESRD** = endstage renal disease; **NUS** = not available in the U.S.

† Ref. for NRTIs and NNRTIs: Kidney International 60:821, 2001

TABLE 17B: NO DOSAGE ADJUSTMENT WITH RENAL INSUFFICIENCY, BY CATEGORY:

Antibacterials		Antifungals	Anti-TBc	Antivirals	
				Non-HIV	Anti-HIV Drugs
Azithromycin	Doxycycline	Amphotericin B	Rifabutin	None	Abacavir
Ceftriaxone	Minocycline	Caspofungin	Rifapentine		Amprenavir
Chloramphenicol	Moxifloxacin	Itraconazole oral solution			Delavirdine
Ciprofloxacin XL	Nafcillin	Voriconazole, **po only**			Efavirenz
Clindamycin	Pyrimethamine				Lopinavir
Dirithromycin	Trovafloxacin				Nevirapine

TABLE 18: ANTIMICROBIALS AND HEPATIC DISEASE

The following alphabetical list indicates antibacterials excreted/metabolized by the liver wherein a dosage adjustment may be indicated in the presence of hepatic disease. Space precludes details; consult the PDR or package inserts for details. List is **not** all-inclusive:

Amprenavir	Efavirenz	Nevirapine
Caspofungin (Table 10B)	Indinavir	Rifabutin
Cefoperazone	Isoniazid	Rifampin
Ceftriaxone	Itraconazole solution	Rimantadine
Chloramphenicol	Metronidazole	Trovafloxacin
Clindamycin	Nafcillin	Voriconazole
Delavirdine		

TABLE 19: TREATMENT OF CAPD PERITONITIS IN ADULTS[1]
(Periton Dial Intl 20:396, 2000)

EMPIRIC Intraperitoneal Therapy:[2] Culture Results Pending

Drug		Residual Urine Output	
		<100 ml/day	>100 ml/day
Cefazolin +	Can mix in	1 gm/bag, qd	20 mg/kg BW/bag, qd
Ceftazidime	same bag	1 gm/bag, qd	20 mg/kg BW/bag, qd

Drug Doses for SPECIFIC Intraperitoneal Therapy—Culture Results Known. NOTE: Few po drugs indicated

Drug	Intermittent Dosing (once/day)		Continuous Dosing (per liter exchange)	
	Anuric	Non-Anuric	Anuric	Non-Anuric
Gentamicin	0.6 mg/kg	↑ dose 25%	MD 8 mg	↑ MD by 25%
Cefazolin	15 mg/kg	20 mg/kg	LD 500 mg, MD 125 mg	LD 500 mg, ↑ MD 25%
Ceftazidime	1000–1500 mg	ND	LD 250 mg, MD 125 mg	ND
Ampicillin	250–500 mg po bid	ND	250–500 mg po bid	ND
Ciprofloxacin	500 mg po bid	ND	LD 50 mg, MD 25 mg	ND
Vancomycin	15–30 mg/kg q5–7 d	↑ dose 25%	MD 30–50 mg/L	↑ MD 25%
Metronidazole	250 mg po bid	ND	250 mg po bid	ND
Amphotericin B	NA	NA	MD 1.5 mg	NA
Fluconazole	200 mg qd	ND	200 mg qd	ND
Itraconazole	100 mg q12h	100 mg q12h	100 mg q12h	100 mg q12h
Amp/sulbactam	2 gm q12h	ND	LD 1.0 gm, MD 100 mg	ND
TMP/SMX	320/1600 mg po q1–2 d	ND	LD 320/1600 mg po, MD 80/400 mg po qd	ND

[1] **All doses IP unless indicated otherwise.**
LD = loading dose, **MD** = maintenance dose, **ND** = no data; **NA** = not applicable—dose as normal renal function. **Anuric** = <100 ml/d, **non-anuric** = >100 ml/d.

[2] Does not provide treatment for MRSA. If Gram-positive cocci on Gram stain, include vancomycin.

January–December 2002 *(MMWR 51:32, 2002) (For overall recommendations, see MMWR 51:RR-2, 2002)*

VACCINE	Birth	1 mo	2 mos	4 mos	6 mos	12 mos	15 mos	18 mos	24 mos	4–6 yrs	11–12 yrs	13–18 yrs
Hepatitis B†	Hep B #1 only if mother HBsAg(–)		Hep B #2		Hep B #3						Hep B series	
Diphtheria, Tetanus, Pertussis§			DTaP	DTaP	DTaP		DTaP			DTaP	Td	
Haemophilus influenzae Type b¶			Hib	Hib	Hib	Hib						
Inactivated Polio**			IPV	IPV		IPV				IPV		
Measles, Mumps, Rubella††						MMR #1				MMR #2	MMR #2	
Varicella§§						Varicella					Varicella	
Pneumococcal¶¶			PCV	PCV	PCV	PCV				PCV	PPV	

—————Vaccines below this line are for selected populations—————

Hepatitis A***											Hepatitis A series	
Influenza†††						Influenza (yearly)						

Range of recommended ages   Catch-up vaccination   Preadolescent assessment

* Indicates the recommended ages for routine administration of currently licensed childhood vaccines, as of December 1, 2001, for children through age 18 years. Any dose not given at the recommended age should be given at any subsequent visit when indicated and feasible. [▒] Indicates age groups that warrant special effort to administer those vaccines not given previously. Additional vaccines may be licensed and recommended during the year. Licensed combination vaccines may be used whenever any components of the combination are indicated and the vaccine's other components are not contraindicated. Providers should consult the manufacturers' package inserts for detailed recommendations.

† **Hepatitis B vaccine (Hep B).** All infants should receive the 1st dose of hepatitis B vaccine soon after birth and before hospital discharge; the 1st dose also may be given by age 2 months if the infant's mother is HBsAg-negative. Only monovalent hepatitis B vaccine can be used for the birth dose. Monovalent or combination vaccine containing Hep B may be used to complete the series; 4 doses of vaccine may be administered if combination vaccine is used. The 2nd dose should be given at least 4 weeks after the 1st dose except for Hib-containing vaccine, which cannot be administered before age 6 weeks. The 3rd dose should be given at least 16 weeks after the 1st dose and at least 8 weeks after the 2nd dose. The last dose in the vaccination series (3rd or 4th dose) should not be administered before age 6 months. **Infants born to HBsAg-positive mothers** should receive hepatitis B vaccine and 0.5 mL hepatitis B immune globulin (HBIG) within 12 hours of birth at separate sites. The 2nd dose is recommended at age 1–2 months and the vaccination series should be completed (3rd or 4th dose) at age 6 months. **Infants born to mothers whose HBsAg status is unknown** should receive the 1st dose of the hepatitis B vaccine series within 12 hours of birth. Maternal blood should be drawn at the time of delivery to determine the mother's HBsAg status; if the HBsAg test is positive, the infant should receive HBIG as soon as possible (no later than age 1 week).

§ **Diphtheria and tetanus toxoids and acellular pertussis vaccine (DTaP).** The 4th dose of DTaP may be administered as early as age 12 months provided that 6 months have elapsed since the 3rd dose and the child is unlikely to return at age 15–18 months. **Tetanus and diphtheria toxoids (Td)** is recommended at age 11–12 years if at least 5 years have elapsed since the last dose of tetanus and diphtheria toxoid-containing vaccine. Subsequent routine Td boosters are recommended every 10 years.

¶ **Haemophilus influenzae type b (Hib) conjugate vaccine.** Three Hib conjugate vaccines are licensed for infant use. If PRP-OMP [PedvaxHIB® or ComVax® (Merck)] is administered at age 2 and 4 months, a dose at age 6 months is not required. DTaP/Hib combination products should not be used for primary immunization in infants at age 2, 4 or 6 months but can be used as boosters following any Hib vaccine.

** **Inactivated poliovirus vaccine (IPV).** An all-IPV schedule is recommended for routine childhood poliovirus vaccination in the United States. All children should receive 4 doses of IPV at age 2, 4, and 6–18 months, and at 4–6 years.

†† **Measles, mumps, and rubella vaccine (MMR).** The 2nd dose of MMR is recommended routinely at age 4–6 years but may be administered during any visit provided at least 4 weeks have elapsed since the first dose and that both doses are administered beginning at or after age 12 months. Those who have not previously received the second dose should complete the schedule by the visit at age 11–12 years.

§§ **Varicella vaccine.** Varicella vaccine is recommended at any visit, at or after age 12 months for susceptible children (i.e., those who lack a reliable history of chickenpox). Susceptible persons aged ≥13 years should receive 2 doses given at least 4 weeks apart.

¶¶ **Pneumococcal vaccine.** The heptavalent **pneumococcal conjugate vaccine (PCV)** is recommended for all children aged 2–23 months and for certain children aged 24–59 months. **Pneumococcal polysaccharide vaccine (PPV)** is recommended in addition to PCV for certain high-risk groups. See MMWR 49(RR-9):1, 2000.

*** **Hepatitis A vaccine.** Hepatitis A vaccine is recommended for use in selected states and regions, and for certain high-risk groups. Consult local public health authority and MMWR 48(RR-12):1, 1999.

††† **Influenza vaccine.** Influenza vaccine is recommended annually for children aged ≥6 months with certain risk factors (including but not limited to asthma, cardiac disease, sickle cell disease, HIV, and diabetes; see MMWR 50(RR-4):1, 2001, and can be administered to all others wishing to obtain immunity. Children aged ≤12 years should receive vaccine in a dosage appropriate for their age (0.25 ml if 6–35 months or 0.5 ml if ≥3 years). Children aged ≤8 years who are receiving influenza vaccine for the first time should receive 2 doses separated by at least 4 weeks.

Additional information about vaccines, vaccine supply, and contraindications for immunization is available at www.cdc.gov/nip or at the National Immunization hotline, 800-232-2522 (English) or 800-232-0233 (Spanish). Copies of the schedule can be obtained at www.cdc.gov/nip/recs/child-schedule.htm. Approved by the **Advisory Committee on Immunization Practices** (www.cdc.gov/nip/acip), the **American Academy of Pediatrics** (www.aap.org), and the **American Academy of Family Physicians** (www.aafp.org).

TABLE 20A (2)

Conjugate pneumococcal vaccine (PCV): The USFDA approved a new conjugate heptavalent pneumococcal vaccine (Prevnar®, Wyeth-Lederle) in 2000. Unlike previous pneumococcal vaccines, this is effective in children <24 months of age. The Advisory Committee on Immunization Practices (ACIP) recommends vaccination of all infants <2 years old and high-risk children (e.g., HIV, asplenia, nephrotic syndrome, sickle cell anemia) between 2 and 5 years of age (*Med Lett 42:25, 2000; PIDJ 19:181, 2000; PIDJ 19:371ff, 2000*).

Immunization schedule:

Age at first dose (0.5 ml)	Total number of doses	Timing
Infants	4	2, 4, 6, and 12–15 months
7–11 months	3	2 doses at least 4 wks apart; 3rd dose after 1 year birthday, separated from 2nd dose by at least 2 months
12–23 months	2	2 doses at least 2 months apart
≥24 months	1*	

* For children ≥24 months old who are chronically ill or immunosuppressed, ICIP recommends 2 doses of PCV administered 2 mos. apart, followed by 1 dose of a 23-valent pneumococcal vaccine 2 or 3 mos. after 2nd PCV dose (*MMWR 50:10, 2001*).

TABLE 20B: ADULT IMMUNIZATION IN THE UNITED STATES[1] *(Travelers: see Med Letter 38:17, 1996)*

AGE GROUP (years)	VACCINE/TOXOID						
	Td[2]	Measles	Mumps	Rubella	Influenza	Pneumo-coccal	Hepatitis B[4]
18–24	x	x	x	x			Individuals at ↑ risk regardless of age. See Table 15, page 120 for post-exposure prophylaxis
25–64	x	x[3]	x	x			
≥65	x				x[5]	x	

[1] From *Guide for Adult Immunization*, 3rd Ed., Am Coll Physicians, 1994. Also see AnIM 12:35, 1996, and IDCP 5:490, 1996.
[2] Td = tetanus + diphtheria toxoids, adsorbed for adult use (contains 5 Fl units tetanus + 2 Fl units diphtheria vs childhood vaccine, which contains 5 Fl u tetanus + 12.5 Fl u diphtheria)
[3] Measles vaccine indicated for persons born in 1957 or later. 9% hospital workers born after 1957 are not immune, serotest and immunize especially during outbreaks.
[4] Screen all pregnant women for HBsAg (give HBIG and vaccine to infants born to HBsAg-positive mothers). Those at ↑ exposure risk: homosexual males, injecting drug users, multiple partner heterosexual exposure, other sexually transmitted diseases, household and sexual contacts of HBV carriers, health care and public safety workers with exposure to blood, residents and staff of institutions for retarded, hemodialysis patients, recipients of Factor VII or IX concentrates, morticians.
[5] See Table 14, page 108 for influenza immunization.

ADMINISTRATION SCHEDULE FOR ABOVE PLUS OTHER SELECTED VACCINES

Hepatitis A (Havrix, Vaqta): 1.0 ml IM & repeat in 6–12 mos. Antibodies detectable >15 days; use immune serum globulin 0.02 ml/kg IM for immediate protection. Indications: Populations at ↑ risk for HAV infection or the adverse consequences of infection [e.g., travelers to endemic areas, children (≥2 yrs of age) in communities that have high rates of hepatitis A, including U.S. states with high incidence (*NEJM 340:644, 1999*), men who have sex with men, illegal-drug users, persons with occupational risk for infection, persons who have chronic liver disease (including hepatitis C) or clotting factor disorders] (*Med Ltr 37:51, 1995; IDCP 5:122, 1996; MMWR 48:RR-12, 1999*). Useful for secondary prevention (*Ln 353:1136, 1999*). (For therapy, see Table 14)
Hepatitis B (Engerix B, Recombivax HB): 3 doses; initial, 1 month, 6 months after 1st. Give IM in deltoid (not in buttocks), use 1½-inch needle; give SC only in pts at risk of bleeding (hemophiliacs). (Seroprotection associated with titers ≥10 mIU/ml). (For therapy, see Table 14)
Combined Hepatitis A & B vaccine (Twinrix): 1.0 ml IM. Repeat 1 & 6 mos. (3 doses total). Each 1.0 ml contains 720 EU inactivated hepatitis A virus & 20 μg recombinant hepatitis B surface antigen. Useful for travelers as long as 2 doses given before departure. Not approved for children. (*Med Lett 43:67, 2001*)
Influenza (killed virus): One dose (0.5 ml) IM. Annual reimmunization with current vaccine recommended (*MMWR 51:RR-3, 2002*).
Lyme disease: 3 doses IM in deltoid: initial, 1 month & 12 months later (0.5 ml; 30 μg). Only for persons 15–70 years old who reside, work or recreate in areas of high or moderate risk (*MMWR 48:RR-7, 1999; EID 5:321, 1999*).
Measles (Attenuvax) (live virus vaccine): Unless contraindicated,[§] one dose (0.5 ml) sc preferably in outer aspect upper arm. Booster not required. Severely immunocompromised patients exposed to measles should receive immunoglobulin prophylaxis regardless of vaccination status because they may not be protected by the vaccine (*MMWR 47:27, 1998*).
Measles + Rubella + Mumps (MMR) (live virus): Unless contraindicated[§] (do not give to pregnant woman), one dose (0.5 ml) sc as with measles. Booster not required.
Meningococcal vaccines: Current vaccines include serogroups A, C (± Y and W135), but not B. No standard guidelines for administration. Usually used for susceptible individuals (terminal complement deficiencies, asplenia) and to control outbreaks (military recruits, college students in dormitories). Dose: 0.5 ml sc (*PIDJ 19:333, 2000; MMWR 49:RR-7, 2000*).
Pneumococcal (Pneumovax 23, Pnu-Immune 23) (pure antigens, 23): One dose (0.5 ml) sc. For adults—revaccination x1 after 5 yrs: (a) immunocompetent pts with anatomic/functional asplenia or age >65 and (b) persons immunocompromised due to HIV, malignancy, meds, or nephrotic syndrome (*MMWR 46:(RR-8), 1997*). However, reimmunization with 23-valent vaccine at 5 years may not produce significant response in patients with AIDS (*CID 34:813, 2002*).
Td (toxoids, not live): Primary: Two doses IM at least 4 wks apart, 3rd dose 6–12 mos after 2nd. Booster every 10 yrs.
Typhoid (Typhim Vi): Single IM dose of 25 μg yields 95% seroconversion. Minimal side-effects. For travelers & lab workers.
Varicella (Varivax): 0.5 ml sc and repeat 4–8 wks later. For susceptible adolescents/adults who are: (1) health care worker, (2) susceptible household contact of immunocompromised person, (3) susceptible in school/day care center, (4) college student/military, (5) non-pregnant woman of child-bearing age. See *MMWR 28:RR-6, 1999*

[§] Review package insert for specific product being administered.

WOUND CLASSIFICATION			IMMUNIZATION SCHEDULE				
Clinical Features	Tetanus Prone	Non-Tetanus Prone	History of Tetanus Immunization	Dirty, Tetanus-Prone Wound		Clean, Non-Tetanus Prone Wound	
				Td[1,2]	TIG	Td	TIG
Age of wound	> 6 hours	≤ 6 hours					
Configuration	Stellate, avulsion	Linear	Unknown or < 3 doses	Yes	Yes	Yes	No
Depth	> 1 cm	≤ 1 cm	3 or more doses	No[3]	No	No[4]	No
Mechanism of injury	Missile, crush, burn, frostbite	Sharp surface (glass, knife)					
Devitalized tissue	Present	Absent					
Contaminants (dirt, saliva, etc.)	Present	Absent					

[1] Td = Tetanus & diphtheria toxoids adsorbed (adult)
TIG = Tetanus immune globulin (human)
[2] Yes if wound >24 hours old.
For children <7 years, DPT (DT if pertussis vaccine contraindicated);
For persons ≥7 years, Td preferred to tetanus toxoid alone.
[3] Yes if >5 years since last booster
[4] Yes if >10 years since last booster

(From ACS Bull. 69:22,23, 1984, No. 10)

(From MMWR 39:37, 1990; MMWR 46(SS-2):15, 1997)

TABLE 20C/2: RABIES POST-EXPOSURE PROPHYLAXIS[1]. All wounds should be cleaned immediately and thoroughly with soap and water. This has been shown to protect 90% of experimental animals!

Post-Exposure Prophylaxis Guide, United States, 2000 *(CID 30:4, 2000)*

Animal Type	Evaluation and Disposition of Animal	Recommendations for Prophylaxis
Dogs, cats, ferrets	Healthy and available for 10-day observation	Don't start unless animal develops sx, then immediately begin HRIG + HDCV or RVA
	Rabid or suspected rabid	Immediate vaccination
	Unknown (escaped)	Consult public health officials
Skunks, raccoons, bats,* foxes, coyotes, most carnivores	Regard as rabid	Immediate vaccination
Livestock, rodents, rabbits; includes hares, squirrels, hamsters, guinea pigs, gerbils, chipmunks, rats, mice, woodchucks		Almost never require anti-rabies rx. Consult public health officials.

* Most recent cases of human rabies in U.S. due to contact (not bites) with silver-haired bats or rarely big brown bats
(MMWR 46:770, 1997; AIM 128:922, 1998). For more detail, see CID 30:4, 2000; JAVMA 219:1687, 2001.

Post-Exposure Rabies Immunization Schedule
IF NOT PREVIOUSLY VACCINATED

Treatment	Regimen[2]
Local wound cleaning	All post-exposure treatment should begin with immediate, thorough cleaning of all wounds with soap and water.
Human rabies immune globulin (HRIG)	20 IU/kg body weight given once on day 0. If anatomically feasible, the full dose should be infiltrated around the wound(s), the rest should be administered IM in the gluteal area. HRIG should **not** be administered in the **same syringe**, or into the **same anatomical site** as vaccine, or more than 7 days after the initiation of vaccine. Because HRIG may partially suppress active production of antibody, no more than the recommended dose should be given.[3]
Vaccine	Human diploid cell vaccine (HDCV), rabies vaccine adsorbed (RVA), or purified chick embryo cell vaccine PECEC) 1.0 mL **IM (deltoid area[4])**, one each on days 0, 3, 7, 14, & 28.

IF PREVIOUSLY VACCINATED[5]

Treatment	Regimen[2]
Local wound cleaning	All post-exposure treatment should begin with immediate, thorough cleaning of all wounds with soap and water.
HRIG	HRIG should **not** be administered
Vaccine	HDCV, RVA or PECEC, 1.0 mL **IM (deltoid area[4])**, one each on days 0 and 3

CORRECT VACCINE ADMINISTRATION SITES

Age Group	Administration Site
Children and adults	DELTOID[4] only (**NEVER** in gluteus)
Infants and young children	Outer aspect of thigh (anterolateral thigh) may be used (**NEVER** in gluteus)

[1] From MMWR 48:RR-1, 1999; CID 30:4, 2000; B.T. Matyas, Mass. Dept. of Public Health
[2] These regimens are applicable for all age groups, including children.
[3] In most reported post-exposure treatment failures, only identified deficiency was failure to infiltrate wound(s) with HRIG (CID 22:228, 1996). However, several failures reported from SE Asia in patients in whom WHO protocol followed (CID 28:143, 1999).
[4] The **deltoid** area is the **only** acceptable site of vaccination for adults and older children. For infants and young children, the outer aspect of the thigh (anterolateral thigh) may be used. Vaccine should **NEVER** be administered in the gluteal area.
[5] Any person with a history of pre-exposure vaccination with HDCV, RVA, PECEC; prior post-exposure prophylaxis with HDCV, RVA, PECEC; or previous vaccination with any other type of rabies vaccine and a documented history of antibody response to the prior vaccination

TABLE 21: ANTI-INFECTIVE DRUG-DRUG INTERACTIONS

Significance/Certainty: ± = theory/anecdotal; + = of probable importance; ++ = of definite importance

ANTI-INFECTIVE AGENT (A)	OTHER DRUG (B)	EFFECT	SIGNIFICANCE/ CERTAINTY
Amantadine (Symmetrel)	Alcohol	↑ CNS effects	+
	Anticholinergic and anti-Parkinson agents (ex. Artane, scopolamine)	↑ effect of B: dry mouth, ataxia, blurred vision, slurred speech, toxic psychosis	+
	Trimethoprim	↑ levels of A & B	+
	Digoxin	↑ levels of B	±
Aminoglycosides— parenteral (amikacin, gentamicin, kanamycin, netilmicin, sisomicin, streptomycin, tobramycin) NOTE: *Capreomycin is an aminoglycoside, used as alternative drug to treat mycobacterial infections.*	Amphotericin B	↑ nephrotoxicity	++
	Cis platinum (Platinol)	↑ nephro & ototoxicity	+
	Cyclosporine	↑ nephrotoxicity	+
	Neuromuscular blocking agents	↑ apnea or respiratory paralysis	+
	Loop diuretics (e.g., furosemide)	↑ ototoxicity	++
	NSAIDs	↑ nephrotoxicity	+
	Non-polarizing muscle relaxants	↑ apnea	+
	Radiographic contrast	↑ nephrotoxicity	+
	Vancomycin	↑ nephrotoxicity	+
Amphotericin B and ampho B lipid formulations	Antineoplastic drugs	↑ nephrotoxicity risk	+
	Digitalis	↑ toxicity of B if K+ ↓	+
	Nephrotoxic drugs: aminoglycosides, cidofovir, cyclosporine, foscarnet, pentamidine	↑ nephrotoxicity of A	++
Ampicillin, amoxicillin	Allopurinol	↑ frequency of rash	++
Amprenavir	Antiretrovirals—see Table 21B		
	Contraceptives, oral	↓ levels of A	++
	Methadone	↓ levels of A & B	++
	Rifabutin	↑ levels of B (↓ dose by 50%)	++
	Rifampin	↓ levels of A	++
Atovaquone	Rifampin (perhaps rifabutin)	↓ serum levels of A; ↑ levels of B	+
	Metoclopramide	↓ levels of A	+
	Tetracycline	↓ levels of A	++

Azole Antifungal Agents[1] [*Flu* = fluconazole, *Itr* = itraconazole, *Ket* = ketoconazole, *Vor* = voriconazole, + = occurs, **blank space** = either studied & no interaction OR no data found (may be in pharm. co. databases)]

Flu	Itr	Ket	Vor			
+	+			Amitriptyline	↑ levels of B	+
+	+	+	+	Calcium channel blockers	↑ levels of B	++
	+		+	Carbamazepine (vori contraindicated)	↑ levels of B	++
+	**+**	**+**	**+**	**Cisapride (avoid all azoles)**	**↑ levels of B (arrhythmias, ↑ Q-T interval)**	++
+	+	+	+	Cyclosporine	↑ levels of B, ↑ risk of nephrotoxicity	++
	+	+		Didanosine	↓ absorption of A	+
	+	+		H₂ blockers, antacids, sucralfate	↓ absorption of A	+
+	+	+	+	Hydantoins (phenytoin, Dilantin)	↑ levels of B, ↓ levels of A	++
	+	+		Isoniazid	↓ levels of A	+
	+	+	+	Lovastatin/simvastatin	Rhabdomyolysis reported; ↑ levels of B	++
+	+	+	+	Midazolam/triazolam, po	↑ levels of B	++
+	+	+	+	Oral anticoagulants	↑ effect of B	++
+	+	+	+	Oral hypoglycemics	↑ levels of B	++
	+			Pimozide	↑ levels of B	++
				Proton pump inhibitors	↓ absorption of A, ↑ levels of B	+
+	+	+	+	Rifampin/rifabutin (vori contraindicated)	↑ levels of B, ↓ serum levels of A	++
			+	Sirolimus (vori contraindicated)	↑ levels of B	++
+	+			Tacrolimus	↑ levels of B with toxicity	++
+	+			Theophyllines	↑ levels of B	+
+				Zidovudine	↑ levels of B	+
Caspofungin				Cyclosporine	↑ levels of A	++
				Tacrolimus	↓ levels of B	++
				Carbamazepine, dexamethasone, efavirenz, nelfinavir, nevirapine, phenytoin, rifampin	↓ levels of A; ↑ dose of caspofungin to 70 mg/d	++
Cephalosporins with methyltetrathiozole-thiol side-chain[2]	Oral anticoagulants (dicumarol, warfarin), heparin, thrombolytic agents, platelet aggregation inhibitors	↑ effects of B, bleeding	+
Cefoperazone (Cefobid)	Alcohol	Disulfiram-like reaction (tachycardia, flushing, diarrhea)	+
Chloramphenicol	Hydantoins	↑ toxicity of B, nystagmus, ataxia	++
	Iron salts, Vitamin B12	↓ response to B	++
	Protease inhibitors—HIV	↑ levels of A & B	+

[1] Major interactions given; unusual or minor interactions manifest as toxicity of non-azole drug due to ↑ serum levels: Caffeine (Flu), digoxin (Itr), felodipine (Itr), fluoxetine (Itr), indinavir (Ket), lovastatin/simvastatin, quinidine (Ket), tricyclics (Flu), vincristine (Itr), and ↓ effectiveness of oral contraceptives.
[2] Cefamandole, cefotetan, cefmetazole, cefoperazone

TABLE 21 (2)
137

ANTI-INFECTIVE AGENT (A)	OTHER DRUG (B)	EFFECT	SIGNIFICANCE/CERTAINTY
Clindamycin (Cleocin)	Kaolin	↓ absorption of A	+
	Muscle relaxants, e.g., atracurium, baclofen, diazepam	↑ frequency/duration of respiratory paralysis	+
	Erythromycin	Mutual antagonism	+
Cycloserine	Ethanol	↑ frequency of seizures	+
	INH, ethionamide	↑ frequency of drowsiness/dizziness	+
Dapsone	Didanosine	↓ absorption of A	+
	Oral contraceptives	↓ effectiveness of B	+
	Pyrimethamine	↑ in marrow toxicity	+
	Rifampin/Rifabutin	↓ serum levels of A	+
	Trimethoprim	↑ levels of A & B (methemoglobinemia)	+
	Zidovudine	May ↑ marrow toxicity	+
Delavirdine (Rescriptor) **NOTE:** Review all pt's meds before starting delavirdine. Interactions with other antiretrovirals, Table 21B, page 141	**Co-administration contraindicated:** Anticonvulsants: Phenytoin, phenobarbital, carbamazepine; Antimycobacterials: Rifabutin, rifampin; Ergot derivatives: Ergotamine; HMG-CoA inhibitors: Lovastatin, simvastatin; Neuroleptic: Pimozide; St. John's wort; Sedatives: Alprazolam, midazolam, triazolam		
	Dose change needed:		
	Antacids, H₂-blockers, proton pump inhibitors	↓ levels of A	++
	Amiodarone, lidocaine, quinidine	↑ levels of B—caution	++
	Calcium channel blockers	↑ levels of B	++
	Clarithromycin	↑ levels of B	++
	Cyclosporine, tacrolimus, rapamycin	↑ levels of B—measure levels	++
	Dexamethasone	↓ levels of A	++
	Methadone	↑ levels of B	++
	Sildenafil (Viagra)	↑ levels of B	++
	Warfarin	↑ levels of B	++
Didanosine (ddI) (Videx)	Cisplatin, dapsone, INH, metronidazole, nitrofurantoin, stavudine, vincristine, zalcitabine	↑ risk of peripheral neuropathy	+
	Ethanol, lamivudine, pentamidine	↑ risk of pancreatitis	+
	Fluoroquinolones	↓ absorption 2° to chelation	+
	Low pH drug solubility: dapsone, indinavir, itra/ketoconazole, pyrimethamine, rifampin, trimethoprim	↓ absorption	+
	Tenofovir	↑ levels of A **(reduce dose of A)**	++
Doxycycline	Aluminum, bismuth, iron, Mg++	↓ absorption of A	+
	Barbiturates, hydantoins	↓ serum t½ of A	+
	Carbamazepine (Tegretol)	↑ serum t½ of A	+
	Digoxin	↑ serum levels of B	+
	Warfarin	↑ activity of B	++
Efavirenz (Sustiva)	Cisapride	**↑ levels of B; do not co-administer**	++
	Clarithromycin	↓ levels of B	+
	Ergot derivatives	**↑ levels of B; do not co-administer**	++
	Methadone	↓ levels of B	++
	Midazolam	**↑ levels of B; do not co-administer**	++
	Rifampin	↓ levels of A	+
Ertapenem (Invanz)	Probenecid	↑ levels of A	++
Ethambutol (Myambutol)	Aluminum salts (includes didanosine buffer)	↓ absorption of A & B	+

Fluoroquinolones (*Cipro* = ciprofloxacin; *Gati* = gatifloxacin; *Levo* = levofloxacin; *Lome* = lomefloxacin; *Moxi* = moxifloxacin; *Oflox* = ofloxacin; *Trova* = trovafloxacin)

NOTE: Blank space = either studied and no interaction OR no data found (pharm. co. may have data)

Cipro	Gati¹	Levo	Lome¹	Moxi¹	Oflox	Trova	OTHER DRUG (B)	EFFECT	SIGNIFICANCE/CERTAINTY
+		+	+	+	+		Antiarrhythmics (procainamide, amiodarone)	↑ Q-T interval (torsade)	++
+	+	+	+	+	+	+	Insulin, oral hypoglycemics	↑ & ↓ blood sugar	+
+					+		Caffeine	↑ levels of B	+
+		+		+			Cimetidine	↑ levels of A	+
+		+		+			Cyclosporine	↑ levels of B	±
+	+	+	+	+	+	+	Didanosine	↓ absorption of A	++
+	+	+	+	+	+	+	Cations: Al+++, Ca++, Fe++, Mg++, Zn++ (antacids, vitamins, dairy products), citrate/citric acid	↓ absorption of A (some variability between drugs)	++
+							Foscarnet	↑ risk of seizures	+
+							Methadone	↑ levels of B	++
							NSAIDs	↑ risk CNS stimulation/seizures	++
+		+	+				Phenytoin	↑ or ↓ levels of B	+
+							Probenecid	↓ renal clearance of A	+
+	+	+	+	+	+	+	Sucralfate	↓ absorption of A	++
+							Theophylline	↑ levels of B	++
+		+	+				Warfarin	↑ prothrombin time	+

¹ Neither gati nor moxi interacts with Ca++

TABLE 21 (3)

ANTI-INFECTIVE AGENT (A)	OTHER DRUG (B)	EFFECT	SIGNIFICANCE/ CERTAINTY
Foscarnet (Foscavir)	Ciprofloxacin	↑ risk of seizures	+
	Nephrotoxic drugs: aminoglycosides, ampho B, cis-platinum, cyclosporine	↑ risk of nephrotoxicity	+
	Pentamidine IV	↑ risk of severe hypocalcemia	++
Ganciclovir (Cytovene)	Imipenem	↑ risk of seizures reported	+
	Probenecid	↑ levels of A	+
	Zidovudine	↓ levels of A, ↑ levels of B	+
Gentamicin	See Aminoglycosides—parenteral		
Halofantrine	Mefloquine	Additive effect: prolong. Q-T interval	++ (avoid)
Indinavir	See protease inhibitors and Table 21B		
Isoniazid	**Alcohol, rifampin**	↑ risk of hepatic injury	++
	Aluminum salts	↓ absorption (take fasting)	++
	Carbamazepine, phenytoin	↑ levels of B with nausea, vomiting, nystagmus, ataxia	++
	Itraconazole, ketoconazole	↓ levels of B	+
	Oral hypoglycemics	↓ effects of B	+
Lamivudine	Zalcitabine	Mutual interference—do not combine	++
Linezolid (Zyvox)	Adrenergic agents	Risk of hypertension	++
	Aged, fermented, pickled or smoked foods — ↑ tyramine	Risk of hypertension	+
	Serotonergic drugs	Risk of serotonin syndrome	+
Lopinavir	See protease inhibitors		

Macrolides [**Ery** = erythromycin, **Azi** = azithromycin, **Clr** = clarithromycin; **Dir** = dirithromycin, **+** = occurs, **blank space** = either studied and no interaction OR no data (pharm. co. may have data)]

Ery	Dir	Azi	Clr			
+	+		+	Carbamazepine	↑ serum levels of B, nystagmus, nausea, vomiting, ataxia	++ (avoid with erythro)
+			+	Cimetidine, **ritonavir**	↑ levels of B	+
+		**+**	**+**	**Cisapride**	↑ Q-T interval; ↑ risk arrhythmias	++
+			+	Clozapine	↑ serum levels of B, CNS toxicity	+
+			+	Corticosteroids	↑ effects of B	+
+	+	+	+	Cyclosporine	↑ serum levels of B with toxicity	+
+	+	+	+	Digoxin, digitoxin	↑ serum levels of B (10% of cases)	+
+			+	Efavirenz	↑ levels of A	++
+			+	Ergot alkaloids	↑ levels of B	++
+			+	Lovastatin/simvastatin	↑ levels of B; rhabdomyolysis	++
+			+	Midazolam, triazolam	↑ levels of B, ↑ sedative effects	++
+	+		+	Phenytoin	↑ levels of B	+
+		+	+	Pimozide	↑ Q-T interval	++
+			+	Rifampin, rifabutin	↓ levels of A	+
+			+	Tacrolimus	↑ levels of B	++
+				Theophyllines	↑ serum levels of B with nausea, vomiting, seizures, apnea	++
+	+		+	Triazolam	↑ levels of B	+
+	+		+	Valproic acid	↑ levels of B	+
+			+	Warfarin	May ↑ prothrombin time	+
			+	Zidovudine	↓ levels of B	+

Mefloquine				ß-adrenergic blockers, calcium channel blockers, quinidine, quinine	↑ arrhythmias	+
				Divalproex, valproic acid	↓ level of B with seizures	++
				Halofantrine	Q-T prolongation	++ (avoid)
Methenamine mandelate or hippurate				Acetazolamide, sodium bicarbonate, thiazide diuretics	↓ antibacterial effect 2° to ↑ urine pH	++
Metronidazole				**Alcohol**	Disulfiram-like reaction	+
				Disulfiram (Antabuse)	Acute toxic psychosis	+
				Oral anticoagulants	↑ anticoagulant effect	++
				Phenobarbital, hydantoins	↑ metabolism of A with ↓ effectiveness	+
Nelfinavir				See protease inhibitors and Table 21B		
Nevirapine (Viramune) *See Table 21B, page 141*				Opiates, including methadone	↓ levels of B (withdrawal)	++
				St. John's wort	↓ levels of A	++
				Tacrolimus	**↓ levels of B**	**+++**
Nitrofurantoin				Antacids	↓ absorption of A	+
Pentamidine, IV				Amphotericin B	↑ risk of nephrotoxicity	+
				Foscarnet	↑ risk of hypocalcemia	+
				Pancreatitis-associated drugs, e.g., alcohol, valproic acid	↑ risk of pancreatitis	+
Piperacillin				Cefoxitin	Antagonism vs pseudomonas	++
Piperazine				Chlorpromazine	Convulsions (occ. fatal)	++
Primaquine				Chloroquine, dapsone, INH, probenecid, quinine, sulfonamides, TMP/SMX, others	↑ risk of hemolysis in G6PD-deficient patients	++

TABLE 21 (4)   139

ANTI-INFECTIVE AGENT (A)						OTHER DRUG (B)	EFFECT	SIGNIFICANCE/ CERTAINTY
Ampren	Indin	Lopinav	Nelfin	Riton	Saquin			

Protease Inhibitors—Anti-HIV Drugs. (Ampren = amprenavir; **Indin** = indinavir; **Nelfin** = nelfinavir; **Riton** = ritonavir; **Saquin** = saquinavir). For interactions with antiretrovirals, *see Table 21B, page 141*

Only a partial list—see package insert   Also see NEJM 344:984, 2001

Ampren	Indin	Lopinav	Nelfin	Riton	Saquin	OTHER DRUG (B)	EFFECT	SIGNIFICANCE/ CERTAINTY
				+		**Analgesics:** 1. Alfentanil, fentanyl, hydrocodone, tramadol	↑ levels of B	+
			+	+		2. Codeine, hydromorphone, morphine, methadone	↓ levels of B	+
+	+	+	+	+	+	**Anti-arrhythmics: amiodarone, lidocaine, mexiletine, flecainide**	↑ levels of B	+
	+	+	+	+	+	**Anticonvulsants: carbamazepine, clonazepam, phenytoin, phenobarbital**	↓ levels of A, ↑ levels of B	++
				+		Antidepressants, all tricyclic	↑ levels of B	+
				+		Antidepressants, all other	↑ levels of B	+
				+		**Antihistamine:** Loratadine	↑ levels of B	++
	+					Atovaquone	↓ levels of B	+
+	+	+	+	+	+	**Benzodiazepines**	↑ levels of B—do not use	++
				+		Beta blockers: Metoprolol, pindolol, propranolol, timolol	↑ levels of B	+
+	+	+	+	+	+	Calcium channel blockers (all)	↑ levels of B	++
+	**+**	**+**	**+**	**+**	**+**	**Cisapride**	↑ levels of B—do not use	++
				+	+	Clarithromycin	↑ levels of B if renal impairment	+
			+	+	+	Contraceptives, oral	↓ levels of B	++
				+		Corticosteroids: prednisone, dexamethasone	↓ levels of A, ↑ levels of B	+
+	+	+	+	+	+	Cyclosporine	↓ levels of B, monitor levels	+
				+		Diazepam, midazolam	↑ level of B—do not use	++
+	+	+	+	+	+	Ergot derivatives	↑ levels of B—do not use	++
+	+			+		Erythromycin, clarithromycin	↑ levels of A & B	+
	+				+	Grapefruit juice (>200 ml/day)	↓ indinavir & ↑ saquinavir levels	++
+	+	+	+	+	+	Ketoconazole, itraconazole	↑ levels of A	+
				+		Metronidazole	Poss. disulfiram reaction, alcohol	+
+	+	+	+	+	+	Pimozide	↑ levels of B—do not use	++
+	+	+	+	+	+	Rifampin, rifabutin	↓ levels of A, ↑ levels of B	++ (avoid)
+	+	+	+	+	+	Sildenafil (Viagra)	Varies, some ↑ & some ↓ levels of B	++
+	+	+	+	+	+	St. John's wort	↓ levels of A—do not use	++
+	+	+	+	+	+	Statins	↑ levels of B, esp. simvastatin & lovastatin	++ (check)
			+	+		Theophylline	↓ levels of B	+
				+		Warfarin	↑ levels of B	+
Pyrazinamide						INH, rifampin	May ↑ risk of hepatotoxicity	±
Pyrimethamine						Lorazepam	↑ risk of hepatotoxicity	+
						Sulfonamides, TMP/SMX	↑ risk of marrow suppression	+
						Zidovudine	↑ risk of marrow suppression	+
Quinine						Digoxin	↑ digoxin levels; ↑ toxicity	++
						Mefloquine	↑ arrhythmias	+
						Oral anticoagulants	↑ prothrombin time	++
Rifamycins (rifampin, rifabutin) *See footnote for less severe or less common interactions*[1] Ref.: ArIM 162:985, 2002						Al OH, ketoconazole, PZA	↓ levels of A	+
						Atovaquone	↓ levels of A, ↓ levels of B	+
						Beta adrenergic blockers (metoprolol, propranolol)	↓ effect of B	+
						Clarithromycin	↑ levels of A, ↓ levels of B	++
						Corticosteroids	replacement requirement of B	++
						Cyclosporine	↓ effect of B	++
						Delavirdine	↓ levels of A, ↓ levels of B—avoid	++
						Digoxin	↓ levels of B	++
						Disopyramide	↓ levels of B	++
						Fluconazole	↑ levels of A[1]	+
						Amprenavir, indinavir, nelfinavir, ritonavir	↑ levels of A (↓ dose of A), ↓ levels of B	++
						INH	Converts INH to toxic hydrazine	++
						Itraconazole[2], ketoconazole	↓ levels of B, ↑ levels of A[2]	++
						Methadone	↓ serum levels (withdrawal)	+
						Nevirapine	↓ levels of B—avoid	++
						Oral anticoagulants	Suboptimal anticoagulation	++

[1] The following is a partial list of drugs with rifampin-induced ↑ metabolism and hence lower than anticipated serum levels: ACE inhibitors, dapsone, diazepam, digoxin, diltiazem, doxycycline, fluconazole, fluvastatin, haloperidol, progestins, triazolam, tricyclics, voriconazole, zidovudine

[2] Up to 4 weeks may be required after RIF discontinued to achieve detectable serum itra levels; ↑ levels associated with uveitis or polymyolysis

TABLE 21 (5)

ANTI-INFECTIVE AGENT (A)	OTHER DRUG (B)	EFFECT	SIGNIFICANCE/ CERTAINTY
Rifamycins (rifampin, rifabutin) *(continued)* See footnote 1 on page 139 for less severe or less common interactions Ref.: ArIM 162:985, 2002	Oral contraceptives	↓ effectiveness; spotting, pregnancy	+
	Phenytoin	↓ levels of B	+
	Protease inhibitors	↑ **levels of A, ↓ levels of B—CAUTION**	++
	Quinidine	↓ effect of B	+
	Sulfonylureas	↓ hypoglycemic effect	+
	Tacrolimus	↓ levels of B	++
	Theophylline	↓ levels of B	+
	TMP/SMX	↑ levels of A	+
	Tocainide	↓ effect of B	+
Rimantadine	*See Amantadine*		
Ritonavir	*See protease inhibitors and Table 21B*		
Saquinavir	*See protease inhibitors and Table 21B*		
Stavudine	Dapsone, INH	May ↑ risk of peripheral neuropathy	±
Sulfonamides	Cyclosporine	↓ cyclosporine levels	+
	Methotrexate	↑ antifolate activity	+
	Oral anticoagulants	↑ prothrombin time; bleeding	+
	Phenobarbital, rifampin	↓ levels of A	+
	Phenytoin	↑ levels of B; nystagmus, ataxia	+
	Sulfonylureas	↑ hypoglycemic effect	+
Telithromycin (Ketek)	Cisapride, pimozide	↑ **levels of B; QT prolongation—AVOID**	++
	Digoxin	↑ levels of B—do digoxin levels	++
	Ergot alkaloids	↑ **levels of B—avoid**	++
	Itraconazole; ketoconazole	↑ levels of A; no dose change	+
	Midazolam	↑ levels of B	++
	Rifampin	↓ **levels of A—avoid**	++
	Simvastatin	↑ levels of B	++
	Sotalol	↓ levels of B	++
Tenofovir	Didanosine (ddI)	↑ **levels of B (reduce dose)**	++
Terbinafine	Cimetidine	↑ levels of A	+
	Phenobarbital, rifampin	↓ levels of A	+
Tetracyclines	*See Doxycycline, plus:*		
	Atovaquone	↓ levels of B	+
	Digoxin	↑ toxicity of B (may persist several months—up to 10% pts)	++
	Methoxyflurane	↑ toxicity; polyuria, renal failure	+
	Sucralfate	↓ absorption of A (separate by ≥2 hrs)	+
Thiabendazole	Theophyllines	↑ serum theophylline, nausea	+
Tobramycin	*See Aminoglycosides*		
Trimethoprim	Amantadine, dapsone, digoxin, methotrexate, procainamide, zidovudine	↑ serum levels of B	++
	Potassium-sparing diuretics	↑ serum K⁺	++
	Thiazide diuretics	↓ serum Na⁺	+
Trimethoprim/Sulfamethoxazole	Azathioprine	Reports of leucopenia	+
	Cyclosporine	↓ levels of B, ↑ serum creatinine	+
	Loperamide	↑ levels of B	+
	Methotrexate	Enhanced marrow suppression	++
	Oral contraceptives, pimozide, and 6-mercaptopurine	↓ effect of B	+
	Phenytoin	↑ levels of B	+
	Rifampin	↑ levels of B	+
	Warfarin	↑ activity of B	+
Vancomycin	Aminoglycosides	↑ frequency of nephrotoxicity	++
Zalcitabine (ddC) (HIVID)	Valproic acid, pentamidine (IV), alcohol, lamivudine	↑ pancreatitis risk	+
	Cisplatin, INH, metronidazole, vincristine, nitrofurantoin, d4T, dapsone	↑ risk of peripheral neuropathy	+
Zidovudine (ZDV) (Retrovir)	Atovaquone, fluconazole, methadone	↑ levels of A	+
	Clarithromycin	↓ levels of A	±
	Indomethacin	↑ levels of ZDV toxic metabolite	+
	Nelfinavir	↓ levels of A	++
	Probenecid, TMP/SMX	↑ levels of A	+
	Ribavirin	↓ **levels of A—avoid**	++
	Rifampin/rifabutin	↓ levels of A	++

TABLE 21B: DRUG-DRUG INTERACTIONS BETWEEN ANTIRETROVIRALS (*I = Investigational)
(Abstracted from Guidelines for the Use of Antiretroviral Agents in HIV-Infected Adults & Adolescents; www.hivatis.org)

NAME (Abbreviation, Trade Name)	Amprenavir (APV, Agenerase)	Indinavir (IDV, Crixivan)	Nelfinavir (NFV, Viracept)	Ritonavir (RTV, Norvir)	Saquinavir—soft gel (SQV, Fortovase)	Efavirenz (EFZ, Sustiva)	Delavirdine (DLV, Rescriptor)	Nevirapine (NVP, Viramune)
Amprenavir (APV, Agenerase)								
Indinavir (IDV, Crixivan)	Levels: APV AUC ↑ 33%. Dose: no change							
Nelfinavir (NFV, Viracept)	Levels of APV ↑, no data on dosage change	Levels: NFV ↑ 80%; IDV ↑ 50%. Dose: IDV 1200 mg bid + NFV 1250 mg bid (I)*						
Ritonavir (RTV, Norvir)	APV AUC ↑ 2.5x. Dose: (APV 600-1200 mg bid + RTV 100-200 mg bid)	Levels: IDV ↑s RTV; RTV ↑s IDV. Dose: RTV 100 or 200 mg bid + IDV 800 mg bid or 400 mg of each bid	NFV levels ↑ 2x; no effect RTV. Dosage: (RTV 400 mg bid + NFV 500-750 mg bid)*					
Saquinavir—soft gel (SQV, Fortovase)	APV AUC ↓ 32%. Dose: Insufficient data	Levels: SQV ↑ 4-7x; no effect IDV. Antiviral antagonism. **Do not combine**	SQV levels ↑ 3-5x; no effect NFV (usual dosage). SQV: 800 mg tid or 1200 mg bid	SQV levels ↑ 20x; RTV no effect. Dosage: 400 mg of each bid				
Efavirenz (EFZ, Sustiva)	APV levels ↓. Dose: (APV 1200 mg bid + RTV 200 mg bid) + EFV standard	IDV levels ↓ 30%; ↑ IDV dose:1000 mg q8h	NFV levels ↑; no effect EFZ. Usual dosage	Modest ↑ levels of both drugs. RTV 600 mg bid	↓ levels of SQV. **Do not combine**			
Delavirdine (DLV, Rescriptor)	APV levels ↑. DLV levels ↓. Correct dosage unclear	IDV levels ↑ 40%; no change DLV. Dose IDV 600 mg q8h	DLV levels ↓ 50%. Usual dosage—watch for neutropenia	RTV levels ↑ 70%. Dosage: Consider ↓ RTV to 400 mg bid	SQV levels ↑ 5x. Dose: SQV 800 mg bid + DLV standard	No data		
Nevirapine (NVP, Viramune)	APV levels ↓, no data on dosage change	NVP levels no effect; IDV ↓ 30%. Dose of IDV: 1000 mg q8h	Standard dose of both	No interaction	SQV levels ↓ 25%. **Avoid combination**	Standard therapy	**Do not use together**	
Lopinavir ritonavir (LP/R, Kaletra)	↓ APV to 600-750 mg bid + LP/R standard	↓ IDV to 600 mg bid	↓ NFV to 750 mg bid	No data	↓ SQV to 800 mg bid + standard LP/R	↑ LP/R to 533/133 mg bid	No data	↑ LP/R to 533/133 mg bid + NWP standard

TABLE 22
SELECTED DIRECTORY OF RESOURCES

ORGANIZATION	PHONE/FAX	WEBSITE(S)
ANTIPARASITIC DRUGS		
CDC	Weekdays: 404-639-3670 Evenings, weekends, holidays: 404-639-2888	www.cdc.gov/ncidod/srp/drugservice/ index.htm
Panorama Compound. Pharm.	800-247-9767/ 818-787-7256	www.uniquerx.com
BIOTERRORISM		
Centers for Disease Control & Prevention	770-488-7100	www.bt.cdc.gov
Infectious Diseases Society of America	703-299-0200/ 703-299-0204	www.idsociety.org
Johns Hopkins Center Civilian Biodefense		www.hopkins-biodefense.org
US Army Medical Research Institute of Inf. Dis.		www.usamriid.army.mil
HEPATITIS C		
CDC		www.cdc.gov/ncidod/diseases/hepatitis/C
Individual		http://hepatitis-central.com
Medscape		www.medscape.com
HIV		
General		
HIV InSite		http://hivinsite.ucsf.edu
Johns Hopkins AIDS Service		www.hopkins-aids.edu
Drug Interactions		
Johns Hopkins AIDS Service		www.hopkins-aids.edu
Liverpool HIV Pharm. Group		www.hiv-druginteractions.org
Other		http://AIDS.medscape.com
Prophylaxis/Treatment of Opportunistic Infections		www.hivatis.org
Treatment of HIV		www.cdc.gov/hiv
IMMUNIZATIONS		
CDC, Natl. Immunization Program	404-639-8200	www.cdc.gov/nip
FDA, Vaccine Adverse Events	800-822-7967	www.fda.gov/cber/vaers/vaers.htm
National Network Immunization Info.	877-341-6644/ 703-299-0204	www.immunizationinfo.org
Influenza vaccine, CDC	404-639-8200	www.cdc.gov/nip/flu
OCCUPATIONAL EXPOSURE, BLOOD-BORNE PATHOGENS (HIV, HEPATITIS B & C)		
National Clinicians' Post-Exposure Hotline	888-448-4911	www.ucsf.edu/hivcntr
Q-T$_6$ INTERVAL PROLONGATION BY DRUGS		www.qtdrugs.org www.torsades.org
SEXUALLY TRANSMITTED DISEASES		www.cdc.gov/std/treatment/toc2002tg.htm Slides: www.hc-sc.gc.ca/pphb-dgspsp/std-mts
TRAVELERS' INFO: Immunizations, Malaria Prophylaxis, More		
Amer. Soc. Trop. Med. & Hyg.		www.astmh.org
CDC, general	877-394-8747/ 888-232-3299	www.cdc.gov/travel/index.htm
CDC, Malaria:		www.cdc.gov/ncidod/dpd/parasites/ malaria/default.htm
Prophylaxis	888-232-3228	
Treatment	770-488-7788	www.who.int/health-topics/malaria.htm
MD Travel Health		www.mdtravelhealth.com
Pan American Health Organization		www.paho.org
World Health Organization (WHO)	(41-22)-791-2122/ (00-41-22)-691-0746	www.who.int/home-page

GENERIC NAME: TRADE NAMES	GENERIC NAME: TRADE NAMES	GENERIC NAME: TRADE NAMES
Abacavir: Ziagen	Dirithromycin: Dynabac	Nitrofurantoin: Macrobid, Macrodantin
Acyclovir: Zovirax	Doxycycline: Vibramycin	Nystatin: Mycostatin
Adefovir: Hepsera	Drotrecogin alfa: Xigris	Ofloxacin: Floxin
Albendazole: Albenza	Efavirenz: Sustiva	Oseltamivir: Tamiflu
Amantadine: Symmetrel	Enfuvirtide (T-20): Fuzeon	Oxacillin: Prostaphlin
Amikacin: Amikin	Ertapenem: Invanz	Palivizumab: Synagis
Amoxicillin: Amoxil, Polymox	Erythromycin(s): Ilotycin	Paromomycin: Humatin
Amox./clav.: Augmentin, Augmentin ES-600; Augmentin XR	*Ethyl succinate:* Pediamycin *Glucoheptonate:* Erythrocin *Estolate:* Ilosone	Pentamidine: NebuPent, Pentam 300
Amphotericin B: Fungizone		Piperacillin: Pipracil
Ampho B-liposomal: AmBisome	Erythro/sulfisoxazole: Pediazole	Piperacillin/tazobactam: Zosyn
Ampho B-cholesteryl complex: Amphotec	Ethambutol: Myambutol	Piperazine: Antepar
	Ethionamide: Trecator	Podophyllotoxin: Condylox
Ampho B-lipid complex: Abelcet	Famciclovir: Famvir	Praziquantel: Biltricide
Ampicillin: Omnipen, Polycillin	Fluconazole: Diflucan	Primaquine: Primachine
Ampicillin/sulbactam: Unasyn	Flucytosine: Ancobon	Proguanil: Paludrine
Amprenavir: Agenerase	Foscarnet: Foscavir	Pyrantel pamoate: Antiminth
Atovaquone: Mepron	Fosfomycin: Monurol	Pyrimethamine: Daraprim
Atovaquone + proguanil: Malarone	Furazolidone: Furoxone	Pyrimethamine/sulfadoxine: Fansidar
Azithromycin: Zithromax	Ganciclovir: Cytovene	Quinupristin/dalfopristin: Synercid
Aztreonam: Azactam	Gatifloxacin: Tequin	Ribavirin: Virazole, Rebetol
Caspofungin: Cancidas	Gentamicin: Garamycin	Rifabutin: Mycobutin
Cefaclor: Ceclor, Ceclor CD	Griseofulvin: Fulvicin	Rifampin: Rifadin, Rimactane
Cefadroxil: Duricef	Halofantrine: Halfan	Rifapentine: Priftin
Cefazolin: Ancef, Kefzol	Idoxuridine: Dendrid, Stoxil	Rimantadine: Flumadine
Cefdinir: Omnicef	INH + RIF: Rifamate	Ritonavir: Norvir
Cefditoren: Spectracef	INH + RIF + PZA: Rifater	Saquinavir: Invirase, Fortovase
Cefepime: Maxipime	Interferon alfa: Roferon-A, Intron A	Spectinomycin: Trobicin
Cefixime: Suprax	Interferon, pegylated: PEG-Intron, Pegasys	Stavudine: Zerit
Cefoperazone: Cefobid		Stibogluconate: Pentostam
Cefotaxime: Claforan	Interferon + ribavirin: Rebetron	Silver sulfadiazine: Silvadene
Cefotetan: Cefotan	Imipenem + cilastatin: Primaxin	Sulfamethoxazole: Gantanol
Cefoxitin: Mefoxin	Imiquimod: Aldara	Sulfasalazine: Azulfidine
Cefpodoxime proxetil: Vantin	Indinavir: Crixivan	Sulfisoxazole: Gantrisin
Cefprozil: Cefzil	Itraconazole: Sporanox	Telithromycin: Ketek
Ceftazidime: Fortaz, Tazicef, Tazidime	Iodoquinol: Yodoxin	Tenofovir: Viread
Ceftibuten: Cedax	Ivermectin: Stromectol	Terbinafine: Lamisil
Ceftizoxime: Cefizox	Kanamycin: Kantrex	Thalidomide: Thalomid
Ceftriaxone: Rocephin	Ketoconazole: Nizoral	Thiabendazole: Mintezol
Cefuroxime: Zinacef, Kefurox, Ceftin	Lamivudine: Epivir, Epivir-HBV	Ticarcillin: Ticar
Cephalexin: Keflex	Levofloxacin: Levaquin	Tobramycin: Nebcin
Cephradine: Anspor, Velosef	Linezolid: Zyvox	Tretinoin: Retin A
Chloroquine: Aralen	Lomefloxacin: Maxaquin	Trifluridine: Viroptic
Cidofovir: Vistide	Lopinavir/ritonavir: Kaletra	Trimethoprim: Proloprim, Trimpex
Ciprofloxacin: Cipro, Cipro XR	Loracarbef: Lorabid	Trimethoprim/sulfamethoxazole: Bactrim, Septra
Clarithromycin: Biaxin, Biaxin XL	Mafenide: Sulfamylon	
Clindamycin: Cleocin	Mebendazole: Vermox	Trovafloxacin/alatrofloxacin: Trovan
Clofazimine: Lamprene	Mefloquine: Lariam	Valacyclovir: Valtrex
Clotrimazole: Lotrimin, Mycelex	Meropenem: Merrem	Valganciclovir: Valcyte
Cloxacillin: Tegopen	Mesalamine: Asacol, Pentasa	Vancomycin: Vancocin
Cycloserine: Seromycin	Methenamine: Hiprex, Mandelamine	Voriconazole: Vfend
Daptomycin: Cidecin	Metronidazole: Flagyl	Zalcitabine: HIVID
Delavirdine: Rescriptor	Minocycline: Minocin	Zanamivir: Relenza
Dicloxacillin: Dynapen	Moxifloxacin: Avelox	Zidovudine (ZDV): Retrovir
Didanosine: Videx	Mupirocin: Bactroban	Zidovudine + 3TC: Combivir
Diethylcarbamazine: Hetrazan	Nafcillin: Unipen	Zidovudine + 3TC + abacavir: Trizivir
Diloxanide furoate: Furamide	Nelfinavir: Viracept	
	Nevirapine: Viramune	
	Nitazoxanide: Cryptaz	

TABLE 23 (2)
LIST OF COMMON TRADE AND GENERIC NAMES

TRADE NAME: GENERIC NAME	TRADE NAME: GENERIC NAME	TRADE NAME: GENERIC NAME
Abelcet: Ampho B-lipid complex	Garamycin: Gentamicin	Relenza: Zanamivir
Agenerase: Amprenavir	Halfan: Halofantrine	Rescriptor: Delavirdine
Albenza: Albendazole	Hepsera: Adefovir	Retin A: Tretinoin
Aldara: Imiquimod	Herplex: Idoxuridine	Retrovir: Zidovudine (ZDV)
AmBisome: Ampho B-liposomal	Hiprex: Methenamine hippurate	Rifadin: Rifampin
Amikin: Amikacin	HIVID: Zalcitabine	Rifamate: INH + RIF
Amoxil: Amoxicillin	Humatin: Paromomycin	Rifater: INH + RIF + PZA
Amphotec: Ampho B-cholesteryl complex	Ilosone: Erythromycin estolate	Rimactane: Rifampin
	Ilotycin: Erythromycin	Rocephin: Ceftriaxone
Ancef: Cefazolin	Intron A: Interferon alfa	Roferon-A: Interferon alfa
Ancobon: Flucytosine	Invanz: Ertapenem	Septra: Trimethoprim/sulfa
Anspor: Cephradine	Invirase: Saquinavir	Seromycin: Cycloserine
Antepar: Piperazine	Kantrex: Kanamycin	Silvadene: Silver sulfadiazine
Antiminth: Pyrantel pamoate	Kaletra: Lopinavir/ritonavir	Spectracef: Cefditoren
Aralen: Chloroquine	Keflex: Cephalexin	Sporanox: Itraconazole
Asacol: Mesalamine	Kefurox: Cefuroxime	Stoxil: Idoxuridine
Augmentin, Augmentin ES-600, Augmentin XR: Amox./clav.	Ketek: Telithromycin	Stromectol: Ivermectin
	Lamisil: Terbinafine	Sulfamylon: Mafenide
Avelox: Moxifloxacin	Lamprene: Clofazimine	Suprax: Cefixime
Azactam: Aztreonam	Lariam: Mefloquine	Sustiva: Efavirenz
Azulfidine: Sulfasalazine	Levaquin: Levofloxacin	Symmetrel: Amantadine
Bactroban: Mupirocin	Lorabid: Loracarbef	Synagis: Palivizumab
Bactrim: Trimethoprim/ sulfamethoxa-zole	Macrodantin, Macrobid: Nitrofurantoin	Synercid: Quinupristin/dalfopristin
	Malarone: Atovaquone + proguanil	Tamiflu: Oseltamivir
Biaxin, Biaxin XL: Clarithromycin	Mandelamine: Methenamine mandel.	Tazicef: Ceftazidime
Biltricide: Praziquantel	Maxaquin: Lomefloxacin	Tegopen: Cloxacillin
Cancidas: Caspofungin	Maxipime: Cefepime	Tequin: Gatifloxacin
Ceclor, Ceclor CD: Cefaclor	Mefoxin: Cefoxitin	Thalomid: Thalidomide
Cedax: Ceftibuten	Mepron: Atovaquone	Ticar: Ticarcillin
Cefizox: Ceftizoxime	Merrem: Meropenem	Timentin: Ticarcillin-clavulanic acid
Cefobid: Cefoperazone	Minocin: Minocycline	Tinactin: Tolnaftate
Cefotan: Cefotetan	Mintezol: Thiabendazole	Trecator SC: Ethionamide
Ceftin: Cefuroxime axetil	Monocid: Cefonicid	Trizivir: Abacavir + ZDV + 3TC
Cefzil: Cefprozil	Monurol: Fosfomycin	Trobicin: Spectinomycin
Cidecin: Daptomycin	Myambutol: Ethambutol	Trovan: Trovafloxacin/alatrofloxacin
Cipro, Cipro XR: Ciprofloxacin & extended release	Mycobutin: Rifabutin	Unasyn: Ampicillin/sulbactam
	Mycostatin: Nystatin	Unipen: Nafcillin
Claforan: Cefotaxime	Nafcil: Nafcillin	Valcyte: Valganciclovir
Combivir: ZDV + 3TC	Nebcin: Tobramycin	Valtrex: Valacyclovir
Crixivan: Indinavir	NebuPent: Pentamidine	Vancocin: Vancomycin
Cryptaz: Nitazoxanide	Nizoral: Ketoconazole	Vantin: Cefpodoxime proxetil
Cytovene: Ganciclovir	Norvir: Ritonavir	Velosef: Cephradine
Daraprim: Pyrimethamine	Omnicef: Cefdinir	Vermox: Mebendazole
Diflucan: Fluconazole	Omnipen: Ampicillin	Vfend: Voriconazole
Duricef: Cefadroxil	Pediamycin: Erythro. ethyl succinate	Vibramycin: Doxycycline
Dynapen: Dicloxacillin	Pediazole: Erythro. ethyl succinate + sulfisoxazole	Videx: Didanosine
Epivir, Epivir-HBV: Lamivudine		Viracept: Nelfinavir
Famvir: Famciclovir	Pegasys, PEG-Intron: Interferon, pegylated	Viramune: Nevirapine
Fansidar: Pyrimethamine + sulfadoxine		Virazole: Ribavirin
	Pentam 300: Pentamidine	Viread: Tenofovir
Flagyl: Metronidazole	Pentasa: Mesalamine	Vistide: Cidofovir
Floxin: Ofloxacin	Pipracil: Piperacillin	Xigris: Drotrecogin alfa
Flumadine: Rimantadine	Polycillin: Ampicillin	Yodoxin: Iodoquinol
Fortaz: Ceftazidime	Polymox: Amoxicillin	Zerit: Stavudine
Fortovase: Saquinavir	Priftin: Rifapentine	Ziagen: Abacavir
Fulvicin: Griseofulvin	Primaxin: Imipenem + cilastatin	Zinacef: Cefuroxime
Fungizone: Amphotericin B	Proloprim: Trimethoprim	Zithromax: Azithromycin
Furadantin: Nitrofurantoin	Prostaphlin: Oxacillin	Zovirax: Acyclovir
Furoxone: Furazolidone	Rebetol: Ribavirin	Zosyn: Piperacillin/tazobactam
Fuzeon: Enfuvirtide (T-20)	Rebetron: Interferon + ribavirin	Zyvox: Linezolid
Gantanol: Sulfamethoxazole		
Gantrisin: Sulfisoxazole		

Bold numbers indicate major considerations. Recommendations in Table 1 not indexed; antibiotic selection often depends on modifying circumstances and alternative agents.

Bold numbers indicate major considerations. Recommendations in Table 1 not indexed; antibiotic selection often depends on modifying circumstances and alternative agents.

Bold indicate major considerations. Recommendations in Table 1 not indexed; antibiotic selection often depends on modifying circumstances and alternative agents.